GLENN AUSTIN, M.D., is a pediatrician in private practice in Los Altos, California, with years of experience both teaching and practicing medicine for children.

THE PARENTS' MEDICAL MANUAL

GLENN AUSTIN

with

Julia Stone Oliver and John C. Richards

PRENTICE-HALL, INC., Englewood Cliffs, New Jersey 07632

Library of Congress Cataloging in Publication Data
Main entry under title:

The Parents' medical manual.

  (A Spectrum Book)
  Includes index.
  1. Children—Diseases.   2. Children—Care and
hygiene.   I. Austin, Glenn.   II. Oliver, Julia Stone.
III. Richards, John C. [DNLM: 1. Medicine—Popular
works.   WB120.3 A935p]
RJ61.P228   618.9′2   78–2759
ISBN 0–13–650317–9
ISBN 0–13–650309–8 pbk.

A Spectrum Book

10   9   8   7   6   5   4   3   2   1

Printed in the United States of America

PRENTICE-HALL INTERNATIONAL, INC., *London*
PRENTICE-HALL of AUSTRALIA PTY. LIMITED, *Sydney*
PRENTICE-HALL of CANADA, LTD., *Toronto*
PRENTICE-HALL of INDIA PRIVATE LIMITED, *New Delhi*
PRENTICE-HALL of JAPAN, INC., *Tokyo*
PRENTICE-HALL of SOUTHEAST ASIA PTE. LTD., *Singapore*
WHITEHALL BOOKS LIMITED, *Wellington, New Zealand*

To my wife, with love.
Her inspiration, faith, and hard work
during both good times and bad
made this book possible.

CONTENTS

PART ONE
BASIC HOME HEALTH RESPONSIBILITIES

1

8

THE MOUTH AND ITS CONTENTS:
TEETH AND BRACES, THUMB AND PACIFIER

9

THE CHEST, ITS CONTENTS, AND COUGHS

10

YOUR STOMACH AND BOWELS

11

KIDNEY, BLADDER, AND BOTTOM

12

THE GROWTH AND DEVELOPMENT
OF FEET, LEGS, AND OTHER BONES

13

BLOOD

20

STINGING, BITING, AND PESKY INSECTS
326

21

OTHER CAUSES OF DISEASE
340

22

POISONOUS PLANTS
344

PART FOUR
MEDICAL LISTS

NOTES
407

INDEX
411

PREFACE

Doctors, especially those in practice, are aware that parents need more than knowledge about health and disease, they need *understanding*. Parents are responsible for their children: They have to make key decisions for them, and they must conscientiously make the effort to acquire and to understand medical knowledge. However, parents, like doctors, are faced with almost more "knowledge" than they can use or absorb. Much of this knowledge is of no practical value to parents and in no way enhances their ability to keep their children or themselves healthy. Therefore, our primary effort here is to increase parents' practical understanding of health and disease.

Just as in our companion volume, *The Parents' Guide to Child Raising*, we started by asking a lot of people, "What would you like to see in a book for parents?" We have the input of over 400 physicians from all over the United States and a few from outside. The response was so great that it took over five years and six manuscript drafts to complete the book. Each chapter was circulated among a wide variety of medical practitioners, parents, nurses, and so on at least five times. From this review, we then concentrated the information we feel can be of most use to you in understanding, preventing, and treating illness. We feel that parents are an integral part of the medical team and that they can and should take a more active role. This book has a greater spectrum of medical and health lore than is usual in a book for nonprofessionals. It took a lot of work from the hundreds of people involved. How can I and my associate editors thank the many contributors and advisors? At least they know who they are and that their efforts are sincerely appreciated. In our companion volume, *The Parents' Guide to Child Raising,* I acknowl-edged the work of my associate editors Julie Oliver and Dr. John C. Richards and recognized the inspiration we received from Dr. Robert F. L. Polley and Dr. Merritt Low, whose effective dedication to children and youth helped guide our efforts. The quality of *The Parents' Medical Manual* is a direct reflection of the efforts of our many contributors and advisors. However, putting these many views together has not been easy. At times the project looked like a scattered jigsaw puzzle, with over-lapping contributions from many different individuals. We are thankful for the talent of Richard Osborne in helping to organize and smooth the text. In the process we took some editorial liberties with our contribu-tors' material in order to develop a consistent and more easily readable style and to avoid duplication. We strove faithfully to retain the mean-ing of each article and the character and identity of each author. Yet, I recognize that the complete view of any single contributor may not al-ways be present—their contributions here were part of a team effort to bring as much pertinent information to you as possible. I wish we could have used all of each article from every contributor, but in the process of condensing and editing the multiple drafts, some of them have been dropped from the authors' list. Actually, the reader may notice that some of the advice given sounds as though it came from his own doctor—and it may well have. Aside from the fact that we don't list all the 400 doctors who helped us, much of the practical knowledge we present comes from physicians in practice who share their day-to-day practical experience with one another. In an indirect way, this book has benefitted from your own doctor's wisdom.

Personally, I learned a lot about medicine from correlating all the advice we received. It left me even more impressed with the excellence of the average pediatrician, family practitioner, and dentist—and of other specialists in private practice. But the greatest reward I had was in work-ing with a really fine lot of understanding, sensitive, and practical peo-ple. I thank you all for your companionship and your contributions to *The Parents' Guide to Child Raising* and *The Parents' Medical Manual.*

CREDITS FOR ILLUSTRATIONS

Illustrations 1, 6, 7, 8, 9, 10, 11, 12, 13, 14, 15, 16, 17, 18, 19, 20, 21, 22, 23, 24, 25, 26, 27, 28, 31, 32, 33, 34, 35, 36, 37, 38, 39, 40, 41, 42, 43, 44, 45, 46, 47, 48, 49, 50, 51, 61, 94 are from the Medical and Graphic Illustration Department, Stanford University Medical Center, Stanford, California.

Illustrations 2, 3, 5, 29, 30 are photographs by Patricia Gough, Los Altos, California.

Illustration 4 is reproduced courtesy of Physicians for Automotive Safety, Irvington, New Jersey.

Illustration 52 is used courtesy of Dr. Judith Carnahan and Dr. Charles Brinton. Reproduced with permission of E. Jawetz, J. L. Melnich and E. A. Adelberg, *Review of Medical Microbiology*, LANGE Medical Publications, Los Altos, California 94022.

Illustration 53 is reproduced with permission of E. Jawetz, J. L. Melnich and E. A. Adelberg, *Review of Medical Microbiology*, LANGE Medical Publications, Los Atltos, California 94022.

Illustrations 54, 55, 56, 57, 58, 59, 60 are from the Center for Disease Control, United States Public Health Service, Atlanta, Georgia.

Illustrations 61 through 92 are reproduced courtesy of Syntex Laboratories, Palo Alto, California.

CONTRIBUTING AUTHORS

ROBERT ALWAY, M.D., F.A.A.P., Professor of Pediatrics, Stanford University School of Medicine

JAY ARENA, B.S., M.D., F.A.A.P., Pediatrician and Professor, Duke University; Chairman, National Poison Control Centers; Past President, American Academy of Pediatrics; Author, *Dangers to Children and Youth. Human Poisoning from Native and Cultivated Plants,* Durham, North Carolina

GLENN AUSTIN, M.D., F.A.A.P., Consultant, American Academy Pediatrics; Pediatrician, Private Practice, Los Altos, California

LEO BELL, M.D., F.A.A.P., Pediatrician, Private Practice; Past President, National Federation of Pediatric Societies, San Mateo, California

FRANK BERRY, M.D., F.A.B.O., Practicing Ophthalmologist; Associate Clinical Professor of Ophthalmology, Stanford Medical School. Los Altos, California

E. E. BLECK, M.D., Chief of Orthopedics, Children's Hospital at Stanford, California; President, American Academy for Cerebral Palsy

RICHARD D. BLIM, M.D., F.A.A.P., Executive Board, American Academy of Pediatrics; Pediatrician, Private Practice, Kansas City, Missouri

JAMES BRAMHAM, M.D., F.A.A.P., Pediatrician, Private Practice; Past President, Sacramento County Medical Society, Sacramento, California

HENRY BRUYN, M.D., F.A.A.P., Past Director, Student Health Service, University of California, Berkeley; Author, *Handbook of Pediatrics,* San Francisco, California

ROBERT BURNETT, M.D.. F.A.A.P., Pediatrician, Private Practice; Chairman, Manpower Committee, American Academy of Pediatrics, Sunnyvale, California

SEYMOUR CHARLES, M.D., Chairman, Physicians for Automotive Safety, Irvington, New Jersey

THOMAS COCK, M.D., F.A.A.P., Bellevue, Washington

WENDELL COFFELT, M.D., F.A.A.P., Pediatrician, Private Practice; Chairman, Public Information, American Academy of Pediatrics, Burbank, California

THOMAS CONWAY, M.D., F.A.A.P., Pediatrician, Private Practice, Terre Haute, Indiana

NANCY COOKSON, reviewing mother, Los Altos, California

WILLIAM CROOK, M.D., F.A.A.P., Pediatric Allergist; President, Child Health Centers of America; Author of *Your Allergic Child* and *Are You Bothered by Hypoglycemia,* Jackson, Tennessee

LEE FARR, M.D., F.A.A.P., Professor of Nuclear Medicine; Medical Director of the Brookhaven National Laboratory, retired, Upton, New York; Author of over 150 articles on environmental hazards, Carmel, California

CLAUDE FRAZIER, A., M.D., Allergist, world authority and speaker on insect allergies; Author, *Insect Allergy,* Ashville, North Carolina

J. W. GERRARD, D.M., F.R.C.P., Professor of Pediatrics, University of Saskatchewan, Canada; Author, *Understanding Allergies,* Saskatchewan, Canada

JOSEPH E. GHORY, M.D., F.A.A.P., Pediatric Allergist; Medical Director, Convalescent Hospital for Children, Cincinnati, Ohio

GLEN C. GRIFFIN, M.D., F.A.A.P., Private Practice, Pediatrician, Bountiful, Utah

BIRT HARVEY, M.D., F.A.A.P., Expert on cystic fibrosis; Stanford Children's Hospital; Past Chairman, Chapter I, American Academy of Pediatrics, Palo Alto, California

A. S. HASHIM, M.D., (Baghdad) F.A.A.P., Pediatrician, Private Practice, Bethesda, Maryland

NEIL HENDERSON, M.D., Pediatrician, Private Practice; Author, *How to Understand and Treat Your Child's Symptoms,* Boca Raton, Florida

ROBERT HERMAN, M.D.. F.A.A.P., Pediatrician-Psychiatrist, Private Practice, Keiser Hospital, Los Gatos, California

CHARLES HOFFMAN, M.D., F.A.A.P., Pediatrician, Private Practice, Flushing, New York

HULL DONALD, D.D.S., M.S., Orthodontist, Private Practice, Los Altos, California

ALVIN JACOBS, M.D., F.A.A.P., Professor of Dermatology, Stanford University, Stanford, California

BLACKBURN JOSLIN, M.D., F.A.A.P., Pediatrician, Private Practice; Chairman, American Academy of Pediatrics Chapter; Socio-economic expert, Bellevue, Washington

RAYMOND KAHN, M.D., Officer, F.A.A.P.; Family Practice, Dayton, Ohio

NORMAN KENDALL, M.D., F.A.A.P., Professor of Neonatology, Temple University, Philadelphia, Pennsylvania

KENNETH LAMPE, Ph.D., Professor of Pharmacology, University of Miami School of Medicine; Author, *Plant Toxicity and Dermatitis,* Miami, Florida

STEPHEN LOCKEY, M.D., Allergist: Exhibit Award Winner, American Medical Association, Lancaster, Pennsylvania

GEORGE LOGAN, M.D., M.S. (Ped), F.A.A.P., F.A.A.A., F.A.C.A., Professor (Emeritus) of Pediatrics, Mayo Medical School; Senior Consultant, Department of Pediatrics, Mayo Clinic, Rochester, Minn.

MERRITT LOW, M.D., F.A.A.P., Pediatrician, Private Practice; Executive Board, American Academy of Pediatrics, Greenfield, Massachusetts

GEORGE B. MARAGOS, M.D., M.Scl., F.A.A.P., Editor of *Pediatrician,* Journal of the International College of Pediatrics, Omaha, Nebraska

MARY ANN MCCANN, Member, American Association of Poison Control Centers; Research Associate, University of Miami School of Medicine

MARVIN MCCLELLAN, M.D., F.A.A.P., Pediatrician, Private Practice; Expert on sports medicine; Past President, National Federation Pediatric Societies; Consultant, American Academy of Pediatrics, Cincinnati, Ohio

FRANK MCDANIEL, D.D.S., Practicing Dentist, Los Altos, California

BEN MCGANN, M.D., Family Practice, Los Altos, California

RICHARD MERCER, M.D., Orthopedic Surgeon, Mountain View, California

ALAN MERCHANT, M.D., Orthopedic Surgeon, Mountain View, California

WILLIAM MISBACH, M.D., F.A.A.P., Pediatrician, Private Practice; Chapter Chairman, American Academy of Pediatrics, Encino, California

JULIA STONE OLIVER, Associate Editor; mother, Los Altos, California

RICHARD M. O'NEIL, M.D., F.A.A.P., Pediatrician, Private Practice, Editor, *The California Pediatrician*, San Jose, California

RICHARD PARKER, D.V.M., Chief, Office of Veterinary Public Health Services, C.D.C., U.S.P.H.S., Atlanta, Georgia

GALE PATE, SR., Chairman of the Board, The Juvenile Shoe Corporation of America, Aurora, Missouri

RUTH POARCH, Reviewing Mother, Woodland, California

ROBERT F. L. POLLEY, M.D., F.A.A.P., Pediatrician, Private Practice; Author, *Call the Doctor;* Columnist, Seattle, Washington

ISAAC M. REID, M.D., F.A.A.P., Kaiser Health Center, Cleveland, Ohio

HENRY RICHANBACH, M.D., F.A.A.P., Pediatrician, Private Practice, Burlingame, California

JOHN RICHARDS, M.D., F.A.A.P., Associate Editor; Pediatrician, Private Practice, Los Altos, California

SAUL ROBINSON, M.D., F.A.A.P., Pediatric Cardiologist; Executive Board, American Academy of Pediatrics, San Francisco, California

DAVID ROSENTHAL, M.D., F.A.A.P., Pediatrics, Private Practice, Sunnyvale, California

SID ROSIN, M.D., F.A.A.P., Pediatrician, Private Practice, Beverly Hills, California

GEORGE RUSSELL, M.D., F.A.A.P., Medical Director, Monon (ghetto) Health Center, Tulsa, Oklahoma

ROBERT SCHERZ, M.D., F.A.A.P., Chairman, Committee on Accident Prevention, American Academy of Pediatrics, Ft. Lewis, Washington

EDWARD SHAW, M.D., F.A.A.P., Professor of Pediatrics and Chairman (retired) University of California Medical School, San Francisco, California

ANNEMARIE SHELLNESS, Executive Director, Physicians for Automotive Safety, Irvington, New Jersey

JACK SHILLER, M.D., F.A.A.P., Pediatrician, Private Practice; Author, *Childhood Illness*, Westport, Connecticut

ERIC SIMS, M.D., F.R.A.C.P., Senior Consulting Pediatrician, Adelaide Childrens Hospital, South Australia

LENDON SMITH, M.D., F.A.A.P., Pediatrician, Private Practice; Author, *The Encyclopedia of Baby and Child Care;* Television program, Portland, Oregon

MARTIN SMITH, M.D., F.A.A.P., Pediatrician, Private Practice; Chairman, Council of Pediatric Practice, American Academy of Pediatrics, Gainsville, Georgia

DAVID SPARLING, M.D., F.A.A.P., Pediatrician, Private Practice; Chairman, American Academy of Pediatrics Chapter, Tacoma, Washington

JAMES STEM, M.D., F.A.A.P., Pediatrician, Private Practice, Clearwater, Florida

LOANA TOMASELLO, mother, swimming instruction, Los Altos, California

HOBART WALLACE, M.D., F.A.A.P., Chapter Chairman, American Academy of Pediatrics; Pediatrician, Private Practice, Lincoln, Nebraska

PAUL WEHRLE, M.D., F.A.A.P., Professor of Pediatrics, University of Southern California, Los Angeles, California

GEORGE WHEATLEY, M.D., F.A.A.P., Medical Director, Metropolitan Life Insurance Company, New York, New York

BURTON WHITE, Ph.D., Senior Research Associate, Harvard Graduate School of Education, Harvard University, Cambridge, Massachusetts

Key to Degrees and Honors

B.S.	Bachelor of Science
D.D.S.	Doctor of Dental Surgery
D.V.M.	Doctor of Veterinary Medicine
D.M.	Doctor of Medicine
F.A.A.A.	Fellow of the American Academy of Allergy
F.A.A.F.P.	Fellow of the American Academy of Family Physicians
F.A.A.P.	Fellow of the American Academy of Pediatrics
F.A.B.O.	Fellow of the American Board of Ophthamology
F.A.C.A.	Fellow of the American College of Allergy
F.R.A.C.P.	Fellow of the Royal Australian College of Physicians
F.R.C.P.	Fellow of the Royal College of Physicians
M.B.	Bachelor of Medicine
M.D.	Doctor of Medicine
M.N.	Masters in Nursing
M.Sci.	Master of Science
Ph.D.	Doctor of Philosophy
R.N.	Registered Nurse

INTRODUCTION

The Parents' Medical Manual covers a broad variety of medical and health information. This information was selected with you in mind. First, several hundred doctors were asked what they would like to see in a medical manual that would be of practical help to parents in preventing disease and in raising healthy children, and in the home treatment of illness and understanding disease. Most health care, and much medical care, of children is in the hands of parents, so as doctors contributed articles, advice, or ideas and these were worked into chapters, they were read by a scattering of parents across the country who were asked if what they read was understandable and what else they would like in a medical manual. Editorially, each piece of information had to be more than generally informative; it had to be *useful* to some of our readers. Everything here will not be useful to you—but some things will. Some areas may not look useful to you at first because we placed a high priority on emphasizing the understanding of disease. Thus, we discuss the differences in size and life style of germs you have probably never heard of and hopefully will never get. However, if you understand these organisms, you will be better equipped to avoid them, to understand their relative contagion, to know why some conditions are not treatable, and to understand and participate in the treatment of those diseases that can be treated. We even included rare bacteria like anthrax, plague, and diphtheria, in spite of questions from some parents about why would they ever need to know about these diseases. During the five years it took to complete *The Parents' Medical Manual* and its companion volume *The Parents' Guide to Raising Children,* there have been cases of plague, anthrax, and diphtheria in the United States. These could have been prevented, or at least more easily recognized and treated, had the people

1

involved read the information in this book. The causes varied from sick squirrels to imported sheepskin bongo drums to neglecting to immunize children. So don't throw up your hands and quit over strange sounding names of germs you never knew existed. Even though it will take time, I suggest that you read the book through so that you can understand the broad spectrum of health care and will at least have been exposed to knowledge that can save the health or life of your child and family.

This book is not an encyclopedia or dictionary of health care. It is designed not just to let you pick out a few facts but rather to help you understand and use medical information. Most pediatricians believe that one of the best things they can do for the health of children is to educate and motivate parents. We have faith that you can increase your understanding and effectiveness in the health care of your child.

One of the first things I believe you should know about health and medical care is that it is not a science. Certainly we depend upon science for a lot of our information—and we attempt to understand the clinical problems we see in practice in as scientific a way as possible—but medicine is a long way from being a science. People who read an article in a medical journal reporting a carefully done piece of research tend to accept it as a scientific truth. However, given five years, probably fifty percent of these research findings are proven to be in error because of factors that were not understood when the work was done; thus, the results are incomplete, misleading, or practically of no help in treating disease. But half of newly discovered medical knowledge does turn out to be valid in five years—thus, there exists a large and valuable store of knowledge discovered clinically or by research over the decades which has survived the test of time and which offers the real basis for medical practice and worthwhile care. But even when it is proven valuable, basic knowledge can be misleading.

The root of the problem is that each of us is different in many ways. Scientific studies usually measure statistical responses. Thus, if you throw a pair of dice on the gambling table in Las Vegas, scientists can tell you your statistical chances of making a seven before you roll two ones and lose. But what counts with each roll isn't the statistics—it is whether you win or lose. Similarly, a scientific study of the benefit of a nasal decongestant may show that it dried up the nose of ninety-two out of one hundred people who took it. But if you are like one of the unaffected eight, it wouldn't work on you. Then, in terms of infection, things become even more complicated. Germs vary in their ability to make us sick, and they change their potency from time to time. On top of that, human variation is even more pronounced. If one hundred people are exposed to a virus, we get almost one hundred different reactions. Some will not become ill at all, some will become mildly ill, some will become severely ill, and some will become seriously ill. If you line up this one hundred people in the order of how sick they are, you can draw a bell-shaped curve representing where they are (See Figure 1). Thus, in understanding illness, the fact that your neighbor's child only caught a mild cold from a virus doesn't mean that the same cold in your child will

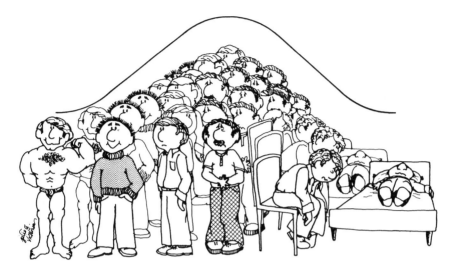

FIGURE 1 *People usually react differently to the same infection.*

be mild. The fact that you had a bad reaction to a drug doesn't mean your spouse will have a bad reaction. So whenever you hear or read about medical care, keep in mind the remarkable variability that occurs in illness and its treatment. Similarly, the time may occur when the best of statistical medical care may not be good for you or your child. All of us in medicine do the best we can, but we are not invincible. Neither are you. Health is fragile. But between you and your doctor and *The Parents' Medical Manual,* you can do remarkably well in keeping your child in good health.

PART ONE

BASIC HOME HEALTH RESPONSIBILITIES

Throughout our companion volume, *The Parents' Guide to Child Raising*, we offered practical knowledge and suggestions on ways to raise children. Here, we concentrate on medical care, and we enter a more professional area with more solid scientific information and experience. Because of the complexities of medical care, we depend heavily upon professionals, including all sorts of specialists, for advice and decisions. But there exists a basic store of rather easily usable medical knowledge that we feel *all* people should have accessible. Perhaps even more important is that some health and medical care can *only* be a home responsibility. The first four chapters emphasize things that you should know so that you can act responsibly at home to prevent or treat many conditions. Some of this may help to keep you out of the doctor's hands, and some of it is designed to get you into a doctor's hands when you need to be there. But these are decisions you have to make. The following chapters will give you information that will help you make such decisions properly—and can help you have a healthier family.

1

PREVENTING
ACCIDENTS
AND POISONINGS

It is a dangerous world, so we must take the problem of "accidents" and poisons very very seriously. We should! Accidents and poisons kill more children than any other single cause—almost as many as *all* other causes together. Most of these deaths are preventable if you anticipate them. In fact, they aren't really accidental, contends Stanford Professor Dr. Robert Alway:

> Parents should *expect* youngsters, especially toddlers, to explore, manipulate, and ingest ANYTHING adult thoughtlessness or *careless*ness has not made unavailable or less intriguing or attractive. The pot pulled off the stove, the gunshot from the "unloaded" firearm, the milky glassful of lye, the paint thinner in the pop bottle, the toddler at the bottom of the pool, the head smashed against the windshield, and so forth and so on, are not accidents.

WHAT CAUSES MOST ACCIDENTAL DEATHS?

An expert who has kept close track of the causes of death in children is Dr. George Wheatley. As Chief Medical Director of the Metropolitan Life Insurance Company, he became appalled at the number of unnecessary deaths, and so founded the first accident prevention committee of the American Academy of Pediatrics. He points out:

> Advances in medical science, better child health services, improved sanitation, pasteurized milk, and sterilized water have cut childhood deaths from disease more than ninety percent in the last thirty

years, leaving accidents, *preventable accidents,* the most likely thing to kill your child. Most of the accidental deaths in babies happen between the ages of three and twelve months when they start rolling over, sitting up, crawling, standing, and exploring their world. This is the first critical time for parents to anticipate their child's development; to foresee chances for accidents, and to prevent them by taking necessary steps. For children between the ages of one and four, the most common causes of accidental death are the auto, fires, drowning, and poisoning. It is mandatory that babies and young children have constant supervision, and good, truly safe play areas.

The HOME is the area of greatest hazard during the preschool years. The state of the family's organization or disorganization and the amount of stress in the home play a large part in the accident-health of the child. During wars, there is a sharp increase in fatal accidents at preschool ages. Families are disorganized by the war, with fathers away and mothers of young children often working. Somewhat similar conditions exist today with the current changes in family roles and the parents' activities. There are fewer accidents among children who attend day care or nursery school facilities than among those who do not.

The AUTO is the major cause of accidental deaths in children. People must become more conscious of the dangers to young passengers riding in motor vehicles. Deaths where the infant under one year is a passenger tend to be evenly divided between boys and girls. However, at a very early age, boys begin to dominate the scene. At nearly every age from one to fifteen, boys more frequently than girls are killed crossing streets or playing in their driveways. Boys are probably either willing or conditioned to take greater risks, and to act out their aggressive feelings by exposing themselves to danger. A large number of deaths in children from one to four occurs in driveways and streets

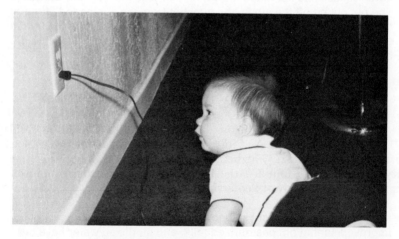

FIGURE 2 *"That looks interesting!"*

close to the child's home. Between the ages of five to fourteen, motor vehicles cause half of the deaths due to accidents. Most of these are due to the child being hit or run over by the vehicle.

Psychologist Burton White points out that you should expect your child to get into all sorts of things. "Curiosity is the birthright of every child," he says.

SPECIFIC DANGERS AND HOW TO PREVENT INJURY AND DEATH TO YOUR CHILD

Merritt B. Low, M.D., Past Chairman of the Accident Prevention Committee of the American Academy of Pediatrics, notes that seventeen million children (one in three) are *injured* in accidents each year. He advises:

Accident prevention must become a way of life. Balance is necessary between overanxiety and carelessness, between over-restriction and ultra-permissiveness. As a parent, you can become a strong activist in this area by alerting yourself to the hazards and by practicing prevention wisely. The hazards are:

For the Young Infant
1. *Falls from the table, bed or bathinette.* From the moment of his arrival, no infant should be left alone on top of anything except the floor. Babies can slide and roll long before some parents seem to realize it.
2. *Crawl-accidents.* Crawling infants can: fall downstairs; pull on cords attached to coffee pots, irons or vaporizers; swallow or choke on tiny objects; cut themselves on sharp objects. Thoroughly check your home with these items in mind. Remember that toys can be a hazard if they are smaller than a baby's mouth or have loose parts, such as eyes, that can be pulled off, or if they have a sharp or pointed edge. Be extra cautious to keep knives and scissors out of reach.
3. *The automobile.* Proper car-restraints and seats are now available for *all* infants and children (see page 14). This is more important at this time than getting immunizations, according to statistics.
4. *Child abuse.* This is unfortunately an important part of the accident picture. Child abuse includes "shaking" and heavy spanking or beating. Such tendencies by a parent are evidence that the parent needs some kind of counseling and help.
5. *Drowning.* Always stay close when the baby is in the tub, even when an infant can sit well. It takes only a split second for him to slip under water.
6. *Accidental suffocation.* More properly called "crib death," this is a rare, and, at the present time, a nonpreventable horror of unknown

cause. True suffocation can result from plastic bags, especially dry cleaners' bags, being left around infants.

7. *Unsafe baby cribs* can kill infants who may:

Become wedged between a poorly matched mattress or spring and the crib or edge pad, or even between closely spaced beds.

Slide under the mattress and hang with the head lodged between the crib slats.

Slide between the edge of the crib and the side of the spring if it is loose.

Strangle from chains or strings hung from the crib or around the baby's neck.

Climb out and fall and hang by the head, caught between the crib and the wall or nearby furniture—or they may land on their heads.

Avoid these tragedies by regularly inspecting the crib:

Make certain it is sturdy and that all latches and the side gates work well.

All spaces between the slats and the side and the head of the crib should be smaller than 2⅜ inches.

The springs should not sag, and the crib mattress should fit snugly. Don't leave toys in the crib so small they can fit in the mouth or so large (later) that the baby can use them to crawl out of the crib.

Never leave plastic bags or sheets in the crib—they can smother a baby easily.

For the One–to–Four Year Group

1. The automobile
   a. Use safe car seats (see page 16).
   b. Do not allow the child to play in driveways or garages, or alone in parked cars.
2. *Poisons*
   a. Keep syrup of ipecac on hand for emergency use (usual dose: one tablespoon).
   b. Use child-proof containers.

All medicines should be locked up. If you don't have a cabinet with a lock, a fishing tackle box makes an ideal place to store medicines. The compartments and shelves make it easy to separate and organize your medicines. An inexpensive padlock on the box will make them inaccessible to the children but convenient for the parents.—*John C. Richards, M.D.*

---

   c. Keep hazardous substances locked up.
   d. Dispose of as many poisons as possible, such as rat poison, roach paste and powder, and ant poisons.
   e. Have the phone number of your physician and poison control center available on or near the telephone.
   f. Lead poisoning presents a serious threat to children: A child

died of lead poisoning every thirty-six hours in 1972 and 6,000 gradually became brain-damaged. One hundred and fifty of these are now *severely* mentally retarded. Although they may be endangered from chewing on windowsills, cribs, or toys that have been coated with lead-based paint, the worst problem occurs in dilapidated housing where old lead-based paint peels off walls and ceilings and is eaten by children up to five years old.

What's the remedy? Parents should be alerted to bring their children to clinics for blood testing and, if necessary, for treatment. Parents and landlords should make old paint inaccessible to children by removing it from all buildings. The cost of doing this is only a fraction of the cost of care for a mentally retarded child. The lead content in new paints is now limited and significant changes in the paint used on toys have been made.

Another sneaky source of lead poisoning comes from lead-containing pottery. Most commercial pottery in the United States is safe, but with home potters' experimentation and large uncontrolled foreign imports, some of those beautiful cups and pitchers may be deadly. Lead is most likely to dissolve into mildly acid liquids such as fruit juices. The amounts are small, but they gradually accumulate and cause symptoms of headache, loss of appetite and weight, weakness and anemia, fatigue, a metallic taste, and if severe, cause abdominal pain, vomiting, diarrhea, black stools, and collapse.

3. *Poisonous Plants*

   Infants first learn about life by tasting whatever they can find. As they get older, their tasting forays may take them to poisonous house plants and outside to the garden where poisonous plants may abound. This hazard continues into school age when uneducated kids will chew on dock sorrel or cook hot dogs on oleander twigs. The number of poisonous plants is so large and the symptoms of poisoning so diverse that, in order to cover the subject adequately, we have an entire chapter and an exhaustive list, about these beautiful hazards (see Chapter 23).

4. *Drownings:*
   a. Teaching babies to swim may give them a false sense of security. Since their judgment and resources are limited, they may panic under unusual circumstances.
   b. Always stay with the child near water.
   c. Watch the child every *second*—not every minute—when around water.
   d. Be sure that pools, ponds, wells, and cisterns are protected. Pools must be fenced.
   e. Empty the bathtub right away when you have finished the bath.

5. *Burns:*
   a. Use flame retardant clothing, especially night wear. The risk of injury from fire far outweighs the unproven risk from fire-retardant chemicals.

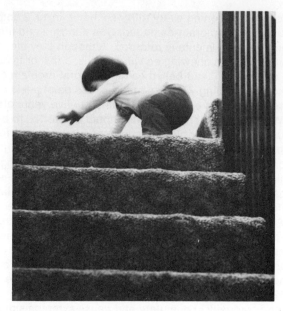

FIGURE 3

    b. Keep matches in places too high for a child to reach, and in closed containers.
    c. Teach the child the concept of "hot."
    d. Turn pot handles toward the wall.
6. *Falls:*
    a. Equip upstairs windows with sturdy screens and guards.
    b. Use gates at top and bottom of stairs until your child knows how to navigate steps.
    c. Use shatter-proof glass wherever indicated.
    d. Door hooks should be high; the play area should be fenced in.
    e. Don't leave a young child alone at home.

For the Five–to–Ten Year Old

1. *Bikes:* Educate as to laws, hazardous streets, driveways.
2. *Cars:* Insist that seat belts are used.
3. *Insects:* If your child is severely allergic, have a sting kit and medication on hand.
4. *Animals:* Teach caution about dogs; report biting dogs to the police.

For the Ten–to–Twelve Year Old

1. *Firearms:* A safety course before handling is mandatory.
2. *Getting lost on trips:* Skills to help avoid getting lost should be developed in advance.

3. *Getting "over one's head"* in activities through errors in underdeveloped, over-aspiring judgment.

For Teenagers

1. The automobile and its driver: Various factors which play a role are affluence, alcohol, marihuana, youth's "need to prove," and the lag between cultural values and technological realities.
2. Motorcycles, motor scooters, and motor bikes: The death rate per mile of motorcycle riding is huge—almost five times as many deaths per distance travelled than for all types of travel (2,500 deaths in one year). Teenagers must be educated about the hazards and taught the concept of defensive cycle driving in relation to autos.

What Can Parents Do to Reduce Teenage Hazards?
1. Insist on driver's training.
2. Set examples of careful driving.
3. Encourage protective legislation, such as laws requiring helmets for motorcycle riders.
4. Encourage scientific engineering improvements, such as improved types of helmets.
5. Encourage improved quality of emergency care in your community from the "moment of injury."
6. Set examples of control in the use of alcohol and drugs.
7. Develop meaningful social roles for adolescents.
8. Help make safety more attractive and manly.
9. Pay special attention to those youths who have a high risk of having accidents—the underachiever, the offensive driver, and those who have deviant behavior or are overaggressive.
10. If you have a "speed demon," help him find better outlets than cars and motor bikes.

Reviewers going over these long lists made some pertinent comments. Mother Ruth Poarch wrote, "I know this is awfully important but it sure gets depressing." Dr. Low replied, "Be positive, a safe life can be a very happy one!" Whether this cheered anyone up or not I don't know, but then pediatrician David Sparling added a few more miscellaneous accident hazards worth noting:

- The sharp edged coffee table in areas where toddlers romp.
- The hot oven door, or its attractive glass window.
- Unprotected hot exhaust pipes.
- The coffee pot with a loose lid that falls off when the coffee is poured or is accidentally tipped over.

I am certain that however extensive our list is, that new items will continue to be added as curious children or thoughtless adults "accidentally" devise new ways to have accidents. They also, however, receive help from some manufacturers who inadvertently produce unsafe household products. Admittedly you can't make everything 100% safe. I had to help a small boy get his head freed from between two innocuous and presumably safe rails that turned out to be close to a turnstile. I am still not sure how the boy managed to get his head in there! But if you find an unsafe consumer product the chairman of the Accident Prevention Committee of the American Academy of Pediatrics advises action:

> Twenty million Americans are injured each year from various manufactured products. Congress established the Consumer Products Safety Commission to help protect the public from unreasonable risks from consumer products. Any consumer may petition the Commission to begin proceedings on safety rules, and consumers are urged to call the Commission to report hazardous products, using the toll free Hot Line number 1-800-638-2666. Fact sheets on safe toys, tricycles and so forth are available. (Consumer Products Safety Commission, Washington, D.C. 20207)

CHILDREN NEED PROTECTION IN THE CAR

A remarkable number of infants and children are seriously hurt or killed each year in often relatively minor auto accidents because they were not in any sort of safety restraint. To many doctors who have to care for the resulting injuries such parental behavior seems akin to criminal negligence. We turned to a volunteer organization to advise you on the details of the important and oft neglected aspects of car safety devices for children, *Physicians For Automotive Safety*. This small group of dedicated doctors has accomplished a lot in upgrading safety standards and in making the public aware of the hazards. The executive secretary, Annemarie Shellness, and the president of P.A.S., Seymour Charles, M.D., write:

> In a car accident there are, in fact, two collisions. The first occurs when a car strikes another vehicle or object and comes to a sudden, violent stop. The second collision involves the vehicle occupants, who keep moving towards the point of impact until they, too, are stopped by the instrument panel, the windshield, or the road surface. It is this second collision that can kill or cause serious injury.
> Safety belts are the single most effective safety device available. The protection they provide by keeping the driver and passengers safely in place significantly reduces the chances of death and injury. Lap belts are a "must," but shoulder belts should also be used to decrease the likelihood of injury to the face and head, particularly in front seats. A shoulder belt must *never* be worn without a lap belt.
> Standard safety belts are not suitable for infants and small children.

The pelvic structure of a small child is insufficiently developed to tolerate the pressure lap belts exert in a crash, and internal injuries could result. Children weighing less than 40 pounds should therefore be protected by special child restraints designed to distribute collision forces over a large body area. *But if no special child safety devices are available, use of standard belts is infinitely preferable to using no restraint at all.*

No child should ever ride on the lap of an adult. *Although this may ordinarily be a most secure place, it is not so in an automobile.* In a collision, the child would be crushed between the adult and the vehicle interior. Even if the adult is wearing a combination lap and shoulder belt, the child would be wrenched from his or her arms by collision forces and thrown against hard, protruding objects inside the vehicle or ejected through the windshield, window, or door. A seat belt must not be fastened around a child sitting on someone's lap; in a crash the weight of the heavier person would press the belt into the child's abdomen—with grave consequences. *Even on the very first ride, the drive home from the hospital, the infant should be transported in an approved car carrier.*

At this time, it is difficult for parents to make an informed choice among a large selection of children's car seats on the market, some of them costing twice as much as others, all of them complying with a government safety standard in effect since 1971.

The federal specifications issued in 1971 have, however, been found to be totally inadequate. Thus, many of the safety devices labeled as meeting or even "exceeding" federal regulations would give poor protection in the event of an accident, and are inferior to the protection that standard belts provide for older children and adults.

The Department of Transportation is in the process of upgrading the standard, but no new specifications have been issued at the time this goes to press. Once the improved standard goes into effect, the label on the device will no longer refer to the year 1971, but to 1978 or possibly an even later date. In the meantime, parents are advised to make a selection from the devices listed and described in Table 1-1. All have performed satisfactorily in crash tests conducted by the University of Michigan Highway Safety Research Institute.

Selection of a safe device is only the beginning. The restraint must also be *used* correctly. This involves (a) anchoring the device to the seat of the vehicle, and (b) putting the harness on the child where one is provided. (Some devices do not have a harness.) In many cases, a top tether strap is also required. (See Figures 3, 4, 5, and 6.)

Unless the instructions given by the manufacturer are faithfully followed, the seat will be virtually useless, even in a minor mishap. Too many parents continue to look upon children's car seats merely as a means of keeping the child in one place and raised up for better visibility. These purposes are secondary: What is required is protection in case of an accident.

TABLE 1-1.   *Crash-tested devices available and where to buy them.*

Name of Device & Manufacturer	Child's Weight	Design Used	Securement and Recommended Location in the Car	Retail Outlets**
American Safety (Swyngomatic)	15 to 40 lbs.	II b	Top of device *must* be anchored.	D & J/S
Astroseat #V† (Internl. Mfg. Co.)	15 to 40 lbs.	II b	Top of device *must* be anchored; use in the center of the back seat.	D & J/S
Bobby-Mac 2 in 1 Bobby-Mac DeLuxe (Collier Keyworth)	7* to 35 lbs. 7* to 40 lbs.	I, II ab	In forward-facing position the 2 in 1 should be used in the center back seat. Easy to install and use.	D & J/S
Child Love Seat (General Motors)	20 to 40 lbs.	II b	Top of device *must* be anchored.	(1) , D & J/S
Dyn-O-Mite Infant Carrier	7–17 lbs.	I		
Infant Love Seat (General Motors)	7* to 20 lbs.	I	Easy to install and use.	(2) , D & J/S
Kantwet Care Seat #785 #885 #597	15– 45 lbs.	II b	Prop up device must be anchored. Use in center of back seat.	
Kantwet Care Seat† #985, #986, #988 (Questor)	7* to 43 lbs.	I, II b	Easy to install and use; optional top strap available.	D & J/S
Little Rider Harness‡ (Rose Mfg. Co.)	15 to 50 lbs.	II c	Top of harness *must* be secured; use in the center of the back seat.	D & J/S
Mopar Child Seat (Chrysler Corp.)	21 to 50 lbs.	II a	Very convenient, requires lap belt only; use in the center of the back seat.	(3)
Positest Car Seat (Hedstrom)	17 to 42 lbs.	II b	With side anchor strap, use on right side of car. Without anchor use in center back.	D & J/S
Safety Shell #74† & 75 (Peterson)	7* to 40 lbs.	I, II ab	With side anchor strap, use on right side of car. Without anchor use in center back.	D & J/S

† Other seats made by the same company not recommended.
‡ Little Rider **Vest** not recommended.
* Suitable for the newborn baby.
Make sure of the model number listed; some devices may look similar, but there could be a considerable difference in their safety performance.
** This column shows where devices are obtainable. Numbers indicate automobile dealerships as follows:
(1) General Motors and American Motors;
(2) G.M., Ford, Chrysler, and American Motors;
(3) Chrysler;
(4) Ford.
D & J/S = Department and Juvenile Specialty Stores
[Researchers and manufacturers are continually improving car safety devices. For the latest update I suggest that you send 25¢ and a stamped self-addressed #10 (business size) envelope to: Physicians for Automotive Safety, 50 Union Avenue, Irvington, New Jersey 07111. Request the latest revision of their pamphlet, "Don't Risk Your Child's Life," which contains a list of car seat safety devices.]

TABLE 1-1. *Continued*

Name of Device & Manufacturer	Child's Weight	Design Used	Securement and Recommended Location in the Car	Retail Outlets**
Sweetheart #11† (Bunny Bear)	7* to 40 lbs.	I, II b	Use in the center of the back seat. Easy to install and use.	D & J/S
Tot-Guard (Ford Motor Co.)	20 to 50 lbs.	II a	Very convenient, requires lap belt only; use in the center of the back seat.	(4)
Trav-L-Guard (Century)	40 lbs.	I, II b	Convertible	
Wee Care #597 (Strolee)	7* to 43 lbs.	I, II b	Top of device *must* be anchored.	D & J/S

For the Infant from Birth

Car carriers for infants are designed to face rearward—never forward. The baby rides in a half upright position, secured with a harness. The carrier is strapped to the seat of the vehicle with a lap belt.

For the Child Able to Sit Up Without Support

The Shield

Safety experts prefer this type of protection, particularly up to the age of two or three. In the event of a crash the child's body is caught by the padded shield which acts as a cushion. The Tot-Guard and Mopar (see chart) are very easy to use—the shield is anchored with a lap belt and no harness is needed— but if your child is overly active and hard to discipline, he or she may climb out or slide through while you are driving. Consider this before making a choice.

The "Traditional" Car Seat

The child is held by a harness which consists of two shoulder straps, a lap belt, and a crotch strap. The seat is strapped down with a vehicle lap

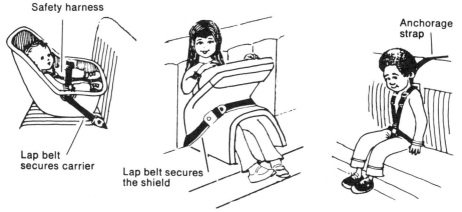

FIGURE 4 *Automobile safety devices.*

belt. Some devices require the belt to be threaded through the back where it can remain permanently buckled. Others must be fastened with the belt around the front of the seat after the child has been put into the harness as shown in the diagram.

A number of seats require additional anchorage: A strap leading from the top must be joined to a lap belt in the seat behind. (This makes one set of belts unusable.) The strap must be pulled taut.

If the device is to be used in the back seat of a sedan, an anchorage assembly will have to be installed on the rear window ledge. (Assemblies can be purchased separately for a second car.) In some station wagons and hatchbacks, installation could present a problem; check this out before you buy.

Securing a top tether may be inconvenient and time-consuming, but seats designed to be secured at the top are believed to provide an extra margin of safety. *If, however, the top strap is not fastened, the seat will lose its protective value entirely.* Unless the top strap is secured every time, your child will be safer riding in a device designed to provide crash protection without the need for a top tether (see chart).

Forward-facing seats should be used in a fully upright position. Use of a "reclining" feature is not recommended.

The Safety Harness

This provides good protection at low cost. The harness is secured with a lap belt and a top tether strap (installation is described above). The child may sit on a cushion.[1]

Children can start using a standard lap belt when they weigh forty pounds. The child should be seated on a firm cushion no more than two inches high, and strapped in with a standard lap belt while sitting upright against the back of the car seat. The cushion will help position the belt across the child's hips, below the belly, with the lower edge touching the thighs. The belt must be adjusted for a snug fit in order to prevent it slipping up across the child's abdomen in the event of an accident. The cushion should be omitted as soon as the child is tall enough to look out of the windows of the car.

Children in the front seat should use the shoulder strap as soon as they are tall enough but *never* without a lap belt. Take into consideration the extra height added by using a cushion—the belt should position across the shoulder and not across the face or neck (consult your car owner's manual).

SKATEBOARD SAFETY

Skateboards have one definite effect. They keep doctors busy patching up children. I suggest that you make your child study this section and pass a 100% test on it before you let him use a skateboard.

1. Keep off of streets, at least those with lots of auto traffic.
2. Don't skate near street corners where an auto driver may not see you in time.
3. Avoid steep hills where control is difficult.

4. Don't use skate boards around dusk when visibility is poor.
5. Check your wheels and make certain that they are not sticking—the bearings may wear out quickly, causing the skate board to stop unexpectedly from mechanical failure.
6. Don't try anything fancy or try for high speed before you have become skilled at the basic use of the skateboard.
7. Wear long pants and long sleeves to reduce abrasions when you fall.
8. Observe the usual traffic rules, including stop signs.

BICYCLE SAFETY

Bike riding is a leading cause of accidents of the school age child: 1,100 deaths in one year. There are 100 million bikes in the United States. In fact, more bikes are sold than cars. In one year there was a 95% increase in bicycle fatalities in California alone.

Lack of proper knowledge of bike safety is a major cause of accidents, even among adults. Study showed that the leading causes of bicycle accidents are:

1. Riding on the wrong side of the road against traffic.
2. Unsafe changing of lanes.
3. Failure of the cyclist to yield when entering a roadway.
4. Ignoring traffic signals and signs.
5. Improper lights and reflectors for dusk or night riding.
6. Mechanical failure.

Cycling on the wrong side of the road is exceptionally dangerous, as drivers often don't see bikes in time, especially when the car makes a right-hand turn. Also, a wrong way bike forces those bicyclists going with the traffic to veer into the curb or the road.

I believe another major cause of bicycle accidents is lack of discipline. An undisciplined and self-centered child is uncaring about anything but immediate gratification. The rest of the world doesn't seem to count. Parents have a duty to teach their children awareness and respect for other people and for the rules we must use to live together. Children under nine should not be allowed to ride in traffic without adult supervision.

Parents should consider the availability in their neighborhoods of areas safe for cyclists before buying a child a bike. There are more fatalities and serious head injuries from falls, particularly from bicycle accidents, in the five to fifteen age group than all other causes combined. To reduce the danger to your child, match the bike to the skill of the rider. *Beware* of hand brakes for younger children. Provide a hard helmet to be worn while bicycling. If there is no safe area in your neighborhood for bicycling, don't buy a bike.

The bicycles themselves should be safe. High rise bikes are particularly dangerous, as shown by an English research study of head injuries. In a population with only twenty percent "high rise" bikes, about seventy percent of severe head injuries were from "high rise" bikes and thirty percent from standard bikes. The high rise has high handle bars and a long seat with a back rest. This arrangement puts the center of gravity over the rear wheel, increasing the accident hazard. Safe bicycles should have:

1. Slip resistant pedals.
2. A solid frame—they can become weak.
3. Modest handlebar-to-seat ratio.
4. Center of gravity in the center of the bicycle.
5. Limited seat heights.
6. Bike flag, raised to car top height to alert traffic to a bike's hidden presence.
7. Good large reflectors for visibility, including spoke, pedal, and leg reflectors.
8. Night lights should be installed, maintained, and used in times of poor visibility (dusk, dawn, rain, and fog).

Dr. Harvey Kravitz has emphasized the often serious injuries from catching the feet between the bicycle spokes and the frame. Usually this is from riding double or from the foot slipping off the pedal. Riding double should be discouraged. Leg guards and shields should be improved and pedals should be made more slip proof.

Bicycle Brakes

The California Medical Association believes that the number of accidents caused by faulty bicycle brakes justifies a public education campaign. They advise:

> The simplest brake to operate is the coaster, which requires only that the direction of the pedals be reversed while the arms are used to push the main weight of the body back from the handle bars and onto the pedals. This bracing action tends to keep the rider from being pitched headlong over the front wheel as the cycle stops.
> The popular multiple speed geared bicycles usually are equipped with brakes operated by special grips applied to the handle bars. Cables transmit the pressure from one hand grip to the front wheel and from the other grip to the rear wheel. If equal pressure is applied to both wheels, the braking action of this system is excellent, but obtaining this result requires a degree of skill not possessed by all children. It too often happens that most of the braking is applied to the front wheel, flipping the bike so that the rider is thrown headfirst to the pavement.

Dr. Hobart Wallace is appalled that:

Parents turn a five- to eight-year-old child loose on a bicycle to ride in the streets with no comprehension of safety regulations and rules of the road. I predict that there will eventually have to be laws regarding licensure to ride bicycles on streets as more and more problems develop.

Pediatrician Donald Blim believes that *most* cyclists have neither the safety, knowledge, or skills to ride bikes on the same roads with cars. He emphasizes two preventable causes of bike accidents:

A tragic cause of accidents is when a parent takes a toddler for a ride "double" on the bike, and the toddler is thrown into the path of a car when a minor bike accident occurs. Another preventable cause of bike accidents is the presence in the streets of storm sewer grates whose slots are just wide enough to trap the front wheel of a bike, which falls into the slot, throwing the rider.

The Evel Knievel Syndrome

Pediatrician Robert Scherz has become alarmed at the number of accidents children have while trying to mimic daredevil heroes:

Parents should be aware of the adverse influence that widely publicized daredevils have on the bike habits of their children. The "Evel Knievel Syndrome" of the mid 1970s produced thousands of injuries to children who tried to imitate the motorcycle escapades of their "hero." In one study of 57 cases treated in hospital emergency rooms (average age ten years), the children were treated for abrasions, cuts—and often fractures—from this sort of misadventure. Those who required hospitalization were more seriously injured, with an average medical bill of $500.00.

Should Your Baby be Taught to Swim?

Dr. Hobart Wallace writes, "No!"

Although some organizations actively push infant swim classes, claiming great benefit with suave assurance, studies so far indicate little, if any, benefit to the infant. Parents may develop a false sense of security regarding the child's ability, which can result in fatalities.

Those who believe that you can teach a baby or toddler under the age of three years to swim overlook a lot of factors. Even if a toddler learns to swim, he has no judgment. It is better that he be afraid of water and avoid it than that he be fearless and jump in. A toddler should never be allowed around unfenced pools, in bathtubs, or around ponds without constant supervision. The only reasonable thing to teach toddlers is how to hold their breath when the head is under water.

There are many other reasons for keeping tiny children away from a pool. It is neither healthful nor appealing to swim in a dilute solution of urine and feces. A child must be well toilet trained before being allowed in a pool. Toddler ponds are, at the least, a health hazard. To put enough chlorine in the water to kill the bacteria (and not all the viruses at that!) creates damaging chlorine irritation. Young children have far less immunity than adults, and they may easily become infected in contaminated water.

Further, young children are unable to conserve heat. Their surface-area-compared-to-weight is larger than that of an adult, so they lose heat easily. Children up to age ten often come out of a pool chilled, shaking, and blue from heat loss.

Most but not all children are ready to learn to swim by age three. First, teach your child how to hold his breath when under water. If he is fearful, the instructor must be very patient. Such children should not be pushed, or they may fear water all their life. Those who "swim like fish" may have less judgment than the finned amphibians, and must be watched closely at all times. All pools must be fenced, with the gate locked, unless a responsible adult is present. The buddy system must be instituted early and the guard never let down—even for adults. In many suburban areas, accidental drowning is the leading cause of death of children. *Pools must be fenced.*

In spite of fencing, babies still drown. A mother in our practice, Lo-ana Tomasello, teaches water safety for infants and children. As you can see, I am skeptical of the "swimming" aspects. However, she has received strong support from Dr. John W. Schieffelin of the University of California Medical Center.[2] He claims that infants over nine months of age can be taught to survive in water twenty minutes by the "aquakinetics" technique. The child is taught first to hold his breath under water and then to float on his back, head out, and finally to roll himself to his back and to bounce upright after being dropped in a pool. They do forget how and need repeated refresher courses. Mrs. Tomasello adds safety tips, "Bright colored bathing suits help identify your child more easily in the water. Keep the water level high so small children will be able to reach the side of the pool." I once pulled out a small child who had fallen un-seen into a pool but hadn't struggled and consequently just floated. Per-haps the "aquakinetics" technique is of worth. Even so, a toddler forgets, lacks judgment, and must always be watched when around water—not just every minute, but every second!

POISONS IN THE HOME

Before Poisoning

1. You *should have* syrup of ipecac on hand at home whenever you have children five years old or under. It is inexpensive and available from the pharmacy without a prescription.
2. Lock your barn door before the horse is stolen. Go through your house room by room, closet by closet, cupboard by cupboard, drawer by drawer—including

purses and bags—and get everything that shouldn't be eaten or played with up and out of your preschooler's way.

In what is probably the best book for parents in existence on the subject, *Dangers to Children and Youth*, Dr. Jay Arena points out that each year in the United States there are over a million cases of poisoning, with over 3,000 deaths. Undoubtedly, many cases are missed, as the symptoms are often misleading, and the cause often undiagnosed. There are over a *quarter million poisonous products* which may be present in the home. Seventy-five percent of all poisoning in small children is caused by *in-sight* drugs or household agents—and thus, such poisonings are due to carelessness or negligence.

The following is a general classification of common household poisons described in detail in Dr. Arena's book.[3] For emergency treatment of poisoning from these substances see page 25. Items followed by X, +, or # require different treatments as outlined on pages 25 to 27:

A. *Common Medications*

Ammoniated mercury	Menthol
Antihistamines	Mercurochrome, Merthiolate, Metaphen
A.P.C. (Anacin, Empirin, etc.)	Motion sickness drugs
Aspirin	Oil of wintergreen
Boric acid	Paregoric
Camphor	Phisohex
Carbolic acid	Potassium permanganate
Cold tablets	Prescription drugs
Cough syrups	Rubbing alcohol
Decongestants	Selenium (Selsun)
Eucalyptol	Sodium fluoride
Gentian violet	Talc (inhaled) #
Hexylresorcinol	Witch hazel
Iodine	

B. *Cleaning, polishing, and bleaching agents*

Ammonia +X	Jewelry cleaners and cement +
Bleach +X	Laundry blue
Carbon tetrachloride +X	Leather polishers and dyes +
Carburetor cleaners +X	Metal cleaners and polishers +X
Chlorinated cleaners +X	Methyl alcohol
Chlorine +X	Shoe cleaners and polishers +
Deodorizer cakes +X	Spot removers +X
Deodorizing tablets +	Strong acids +X
Detergents +	Strong alkalis +X
Drain cleaner unclogger +X	Toilet bowl cleaners +X
Dry cleaning fluids +X	Typewriter cleaner +

C. *Cosmetics*

After shave lotion
Catnip
Clove oil
Colognes
Cuticle removers
Depilatories
Hair dyes, tints, and colorings
Hair lotions
Hair preparations
Hair sprays

Lacquers, plasticizers, resins
Nail preparations
Neutralizers
Organic solvents X
Perfumes
Permanent wave solutions
Skin preparations
Styptic pencil
Sun tan lotions

D. *Food products taken in excess*

Ethyl alcohol (gin, rum,
    vodka, whiskey)
Honey from toxic sources
Licorice
Saccharin

Salt
Vegetable dye
Vitamin A
Vitamin D

E. *Garden supplies*

Ant poison
Cockroach poison
Earwig bait
Fungicides
Fumigants
Herbicides

Insect sprays
Mice poison
Rat poison
Snail bait
Weed killer

F. *Paint and solvents*

Barbecue lighter fluid +X
Cigarette lighter fluid +X
Gasoline +X
Kerosene +X
Paint +
Paint brush cleaner +X

Paint remover +X
Paint thinner +X
Putty
Turpentine +X
Varnish +

G. *Others*

Airplane glue
Antifreeze
Anti-rust products
Brake fluids +
Carbon monoxide #
Christmas bulb fluid X
Cigarettes
Epoxy glue
Fiberglass and resin plastics

Fire extinguishing fluids
Holly berries
Inks
Mistletoe
Mothballs
Plastic menders and glues
Propane gas
Rug adhesives
Spray de-icer

What to Do for Poisoning

1. Identify the poison. Keep the container or label, its contents, or some of the vomitus for analysis if needed.
2. Estimate how much the child took.
3. Have someone *call the doctor* or poison control center while you:
4. Check the above list and follow the procedure below A, B, C, D, or E.

   A. For the list on pages 23 to 24, if the item marked with (X):

     1. *Give two glasses of milk or water at once.*

     2. Do *not* give ipecac or induce vomiting if the child has drunk paint thinner type material, oven or brush cleaners, alkalis, and drain cleaner caustics.

        Doctors disagree: There are two schools of thought on the use of ipecac for the treatment of ingestion of petroleum products (kerosene, turpentine, etc.). Because of the possibility of aspiration of these substances during vomiting and getting them in the lungs, many physicians recommend against ipecac use for this type of poisoning. However, because petroleum products are absorbed in the intestine and can poison the liver and lung indirectly anyway, other physicians recommend that ipecac be given. They point out that children frequently vomit spontaneously after ingesting petroleum products. If the child is kept in a head-down chest-down position when vomiting is likely, there is little likelihood of aspiration. With or without ipecac, a child who has ingested petroleum products should be kept on his stomach with the head down for the first two hours or so. If the petroleum product contains another poison, such as an insect killer, ipecac should be given anyway to eliminate the poison.

   B. Do not give ipecac or induce vomiting if the child is very sleepy, or if he is sleeping, convulsing, or in coma.

   C. For the above list, unless marked with (X):

     1. *Give syrup or ipecac 1 ounce (or six teaspoons or two tablespoons) at once* (Catch the vomitus with pan or towel).

     2. Repeat the same dose of syrup of ipecac in ten minutes if vomiting has not occurred. Give large amounts of water and stick your finger down the child's throat to gag him and induce vomiting.

     3. If no ipecac is in the house, give mustard water (one teaspoon of wet or dry mustard to a tall glass of water).

     4. Check with your doctor or poison control center.

     5. If vomiting has not occurred within fifteen minutes, take the child to the nearest doctor's office or emergency room after *calling your doctor.*

   D. If the substance is marked (+):

     1. *Give two glasses of milk or water at once.*

     2. Again, call the doctor at once, and if he isn't available call the poison control center or hospital emergency room.

   E. If the substance is marked (#):

     1. *Move the victim out of the area of gas or vapor and give artificial respiration if he is not breathing, or:*

     2. Assist his respirations if he is breathing but dusky or blue. If a poisonous fluid such as carbon tetrachloride is on the clothes, *remove the clothes and wash the skin.*

F. If there is a possibility that some of the poison is left in the stomach after ipecac has been given, especially if it is a slow acting poisonous plant, your doctor may give an activated charcoal slurry ("solution") to absorb the remaining poison.

In all cases, start one of the above treatments at once. Then call your doctor—or the poison control center, if the doctor is not available. If neither is available, call the nearest hospital emergency room.

If you go to the doctor's office or emergency room, take the poison container with you.

Soaps, Detergents, and Cleansing Agents

Severely poisonous cleansing agents include sink unpluggers, such as Drano, Saniflush, and Liquid Plumber; dishwasher detergent; lye; oven cleaners; and some wall and floor cleaners, as well as bleaches—as Clorox—and disinfectant cleaners. They all cause severe chemical burns.

First Aid
If these substances get in the eye:
Flush out the eye with continuous running water, holding the eyelids open and the head under the faucet or hose.
If swallowed, they may severely burn the mouth and esophagus:
Immediately give milk, or soup, gravy, or water. Do not give acid citrus juice or vinegar: If the detergent contains carbonates, these may release carbon dioxide gas in the stomach.

Symptoms of Ingestion of Various Cleaning Agents
• Nausea, vomiting, and abdominal pain
• Burning of the mouth, esophagus, and stomach
• Lethargy, coma, or convulsions
• Fever, pneumonia, and respiratory distress
• Dizziness and low blood pressure

Cleaning products account for five percent of all "accidentally" ingested substances in children under five years of age. If the use of soaps and detergents is a hallmark of civilization, we are a *very* civilized society. Soaps account for fifteen percent of cleaners, and detergents for eighty-five percent. Generally, three to four swallows of detergent are not likely to be severely poisonous.

In case of detergent ingestion, call your doctor or local poison control center to see how toxic the particular brand is. The Soap and Detergent Association has emergency telephone numbers available for information from companies on their products.

Is Your Purse Dangerous?
Infants and toddlers love to explore purses. Your purse is a bag of poisons—at least if you're among that half of women who carry pills in their purses. Most of these can kill a child, who may be attracted to the

various "candy colored" tablets. Although each purse is as different as its owner, most pills in purses are either aspirin, pain pills, or sedatives. These medications can easily be lethal, so don't put pills in your purse, and always put your purse out of reach of children.

IS YOUR CHILD ACCIDENT PRONE?

If your child has repeated accidents, is he accident prone? Even the experts are not able to agree on what "accident proneness" really is. Dr. Merritt Low points out that:

We do know that some children are more "accident prone" than others. Usually they are more compulsive: They are doers instead of thinkers. Another group of accident prone youngsters are those with behavioral maladjustments. These children take more risks because their self-image is low. They need to "prove" something.

For both of these groups, preventive education is very important. It is too easy to say, half in jest, "Oh, that child is just accident prone and can't help it." An accurate analysis of each situation is needed so that some preventive steps can be taken.

Unfortunately, statistics prove that if a child has had a number of accidents, his chances of having more accidents are greater than those of a child who has never had one. Certain children have recurrent accidents, whether falling, breaking bones, or cutting themselves.

Pediatrician Jay Arena, Chairman of the National Poison Control Center offers some good positive advice to parents.

Your methods of handling your child may do more to induce safety than simply removing hazards. It is important to recognize that a child is ever-changing, with ever-increasing capabilities. Adults frequently make one of two mistakes: Either they credit the child with more intelligence than he possesses, or they assume that he is quite unable to think for himself. In both situations, they fail to appreciate that they are dealing with a mind and body in constant development.

There Are Three General Lines of Safety Education
1. Teach the child to distinguish between the risks he may take and those he had better avoid.
2. Teach him the best ways of dealing with dangers that cannot be absolutely escaped.
3. Teach him the discipline of obedience. Discipline is setting limits on behavior and maintaining these limits through education; parental example; encouragement; cooperation; insistence; temporary isolation, if necessary; and, sometimes, punishment.

If parents are to provide their children with a judicious blend of advice, reprimand, and prohibition, they must learn to know themselves and their children better. They should, for instance, be familiar not only with the complex problems responsible for home accidents, but also with the strains and causes that may bring about accidents.

Stresses and Pressures May Increase the Risk of Childhood Accidents

1. Hunger or fatigue, particularly during the hour before a scheduled meal, during late afternoon, or before bedtime.
2. Hyperactivity.
3. Parental lack of understanding of what to expect at various stages in childhood development.
4. Illness, pregnancy, or menstruation of the mother.
5. A recent substitution of the person caring for the children—as where responsibility is shifted from mother to sister.
6. Continually tense relationship between parents.
7. Illness or death of other family members which takes most of the mother's attention.
8. Sudden change of the child's environment, as in moving or at vacation time.
9. A mother who is rushed or too busy. Saturday is the worst day for accidents, particularly between 3:00 and 6:00 P.M.

To Raise Your Child Safely

1. Ask what you would need to do if you were going to leave your child alone for one hour.
2. Realize that children want to obey, and that they expect the leadership of rules.
3. Tell the truth.
4. Ration your commands.
5. Enforce your commands.
6. Be consistent.
7. Agree on commands.
8. Punish the child in some appropriate manner when he violates obedience rules.
9. Do not set goals too high to reach.
10. Forbid dangerous games, tricks, and sports. Have your child taught to swim at an early age (four years).
11. Reward obedience.
12. Make sure children understand your meaning.
13. Love and enjoy your children: Their response is effective discipline.[4]

NOW THAT YOU KNOW HOW TO PREVENT ACCIDENTS, WHAT WILL YOU DO ABOUT THEM?

There is a temptation to protect small children by keeping them safely in a play pen. That, however, can have adverse effects, cautions psychologist Burton White:

An infant is a very curious human being. Ideally, that curiosity should get deeper and stronger; but many mothers stifle curiosity because they

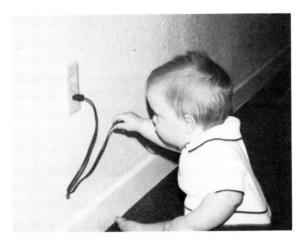

FIGURE 5   *"I think I will see what happens!"*

are protecting the child and/or the house. If curiosity is stifled, it can lead to the child's having undue interest in the mother or too little interest in the mother.[5]

On the other hand, Dr. John Richards believes that play pens can be reasonably used for short periods of time to keep the explorer out of trouble while mother performs some necessary functions.

As they get older and protection becomes more difficult we have to educate them that this is a dangerous world. Yet with all the facts available there are still over 16,000 child deaths from accidents each year in the United States. Why? Partly, contends pediatrician Merritt Low, because we suffer from a series of myths we take for facts:

Myth 1: "Education can solve the problem." Knowing just isn't enough. Attitudes have to be changed and myths abolished before education can be effective.

Myth 2: "Accidents will happen," is the common excuse. At least ninety percent of accidents could be prevented.

Myth 3: "Protection and restriction will prevent accidents." Not forever. As the child matures, a delicate balance must be established between protection and education. The overprotected child is at risk when he does get loose.

Myth 4: "You must make them afraid of hazards." Anxiety does not prevent accidents; it may encourage them.

Myth 5: "It can't or won't happen to me or my children." We all tend to believe in or hope for "good luck" and a charmed life. There is need for such feelings of security, but a balance must be struck with the realities of life.

The real fact is that accidents almost always could have been prevented. To accomplish such prevention requires a change of attitude toward accidents so that we can abolish the myths and substitute rational actions. To accomplish this, we should:

1. Apply the successful accident prevention techniques of industry to school, recreational, and home activities.
2. Recognize the increased risks of modern technology and alter our attitudes in order to take them into account.
3. Insist upon public action to force legislation and engineering for safety.
4. Change our emotional attitudes and social actions so we stop acting as if risk is virile.
5. Teach our children to analyze situations in advance so they can anticipate hazards.
6. Use consistency and love to teach our children the anti-accident character traits of obedience and responsibility.

2

FIRST AID,
SECOND AID,
AND EMERGENCY MEDICAL CARE

It is your job at home to be ready for those emergencies that you cannot or do not successfully prevent. The first requirement is knowledge, so it will be best for you to read this chapter now—then you will be more familiar with the material and can locate it more easily if an emergency occurs. Of course, most injuries are not emergencies, and one of the key factors in efficient home care is deciding what does and what does not need a physician's attention. Over twenty physicians from different parts of the nation contributed to and reviewed this chapter. They include twelve different specialties, from allergists to urologists, from pediatricians and family practitioners to neurosurgeons. We found that we were not always in agreement, but we settled on one way even though other methods may be equally good—there is no time to debate in an emergency. But if you study this chapter before an emergency, it is a good idea to ask your own doctor's opinion on the advice we present. He may recommend some other techniques and methods. After first aid has been given, there are still many things you can do at home to aid healing and prevent complications. Here again, you may find differences in advice on how to offer "second aid." If there is doubt in your mind, or if the advice offered here doesn't work for you, call your doctor. For further information about the diseases and care of problems discussed in this chapter, see section on "Illness: The Location" (page 123).

If you have moved to a town new to you or if you have never bothered thinking about what to do in case of an emergency, start by picking a doctor for your children and for yourselves (see page 116). Ask him how he wants emergencies handled: What telephone number do you use when the office is closed; what doctor covers his practice when he is gone; when should you go to his office and when to the emergency room;

and should you call him first? Have the telephone numbers of the fire department emergency squad and a reliable ambulance company handy. Instruct your children on what to do in case of emergency—how to get a hold of you or a neighbor or a block mother. It is a good idea to sign an emergency care authorization in the doctor's office so that, if you are unavailable in an emergency, the doctor is legally authorized to do what is required. The school should know who your child's doctor is and have authorization to take the child to the doctor or hospital for emergency care when they cannot find you.

SKIN

Mild Sunburn

First, sunburn should be prevented, for repeated and chronic sunburn causes early skin damage which can lead to later skin cancer.

A mild sunburn is red and without blisters. A tepid corn starch bath is soothing (½ cup of Linit or Argo corn starch mixed to a paste and put in a tub of water). Keep cool and use smooth clothing. Apply bland lubricants, such as cold cream, hand lotion, vaseline and so forth.

A small area of sunburn which is swollen and blistered is relieved by a starch bath, but better relief can be obtained from cool wet dressings. Use Burrows solution (non prescription), salt solution (2 tsp/quart of water), or fresh milk, to soak smooth thin fabric strips made out of old diapers, sheets, or muslin. Lay the wet cloth over the burn area and replace every ten minutes with a fresh wet cloth. Rinse them well and wring dry the used cloths and put them back into the solution for the next change. Use these dressings intermittently, a few hours at a time. Once the swelling and oozing has subsided, coat the area with antibiotic ointment to help prevent infection. Do not break blisters unless they contain pus. If there is pus or other signs of infection (foul odor, red streaks radiating from the burn area), call your doctor.

Severe Sunburn

A large area of sunburn can be as dangerous as any other burn. Medical attention must be sought. Be certain to take plenty of fluids, keep the urine output high, and watch for red or tea colored urine and report it at once. Check for fever, and look for any swelling of the feet. Kidney damage, dehydration and shock, blood poisoning and local infection can all complicate a large or severe sunburn.

First Aid for Burns

Severe Burns
1. *Immediately douse burns with cool liquid.*
2. Don't take time to take off the clothes.

3. Use any cool liquid at hand, quickly:
   A coke or Koolaid
   A glass of milk
   Plop a small child in the sink or a teenager or adult in the nearest tub or shower or creek or use a garden hose or spigot.
4. Keep the burn in the cool water at least five minutes—longer if it is painful.
5. Ice is not usually required.
6. Do not take the clothes off.
7. Keep the burn in water (or the clothes wet) on the way to the hospital or office. Cover with a clean sheet if needed, but don't waste time.
8. Do not use ointments or grease.
9. Wrap the unburned area in a blanket if the weather is cold.

Minor Burns

1. Put in cold water immediately.
2. If dirty, wash gently with soap under cold running tap water; rinse well.
3. Pat dry with a clean towel.
4. Coat with: antibiotic ointment, vitamin A & D ointment, butysin picrate ointment or petroleum jelly (listed in order of preference). (Ask your pharmacist to help you stock a first aid kit with these non-prescription items.)
5. Cover with a non-sticking sterile dressing.
6. Wrap with gauze.
7. Change dressing daily; if infection occurs, call your doctor.

Minor Abrasions ("Skinned")

Wash well with soap and water. The bathtub is the best way to soak and soap children's scrapes and bruises. The child will relax in the soothing, warm, soapy water, and will be more cooperative as you cleanse him. Dirt left in the skin can cause infection, and occasionally the skin will heal over the dirt, leaving an unsightly tattoo or scar.

An antibiotic ointment or spray may be applied after the tub bath. If the abrasions are deep or may stick to the clothes or get dirty again, use a non-stick dressing to cover the area and change it every day. Minor shallow abrasions may be left open to the air. Even deeper abrasions should rarely be bandaged for over two days.

Cuts

1. Stop the bleeding by applying a clean dry cloth directly over the wound for at least five minutes without releasing the pressure. Tourniquets are only needed in very large deep wounds; enough local pressure will usually suffice.
2. Scrub the wound thoroughly with soap and water with a clean wash cloth, cotton balls, or gauze pads. Pull the wound open and irrigate it well inside with water. Make certain that all dirt is out of the wound. Then stop the fresh bleeding with pressure over a sterile or clean cloth. Do not be afraid to cause a little crying during the scrubbing: This is better than treating a later infection due to retained dirt.

3. If the wound is large, deep, gapes open, is on a joint or on a cosmetically important area, see the doctor.
4. Apply an antiseptic in and around the wound. Doctors differ in what they recommend, but Betadine or Mercurochrome are advocated by some. Antibiotic ointments work but they tend to loosen the adhesive so the bandages won't stick. (Local antiseptics such as Mercurochrome or local antibiotics containing Neomycin or Furacin may cause rashes in some sensitive individuals.)
5. Dry the wound well and close with a bandaid, steristrips, or a butterfly.

Butterfly Dressings

Minor cuts can be held together with a "butterfly" tape, which is adhesive tape with a non-sticking center bridge. These can be purchased in the drug store or made at home:

1. Wash and dry your hands and scissors well.
2. Make four cuts in the tape as shown by the marks in Figure 6.
3. Fold the flaps onto the adhesive side as shown.
4. Put a small amount of antiseptic on the flaps to kill possible contaminating skin germs from your hands.
5. After the wound is clean and dry, and painted with antiseptic, stick one side of the butterfly on one side of the cut.
6. Pull gently, in order to bring the edges of the cut together, and stick the other side of the butterfly to the skin.
7. Then bandage over the area.

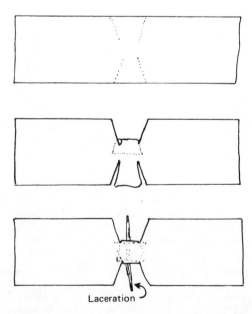

Laceration

FIGURE 6   *A homemade butterfly adhesive bandaid.*

Butterflys can be used for minor lacerations which are not too deep, and which are on a flat surface where you are not worried about a scar. They rarely work well on small children (who pull them off), in hot sweaty weather, or on a surface where the skin or underlying tissue moves—such as near joints.

Frostbite

A committee of physicians from The California Medical Association offers the following health tips on frostbite:

When frostbite occurs, begin rewarming as soon as possible. A hot bath is excellent, but avoid scalding. Hot wet towels, changed frequently and applied gently, will help. If no fire or hot water is available, place the victim in a sleeping bag or cover him/her with coats and blankets. Hot liquids help raise body temperatures.

In first aid for frostbite, do not rub or massage the affected part with snow. In fact, don't touch it at all! Rapid thawing is the most important need.

For any frostbite, even a mild case, prompt medical attention is important. The depth and degree of the frozen tissue cannot be readily ascertained, and the treatment will vary with the severity of the injury.

True frostbite means that the tissues are frozen. Crystals of ice form between the cells. Nerves, muscles, and blood vessel tissues are most susceptible. The wind plays an important part in frostbite. The chilling effect of air at 20° moving at 45 miles an hour is the same as forty-below-zero air on a still day.

One of the dangers of frostbite is that you often don't feel it. Someone else may notice that your nose or ear is turning *white*. The frozen part becomes hard to the touch and loses feeling. Many sports leaders advocate a buddy system for outdoor winter sports, whereby two persons are paired off, each watching the other for signs of frostbite.

In order to prevent frostbite, first be certain that you are properly dressed for the temperature. Avoid overexertion and excessive perspiration. Avoid contact of bare flesh with cold metal. Don't smoke or drink alcohol.

HEAD INJURIES

Local bumps or swellings do not necessarily indicate that an injury is serious or that there is an internal injury. RX: Use a cold wet cloth or ice pack for the first several hours in order to reduce the swelling and discomfort.

Soft mushy bumps in infants are more likely associated with fractures than are hard lumps.

Forehead blows often swell, and the blood in the resulting bruise may seep to the eye area below after a day or so, resulting in a black eye. A black eye on the *opposite* side from the injury might indicate a fracture, and your physician should be notified. RX: Early use of cold packs helps; then just wait for the bruise to be reabsorbed.

Temple blows above or in front of the ear may be more significant. RX: Observe; and call the doctor if the signs below appear.

Most important, watch the patient for increasing signs and symptoms. Watch especially for *increasing* confusion, lethargy, or irritability.

Call the doctor if:

1. The individual was or is unconscious, confused, or delirious.
2. He has amnesia; (cannot remember the injury or the events leading up to the injury).
3. There is repeated vomiting.
4. He will not arouse and act normally after sleep. Awaken every half hour for two hours, then every two hours for twenty-four hours.
5. There is a bloody or watery discharge from an ear or nostril, or from the mouth.
6. There is a disturbance in vision, balance, or coordination.
7. The pupils are not equal in size when there is equal light on both eyes.
8. There is double vision or crossed eyes.
9. There is significant personality change.
10. He cannot move or has definite weakness in an arm or leg.
11. He cannot keep his balance.
12. It is a baby, and the soft spot on the top of the head swells.
13. The neck is stiff.

Home RX: If the individual is alert, not vomiting, not pale, and has not been unconscious, you can feel secure. Let him go to sleep if he desires, propped up so the head is elevated. Wake him from sleep according to the above schedule. Some children will vomit just from excitement, but if it persists, you should call. Continue to watch the patient for odd or unusual behavior, especially in the first twenty-four hours; but be observant for several days for the unlikely but possible delayed symptoms or signs of brain disturbance. Keep the patient quiet for a day or two and on a light diet.

If the injury involves an athlete, encourage rest, withhold all stimulating medicines or liquor, and elevate the head. The coach or manager involved in the team should be notified. Generally, there should be no further vigorous competition until at least five days after the headache has gone.

BACK AND NECK INJURIES

Back and neck injuries require careful assessment before handling. Make certain that the victim can grip with his hands, wiggle the toes, or raise the knees, and that he has good feeling in the feet and inner legs. If he has urinated (wet himself) or soiled himself with stool, the injury may be quite serious. Every effort must be made to avoid making the injury worse by bending or moving the back, head, or neck. Do not forget to keep the patient covered with blankets while waiting for a stretcher.

EARS

Foreign bodies. Children can get a large variety of objects lodged in their ears. These foreign bodies can occasionally be jarred loose from an ear by gently pounding with your hand on the opposite side of the head with the affected ear held down. Do not go into the ear canal to remove foreign bodies. (One try with tweezers may be justified for paper or cotton if you don't push it into the canal.) Do not try to wash the object out, for it may swell with water, especially if it is a bean in the ear.

Buzzing insects in the ear canal can be stilled and killed by filling the ear with oil (mineral, baby, or olive oil). Sometimes they will float out; at other times, they require removal by the doctor.

Pus or blood from an ear canal requires a visit to the doctor.

Pain when wiggling an ear, or tenderness or swelling in front of or below an ear, along with a history of water exposure (swimming, baths with the head dipping under water, hair washing, and showers), may be a skin infection inside the ear canal called "swimmer's ear," which almost always needs a doctor's attention.

Pain from a slap with an open palm on the ear, or from faulty swimming dives, falls from water skiing, air blasts from shot guns, BB guns, or air hoses may mean a *rupture* of the ear drum (perforation). Pain, a "plugged ear" sensation, or bleeding may be present.

Another cause of earache occurs when diving or descending in an airplane when you have a "cold." The sudden pressure may put undue stress on ear drums, causing pain because of congestion in the Eustachian tube or rupture of the ear drum. RX: Keep water out of the ear; do *not* use ear drops; do see your doctor.

Treatment of Earaches

While there are a few stop-gap measures a parent may take, every earache deserves a call to the doctor. Earache may be the result of a plugged or an infected ear, but it is hard to tell. The pain can go away, but the ear may be infected or left full of mucus. If the hearing is affected, or if there is pus in the ear canal, the child *must* be checked by a physician. Treat ear infections early in order to save both ears and money. Early treatment prevents abscessed ears, ruptured ear drums, and mastoid infections. Most earaches start in the middle of the night, and they can wait until morning for a check. While waiting give aspirin. (Aspirin dosage: One grain per year of age up to ten grains every four hours. Anacin or Emperin: One tablet per three years up to two tablets.) A heating pad on the ear may help, or try a few drops of warm mineral oil. A hair dryer with a bonnet can be used to get heat into the ear drum in order to help relieve acute pain. It may help to use nose drops (in the nose), and then to repeat them again ten minutes later. This will often open the Eustachian tube to the ear and relieve the pressure and pain. Prescription ear drops for pain often help, but shouldn't be confused with drops for a swimmer's ear infection—which don't help this sort of pain. If the pain persists, it may be eased by two or three teaspoons of a cough syrup containing codeine. A dose of sedative for sleep is worthwhile if it is in the middle of the night. (For more detailed information see page 154. Also, see Chapter 7 on ears, nose, and throat for other problems.)

EYE

When there is an eye injury, watch for the 4 "P's";

1. Pain
2. Pupils (are they equally round and regular?)
3. Perception (can he see as well as usual?)
4. Personality (has it changed since the injury?)

Chemicals in the Eye

For any liquid or powdered substance in the eye:

1. *Immediately wash thoroughly* with copious amounts of cool or warm water. If water is not available and milk is, pour milk into the eye, holding the lid open, and then wash the milk out with water later. Hold the eyelids open to make certain that the water gets under the lids. Do not try to neutralize chemicals. If the child will not cooperate by holding the eye lids open, run water over his head. The water will run into the eyes, and blinking will allow contact.
2. *Do not rub.*
3. Patch the eye with a cloth and *get medical attention at once.*

Foreign Bodies

Symptoms: a "scratchy" feeling, burning, pain, tears, sensitivity to light. The initial pain may subside, only to recur hours later—especially if the foreign body is imbedded in the cornea, where it is very difficult to see.

RX:

1. Gently hold the lashes of the upper eyelid, then pull the eyelid out and down over the lower lashes. This may dislodge specks in the eye.
2. Hold the eye open under water—in a basin, a drinking fountain, shower, or stream.
3. Pull the lower eyelid down gently and look for foreign bodies in the cup it makes. Have the patient roll the eye around slowly and look at the cornea and white of the eye. If the speck will not wash out, try to remove it gently with a cotton tipped applicator or the corner of a clean handkerchief.

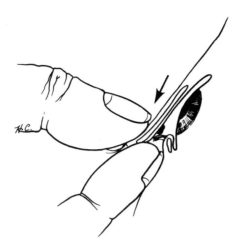

FIGURE 7   *Scraping a foreign body off the inside of the upper eyelid*
by pulling the upper lid out and down over the eyelashes
of the lower eyelid. Then scrape the inner side of the
eyelid on the eyelashes as you push the lid up.

4. Most cinder or dust specks usually end up under the upper lid. If a parent
is at all adroit, and if the child is not too sensitive, this lid can be lifted up
and turned out and the foreign body removed. Have the victim sit with his
head braced against the wall. He must look only at his toes. Grasp the lashes
of the upper lid, and pull the lid down toward the cheek. At the same time,
put a match stick or similarly shaped rod horizontally on the outside of the

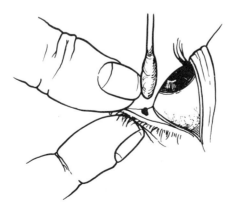

FIGURE 8   *Removing a dirt speck from the lower eyelid with a cotton*
tipped applicator.

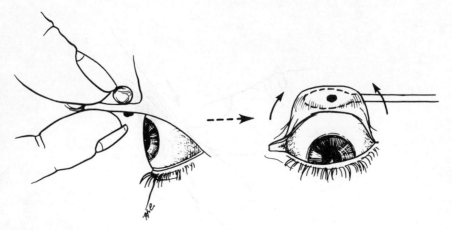

FIGURE 9   *Everting the upper eyelid using a cotton tipped applicator on the outside to expose a foreign body.*

upper lid. Roll the eyelid back over the match stick. The stiff cartilage in the upper eyelid (the tarsal plate) will flip over the stick, exposing much of the inner side of the upper eyelid—and a foreign object can usually be seen against its pink surface. A wisp of cotton or tissue may then be used to tease it off the surface.

5. Do not allow the eye to be rubbed. If it is irritated, tape a handkerchief over the eye.

6. *If pain persists after an eye injury, or after a foreign object has been removed, the child should have an eye examination by the doctor to rule out a corneal abrasion.* A fluorescent dye is dropped in the eye. It stains areas from which the conjunctiva has been eroded. Antibiotic ointment, eye-patching, and a follow-up examination are usually all that is required. Sometimes the foreign body is impossible to see and may still be in the eye. If pain persists, examination by an ophthalmologist is suggested.

Burns in the Eye

Burns in the eye may result from sunlight (often reflected from water or snow), flash burns, or welding arcs. Symptoms may not appear right away, but when they do, there will be pain, tearing, and, usually, redness of the eyelids.

Treatment

1. Cold water compresses held over the eyes.
2. Vaseline or baby oil on the lids.
3. Aspirin may be given by mouth.
4. If symptoms persist, see a doctor.

Black Eye

Put cold wet compresses over the eye lids and eat the proverbial steak. After a day or two, alternating cold and hot compresses will help speed up the healing of the bruise. See the doctor if vision is poor or if pain persists.

Eye Damage from Facial Blows

The bones around the eyeball are difficult to break. If they should break, it will be the result of more than the usual childhood fall or an ordinary blow to the head. If the child complains of double vision, or if one eye does not move well after a face injury, there may be a "blow-out" fracture of the bones below the eye. This fracture will snag one of the muscles and limit eyeball motion. This requires immediate medical attention and possibly surgery.

Pink Eye

Redness of the white of the eye can be due to infection of many sorts, or to a foreign body, eye injury, or even a sinusitis. Check with your doctor by phone. He will want to know if there is pus coming from the eye, what the color of the pus is, and whether the patient has a cold, stuffy nose, fever, or earache.

Pain

Eye pain from sensitivity to light is often associated with viral infections. Pain can also be caused by eye strain, sinusitis, or injury. Notify the doctor.

Styes

Small boils or plugged-off oil glands on the eyelids may be due to staphylococcal infection. Frequently, they respond to local antibiotics applied on the eyelid and local hot soaks with a washcloth covered by a dry towel to keep in the heat. If they persist beyond a few days, call the doctor. (See Chapter 6, on the eyes, for other problems.)

NOSE

Nose Bleeds

Press the entire soft lower part of the nostril against the middle of the nose on the side that is bleeding, or pinch the nostrils, and hold at

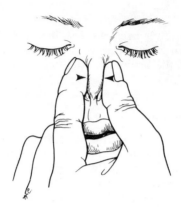

FIGURE 10   *Pinching the nostrils in against the center septum of the nose to control nose bleed.*

least five minutes. Have the patient sitting up and leaning forward. If the bleeding continues down the throat or out the other side of the nose, try putting a small cone of cotton or soft tissue into the side of the nose that is bleeding. Ice packs over the bridge of the nose will help. Some regular nose drops on the packing before inserting into the nose may help. Again, press the side of the nostril against the middle of the nose for five minutes. After the bleeding is stopped, leave the packing in place for several hours or until you can see your doctor.

Foreign Body in the Nose

Foul odor or a bloody or purulent discharge from the nose may mean that there is a foreign body in the nostril. If you know a child has just put a foreign body in the nostril, try to have him blow it out as you compress or squeeze the opposite nostril. If it is easily visible and you can grab it with tweezers, pull it out. Sometimes it can be sneezed out. Try a little pepper. Be careful not to push on it and lodge it further in the nostril. If it doesn't come out easily, or if there is evidence of infection (pus or blood or odor), have the doctor take care of it.

Broken Nose

If a child has been hit hard on the nose, there is a possibility of a break, in which case there sometimes is bleeding. Cold packs are helpful in order to reduce swelling and pain. If seen early, the doctor may be able to reduce a fracture immediately, but once much swelling has occurred, it may have to subside before reduction is possible. If there is a question of cosmetics, take a recent photo of the child with you to the doctor to help him judge the proper position of the nose.

MOUTH AND THROAT

Foreign Body: Choking (Unable to speak or breathe)

Occasionally, a foreign body will lodge in the back of the throat over the opening of the windpipe. Rarely, the foreign body will be inhaled and pass below the vocal cords into the lungs. Have someone call an ambulance or the fire department.

If the victim is choking or turning blue, turn him over your lap with his chest and neck angled downwards and with the head extended. Vigorously pound between the shoulder blades with the flat of the hand three to five times. If the choking is not *immediately* relieved, keep him face down and run your index finger along the outside of the teeth clear to the back of the throat—if you feel the foreign body, quickly flip it forward. Do not push the object back toward the windpipe. If this doesn't work, try to pop the foreign body out of the windpipe by suddenly squeezing the air out of the chest:

1. For a child over age two to five years, or for an adult:
   a. Hold the victim from behind with your arms encircling the upper abdomen just below the rib cage.
   b. The victim should be bent forward, hanging down some from your arms.
   c. Make a fist with your hand between the belly button and the lower end of the breast bone and put your other hand over your fist.
   d. Now quickly push your fist sharply upward and in toward his backbone at about a 45° angle toward the heart.
   e. Do not press the rib cage.
   f. Do not *squeeze* with the arms, but press the fist quickly upward, pushing against the diaphragm.
2. For a smaller child or infant:
   a. Lay him on his back, with the heel of your hand placed between the belly button and the bottom of the breast bone.
   b. Push quickly and sharply toward the heart at about a 45° angle.
3. The victim can do this himself if no help is available by pressing his fist into and up onto the upper abdomen or rolling against an edge of the back of a chair or a counter. The principle involved it to force the diaphragm up suddenly, compressing the remaining air in the lungs, and pop the foreign body out of the windpipe like a cork can be popped out of a plastic bottle.
4. If you are unable to remove the foreign body this way, and if the child's color is poor, lay him on his back and start mouth to mouth resuscitation (page 45). If you cannot blow air into his lung and he is unconscious, it means that the obstruction is still present. Reach way down the throat again, immediately behind the tongue, to try to move—or remove—the obstruction. It is frequently caught at the larynx (voice box). Restart mouth to mouth resuscitation.

If his color is good and he is breathing reasonably well, keep him face down and head down, or in whatever position he breathes best, and take

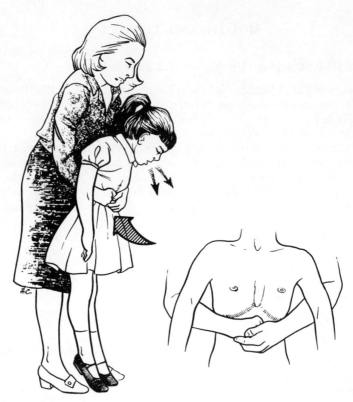

FIGURE 11   *Sharply and forcefully push your fist into upper abdomen toward the heart to pop out the food.*

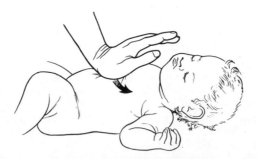

FIGURE 12   *Push sharply toward the heart with the heel of the hand between the belly button and bottom of the breast bone to dislodge an object in the windpipe.*

him to the nearest hospital emergency room. Have someone call your doctor to tell him that you are on your way.

Small children should not walk around eating, especially carrot and celery sticks, popcorn, peanuts, and so forth. If they fall or cry, they may breathe a piece of food into the lungs or windpipe and choke.

RESUSCITATION

Drowning

1. Lay patient face down on abdomen.
2. Lift hips enough that chest is at a 45 degree angle, then put hips down.
3. Repeat lifting every five seconds to empty lungs of water and possibly start breathing.
4. If breathing does not start after three lifts, do mouth to mouth resuscitation.

Mouth-to-Mouth Resuscitation

1. If there is vomit or other material in the mouth, wipe it out quickly.
2. Tilt the head back so that the windpipe is stretched.
3. Pull the chin forward.

For Children

1. Open your mouth widely and place it tightly on the child's face, covering the nose and mouth.
2. For infants, most of the air should come from pushing with your checks; **for** toddlers and older children, some of the pressure is from the lungs—but don't blow too hard.

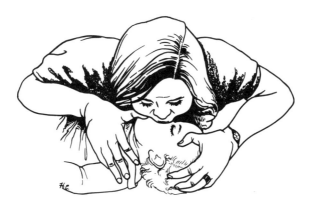

FIGURE 13 *Mouth-to-mouth resuscitation for infants or small children.*

3. Watch as you blow to see if the air expands the chest.

4. Remove your mouth and listen to the air rush out.

5. Reapply your mouth and blow and release every three seconds—twenty times per minute.

6. If air does not get into the chest, turn the child over, head and chest angled down, and slap sharply on the back. Restart mouth to mouth breathing.

For Adults

1. Open your mouth wide and place it tightly over the victim's open lips.

2. Pinch the nostrils shut.

3. Blow into the mouth—watch to see if the air expands the chest.

4. Remove your mouth and listen to the air rush out.

5. If air does not get through, turn the victim over and slap the back sharply to dislodge obstruction. Be sure the head is turned to the side.

6. Repeat blowing every five seconds, twelve times a minute.

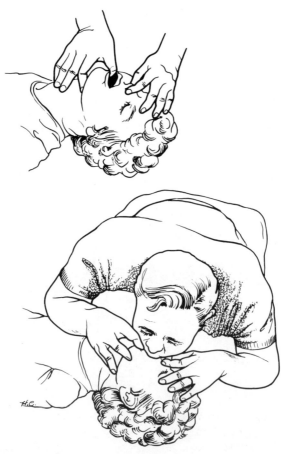

FIGURE 14   *Mouth-to-mouth resuscitation for larger children or adults.*

Heart Massage

1. To tell if the heart has stopped, hold your ear tightly to the bare chest, or feel for a pulse with your fingers high in the neck deeply behind the adam's apple or voice box, or in the groin.
2. Have someone give mouth to mouth resuscitation while you massage the heart.
3. Lay the victim on the back on a firm surface.
4. Give a sharp blow with the flat of your hand to the heart area and re-check to see if that started the heart beating.

For Small Children
1. Push the breast bone in an inch, using the tips of two fingers, and release.
2. Repeat rapidly, around one hundred times a minute.

For Adults
1. Push the breast bone in two inches, using the heel of your hand and pushing it with your other hand, elbows straightened. If the patient is heavy, you may have to lean on the chest, using the weight of your shoulders: then release.
2. Repeat about once a second; sixty times a minute.

Training

Citizen training in resuscitation techniques is available in many communities through fire departments, Red Cross, Boy Scouts and other organizations.

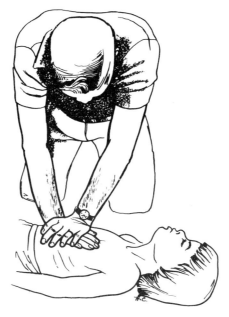

FIGURE 15   *Heart massage for a child. Pressure point should be just above the bottom of the breast bone.*

CROUP

Croup is a dry barky cough, hoarse voice or cry, and possibly a wheeze when the child breathes in.

How You Tell If Croup Is Serious

1. Increasing restlessness in a sick, croupy child is an early sign of possible serious croup.
2. An increasing rate of breathing is an early sign. The normal respiratory rate is twenty breaths a minute when quiet or asleep. Children with croup and colds often breathe above forty times per minute. If the rate increases steadily above fifty when the child is quiet, it may indicate problems.
3. Retracting, or "sinking in" between the ribs, below the ribs, and in the neck with each inspired breath is another signal. Mild retractions are not unusual, but if severe, they should be reported. To experience retraction, pinch your nostrils shut, close your lips tightly, and attempt to breathe in; no air can get in. You will sink in between the ribs as described. Doing this, you understand the restlessness and panic that can occur in a child with severe croup.
4. Fever above 102–104° F with croup may occasionally indicate bacterial infection requiring antibiotic treatment, especially if the child looks ill.
5. Recurrent vomiting with coughing.
6. Episodes of choking unrelieved by vomiting should be reported at once to the doctor.
7. Extremely pale, dusky, or bluish color can indicate lack of oxygen.
8. Croup so severe that the child can't lie down or sleep requires treatment.
9. An uncontrollable cough and labored breathing deserve a call to the doctor.

Treatments for Croup

1. Routine use of moist air to breathe with a cold mist humidifier or steam vaporizer and croup tent.
2. Expectorant or loosening cough syrups.
3. Intensive hot steam inhalations for five to ten minutes. Hold the child up high in the bathroom where the hot steam from the shower accumulates.
4. Put him face down, pat him on the back, or gag him with your finger in the throat to aid him in vomiting and spitting up mucus.
5. Wrap him up well and take him outside in the cool night air for five to ten minutes.
6. An ice bag or cold cloth held on the adam's apple area may help (See p. 151 for more details on croup.)

INGESTION OF FOREIGN OBJECTS

Small children are prone to grab any object within their reach and put it in their mouths. The usual objects that children swallow are coins, beads, and pieces of toys. If the object is small enough and is not sharp, and if it is successfully swallowed, it will usually pass on through the intestinal tract with the normal contents and will be excreted. Dimes and pennies will usually pass without trouble; nickels and quarters will often lodge in the esophagus. If a child has swallowed a small rounded object without projections or sharp areas, and if he is having no symptoms of any distress, you should examine each bowel movement during the one to ten days that is required to pass the object.

If there is doubt that the child has successfully gotten the object down to the stomach, test him by giving a few sips of clear water. If he can swallow the water and later can eat without discomfort, he does not have anything lodged in the esophagus. If the child is unable to swallow the sips of water or swallow his saliva, the esophagus is blocked, and he should see his doctor at once. If the object is a sharp one, such as a pin, you should take him to the doctor at once anyway. If the child choked and gagged while swallowing the object, and then has any respiratory difficulty or coughing, the object may have been sucked into his windpipe. In this case, see a doctor at once.

Knocked-out Tooth
Wash with tap water and immediately re-insert the tooth, pushing it gently but firmly into its socket. Call your dentist.

Chemicals in the Mouth
Wash out immediately with milk, water, or bottled drinks and call your doctor.

Poison Ingestion
1. *Caustic agents* (such as Drano, Liquid Plumber, Lye, Clorox, strong detergents, cleaning agents such as ammonia, etc.). RX: Give milk, water, or soup immediately, at least one large glass full for a small child or a quart for a larger child.
2. *Petroleum products* (gasoline, kerosene, furniture polish, lighter fluid, etc.). Do not force the child to vomit, as the petroleum substance may be aspirated into the lungs, causing pneumonia (See page 25). RX: Keep the child face down, head down, so that if he vomits, the vomitus will not get into the windpipe.
3. *Other poisons.* RX: Give syrup of ipecac one tablespoon immediately. Give two glasses of milk or water. Repeat syrup of ipecac if no vomiting has occurred within ten minutes.

   If you have no ipecac on hand, induce vomiting by inserting your finger clear to the back of the throat. If this doesn't work, give a glassful of warm mustard water (one teaspoon to a full glass) or warm salt water (two tablespoons to a full glass). If immediate vomiting does not occur, take the child with you (and bring a pan and towel) into the nearest physician's office, emergency room, or drug store, for treatment with syrup of ipecac or gastric lavage. Call the doctor as soon as you have instituted the above. *Check page 25 for details.* If the doctor isn't in, call your nearest poison control center or emergency room.

4. *Poisonous plants.* If there is a possibility that the plant was not all vomited out, your doctor may advise that a cup of activated charcoal in water be given in order to help absorb remaining toxins (see page 26).

ABDOMINAL INJURIES

Children suffer severe abdominal injuries relatively easily. Even trivial injuries, such as a bicycle handle poking the abdomen as the child falls, may cause rupture of the spleen, liver, stomach, or intestine. For an injury in this area, especially if he had the wind knocked out and complains of abdominal pain, be sure to take the child to the doctor if:

1. The pain lasts for over five to ten minutes.
2. The abdominal wall becomes rigid and tender.
3. Shock occurs, initially or delayed, with pallor; cool, clammy skin; and faintness.
4. Vomiting occurs.
5. The urine turns red or coffee colored.
6. If there is pain in the shoulder at the same time.
7. If the jar of walking hurts the abdomen.

Although there could be a ruptured spleen, ruptured bowel, injured kidney, or damaged liver, it more likely is a small bruise in the abdominal muscle. But don't take chances.

Blood in the Urine

If hit in the kidney or bladder area, there may be a contusion or bruising of the tissue, which then leads to bleeding. A person of any age with blood in the urine may have a kidney or bladder infection, so the circumstance must be investigated before the answer can be given. Blood in the urine warrants prompt medical attention.

Stomach Aches and Nausea

Stomach aches and nausea result from a large number of causes. The majority are due to tension (nervousness) or viral intestinal infections. Some of the causes and symptoms which should alert you to seek prompt medical help are:

- Vomiting fecal matter.
- Vomiting fresh blood or coffee ground colored material.
- Bloody or tarry black stools.
- Prolonged diarrhea.
- Diarrhea with green mucus.
- Distended abdomen.

- A hard abdomen very tender to the touch.
- Consistent pain on walking, with inability to straighten up fully because it hurts more.
- Recurrent colicky pain.
- Pain associated with pallor; cold, clammy skin; faintness; and thready pulse.
- Abdominal pain associated with shoulder pain.
- Coffee colored or red urine.
- Pain when urinating or excessively frequent urination.
- Jaundiced or yellow skin, or yellow eyes.
- Backache in the kidney area, especially with fever.

Nausea and/or abdominal pain may be caused by:

- Streptococcal throat in children.
- Pneumonia.
- Migraine headache.
- Back ache with pain referred to the stomach.

Infections
- Viral enteritis, for example, intestinal "flu," and so forth.
- Hepatitis.
- Gall bladder infection.
- Childhood diseases (e.g., measles, mumps, chicken pox, etc.) .
- Worm infections (e.g., roundworms) .
- Protozoa infections (e.g., amoeba) .
- Bacterial infections (e.g., Salmonella) .

Intestinal problems
- Ulcers (relieved with antiacid) .
- Bowel obstructions (distended abdomen) .
- Colitis (loose bowels) .
- Constipation.
- Appendicitis.
- Hemorrhoids.

Genito-urinary problems
- Ovarian cysts.
- Menstrual cramps.
- Prostatitis.
- Pelvic inflammatory disease (infection of the vagina, uterus, or tubes) .
- Urinary infections.

Injuries

Emotional upset

Black Widow spider bite

Poison ingestion

See chapter 10 on Your Stomach and Bowels for further information.

GENITALIA

Penis and Vagina

Injuries to the penis or vulva (vaginal area) causing swelling or difficulty in urination should be checked by the doctor. Any painful urination, difficulty in passing the urine, blood in the urine, very frequent urination, coffee or tea colored urine, or a discharge from the penis or vagina (the clear or white midperiod discharge or expected menstrual bleeding discharge is normal) also require a visit to your doctor. If possible, collect a fresh urine sample in a clean container and take it with you.

Groin

A lump in the groin may mean a hernia in either boys or girls. The swelling may go down into a boy's scrotum. Usually, such lumps are soft and will go away when the child lies down. If possible, get the child to the doctor when the swelling is present, but have him seen anyway. Firm lumps at the crease of the groin or below it may be swollen lymph glands. If they are sore or readily visible, they should be checked.

Testicles

Pain or swelling in the scrotum (the sack which holds the testicles) should always be checked, whether there is an injury or not. On occasion, the testicle can twist around for no known cause, shutting off its blood supply, and the testicle will become gangrenous inside the scrotum. This usually starts suddenly with severe pain. An operation is often done within hours to untwist the testicle in order to prevent gangrene. Usually the cremaster muscles pull the very tender testicle up into the edge of the canal, and the scrotum on that side is higher than the other. A small tag of tissue normally on the testes can twist and cause pain. Mumps can infect the testicle and cause swelling, pain, and soreness. All testicular pain or swelling deserve prompt medical attention.

A diffuse "wormy" mass above the testicle in the scrotum, usually on the left side, is frequently caused by dilated veins, and is called a varicocele. Inform the child's doctor if this is noted. There is no urgency. A loop of bowel from a large hernia may get into the scrotum, but this can also be felt in the area of the groin in which a hernia starts.

Infant boys frequently have a sack of water around or above the testicle called a hydrocele. A flashlight will shine through the clear fluid. Most hydroceles will spontaneously vanish, but a few may persist and be associated with a hernia.

BONE, JOINT, AND MUSCLE INJURIES

Fractures (Broken Bones)

Fractures are not always easy to diagnose. It is often possible to move the fingers or walk on a "mildly" broken leg or foot. Obvious fractures require immediate care, but minor fractures do not usually warrant the same degree of urgency. If the soreness, pain, or limp from an injury do not go away after three to four days, then it is wise to check, even if you don't think the bone is fractured. With children, it is difficult at times to assess just how much pain they feel. Pinpoint tenderness is more often associated with a fracture than vague tenderness. A good rule of thumb is "Low's sign": If an injured extremity keeps a child awake a lot, it is probably a fracture; if it doesn't, it is probably a sprain or bruise. A swollen wrist is more likely to be fractured than a swollen ankle.

Strains, Sprains, and Ruptures

- A strain is a pulled ligament that is painful but usually not swollen.
- A sprain is a partially torn painful and swollen ligament.
- A rupture is a complete tear of the ligament.

How can you tell a fracture from a sprain? An x-ray is the only sure way to make such a differentiation. This doesn't mean we will always x-ray. Often the doctor gives a trial of time, with or without a splint, before resorting to x-ray if it is a minor injury, even a slight fracture. Twenty-four hours of rest, elevation, and ice packs for injured areas gives minor soft tissue injuries time to recover.

Collar Bone

Fractures of the clavicle can occur if a child's arm is jerked up suddenly or if he falls or is hit on the shoulder. Usually he cannot raise that arm well and cries if one attempts to pull off a pull-over shirt or sweater. There is tenderness to direct pressure on the bone. A physician's examination—and possibly x-ray—are indicated. RX: Hold the forearm horizontally across the lower chest with the other hand or with a sling from the neck to the wrist.

Ribs

Fractures of the ribs are tender to touch and often hurt with a deep breath or arm motion. Check with you doctor. Rarely the fracture may puncture the lungs and make breathing very difficult, requiring emergency treatment.

Shoulder

Injuries in the shoulder area may involve the clavicle, the scapula, and the upper arm. They are often difficult to diagnose and may require x-rays. Treat for emergency, as with the collar bone.

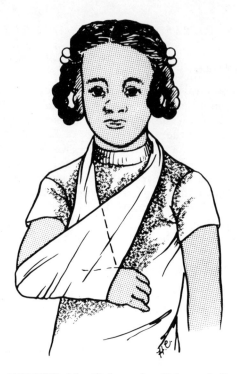

FIGURE 16   *Triangular dishtowel sling.*

When pain in the shoulder is associated with an abdominal blow or shortness of breath, it may be an ominous sign and requires prompt attention for abdominal bleeding or a puncture of the lung.

Upper Extremity First Aid

If there is distinct distortion or severe pain, call the doctor at once. For mild injuries, put the forearm in a triangular sling (a dishtowel will do). For severe injuries, wrap the extremity with corrugated cardboard or stiff magazines long enough to cover and support the forearm, hand, elbow, or upper arm and elbow. Then, put it in a sling. A bathtowel or handtowel will suffice for padding.

Upper Arm
Injuries close to children's shoulders or elbows may involve growth centers. Occasionally, there are muscle pulls rather than fractures. X-rays are usually required.

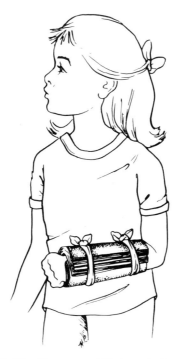

FIGURE 17   *Forearm splint made from a magazine.*

Elbow

Elbow injuries may involve the humerus, radius, or ulna. Severe injuries may be difficult to treat, and residual disability is not uncommon.

Nursemaid's Elbow

Toddlers frequently suffer a dislocation of their very shallow elbow joint when someone pulls them up by one arm. They are unable to use the arm and cry when the forearm is twisted or bent, even though there may be no swelling. Your doctor may show you how to reduce the dislocation if it is recurrent. These "nursemaid's elbows" are preventable if one avoids pulling children off curbs, into the air, or swinging them by one arm.

Forearm

The most common fracture is in the radius on the thumb hand side of the arm just above the wrist. Often, there is very little swelling with this fracture. Greenstick fractures often occur in children, where the bone is cracked but not out of place.

Wrist

A swollen painful wrist may be caused by a sprain, a Colle's fracture, or a hard to diagnose fracture of the small navicular wrist bone on the thumb hand side of the wrist. Persistent pain in the wrist several days beyond a seemingly minor injury may be significant and requires medical attention. A persistence of swelling in the wrist from any cause may squeeze the nerves and blood vessels and cause swelling, weakness, numbness, or tingling of the hand and must receive medical attention. RX: If it is not too painful or swollen, and the hand can be used and is not numb, you can afford a night's trial at home with rest, cool packs, and, possibly, a splint. If it is swollen, really painful to touch, or persists the next day, call your doctor.

Hand and Fingers

The most frequent injury is a sprain or subluxation or dislocation of the finger joints from "jamming" (a blow on the end of the finger) in which the finger goes back into place by itself. Occasionally, the joint capsule is torn and bleeding, and swelling occurs. A fracture or ruptured tendon at the joint at the end of a finger may result in a finger drop: The finger cannot straighten out thoroughly, and this can result in a permanent disability. RX: Minor injuries will usually respond to initial cold applications, rest, and temporary splinting. Physicians may splint such an injury for a week in a position of function without an x-ray. Marked bruising and swelling often indicates a fracture and requires medical attention. A handy way to "splint" a sprained finger is to tape it to the adjacent finger beyond the injured site. Fractures of the fingers are frequently missed. Swelling and pain are often minimal. Popsicle sticks or tongue blades make excellent temporary finger splints.

Hips and Thighs

Hip Pointer

There are several injuries called hip pointers:

1. One is a bruise of the front projection of the hip bone (the anterior iliac spine), usually from falling on it—resulting in bleeding under the bone covering.
2. A second type is a strain or tear of the muscle or ligaments where they attach to this bone projection.

Both of these are painful, incapacitating injuries because every walking, stepping motion pulls on this area.

Another bruise sometimes called a hip pointer is on the side of the hip where the trochanter (a lump at the top of the leg bone, the femur) can be felt on the side of the top of the leg. This is best treated with ice and rest, and then with medical attention, if it does not improve in two or three days.

A Hard Sore Spot in the Thigh

This condition is caused by bone being formed in a bruised muscle. Usually, recovery is spontaneous with limited activity and by graduated and consistent exercise. Repeated injury to the same area should be avoided. If a large mass is formed in the muscle you may be advised to wait and see if it will resorb. Early surgery could make the condition worse. For athletes, special foam pads can be used for protection in order to avoid repeated injury.

Early treatment of severe bruises with rest, elevation, and ice can often prevent this type of injury. Overenthusiastic passive or active exercising of an injured muscle can aggravate the process. If bone formation occurs, even greater patience is required. Rest with limited activity is indicated, avoiding sports—especially contact sports—for up to a year. Most children can continue in contact sports after the bony area has completely healed, but if this type of injury occurs more than once, the child may be advised to quit contact sports.

Lower Extremity First Aid

Severe upper leg or hip injuries: Splint on the outside with a padded board from well above the hip to the ankle, and on the inner thigh from the crotch to the ankle. It is best to transport by stretcher. An ironing board will do for small children. Mild leg, foot, and ankle injuries: Simply support the child, and do not allow him to bear weight. Severe lower foot and ankle injuries: Splint with cardboard or boards padded with towels or a pillow and wrapped with gauze, rope, towel, or strong string and do not allow the foot to bear weight. Carry the child to the physician.

Knee Injury

The most common knee injury is a simple contusion or blow to any part of the knee. Most of these can be treated at home with rest,

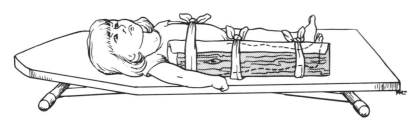

FIGURE 18 *Padded board splint (and transportation) for severe upper leg injury.*

elevation, ice, and crutches for a few days before consulting a physician providing:

1. The knee has a normal range of motion equal to the other knee.
2. The knee does not tend to collapse with weight bearing.
3. There is no acute pain with weight bearing.

If the range of motion is limited by a feeling of something mechanically catching, or if the knee will not bear weight because of instability, this requires prompt attention. A ligament injury will give such a feeling of instability with weight bearing.

Even a modest amount of swelling about the knee and lack of full range of motion from tightness can be tolerated and watched for a few days. If there is a catching or "slipping a cog" somewhere after the pain subsides, it may represent a torn cartilage or a kneecap problem and should be seen. Injuries to the kneecap which give continued pain with activity should be seen initially. If there is just a little discomfort, and if that subsides in a day or two, there may be no necessity for a physician's examination.

Serious Knee Injuries

The most common serious injury to the knee is a stretch or rupture of the inner ligament of the knee joint (medial collateral ligament). An examination just after the injury will reveal an unstable knee. If this ligament is ruptured completely, surgical repair should be done within the next day or two. Sprains can be treated in a plaster cast or splint. This ligament injury can be accompanied by ruptures of the central ligament of the knee and a tear of the cartilage. (The cartilage is a piece of tough fibrous tissue, a cushion between the joint surfaces.) Usually major ligament or cartilage tears bleed into the joint and cause massive swelling.

Occasionally, the injury will fracture the joint surface, loosening a piece of cartilage and underlying bone which may break off and float in the joint. The diagnosis can be difficult. Surgery is indicated to remove or replace the loose fragment of bone and joint cartilage.

Leg and Foot Shin Splints

There are several types of leg pain loosely called "shin splints." Typical shin splints are in the muscles in the front and outer side of each lower leg. These muscles are in a tight compartment, and the swelling causes pain. The muscles are injured by overuse on hard floors or surfaces during track, basketball, football, and baseball. If the injury is mild, it will get better with rest. Swelling in the tight muscle compartment may decrease the blood supply with resulting very severe pain, and at times surgical decompression is necessary. Medical attention is needed if:

1. The pain persists.
2. There is numbness over the top of the foot.
3. It is hard to bend the foot upward toward the leg.

Other lower leg pains may be due to muscle fatigue, muscle strain, or a fatigue fracture of the bone. Pain in the calf that subsides with rest is usually muscle fatigue. Pain with tenderness over the bone may be a stress fracture, and this should be checked by the physician before further sports. The treatment for fatigue fractures is complete rest until healing occurs. Fatigue fractures can also occur in the hip and the heel bone.

Sprained Ankles

Sprained ankles and fractures are difficult to differentiate and at times complicated to treat. Often x-ray is required. The swelling of most sprained ankles is below and in front of the outside ankle bone, not in front of the ankle over the top of the arch or above the ankle bone. You should see your doctor for:

- Recurrent sprains.
- Gross distortions or swelling.
- Extreme tenderness.
- Inability to walk on the foot.

If there is no gross swelling, and if weight can be borne on the foot immediately after the injury and the tenderness and swelling are not severe, it is usually reasonable to try a few days of home treatment:

1. Don't bear weight—use crutches or a cane.
2. Elevate the leg.
3. Use cool cloths or ice packs for the first two days. Crushed ice put in a plastic bag will do.
4. Use a heating pad on low after two days.
5. Try to bear weight after a day or two. If it hurts too much, call the doctor.
6. Apply a firm elastic bandage. Start wrapping at the toes in order to prevent swelling below the bandage.

If the sprain is severe, and if one continues to walk and play on it, the ligament may not heal at all, or else it may heal with excessive length, causing a chronically unstable ankle. A cast may be necessary.

Foot

Pain in the foot may represent a fracture or torn ligament, and can require crutches, taping, or casts as well as elevation and rest.

Stubbed Toes

If the injury results in a blood clot under the toenail, the pain may become more severe after a few hours. Your doctor should be consulted. If the toe is broken but is not out of place, and if it is not too swollen or tender, no treatment may be required except to hobble on your heel for a week or so until it heals. The injured toe can be taped to the adjacent toe.

How to Use Crutches

Crutches must be adjusted to the size of the individual. When standing up with the arms relaxed, the top of the crutches should be one to two inches below the armpit. Do not bear weight on the top of the crutches. Weight bearing should be with the hands on the crossbar, which should be near the top of the hips at about the level of the belly button so that the elbow is held at near a 90° angle.

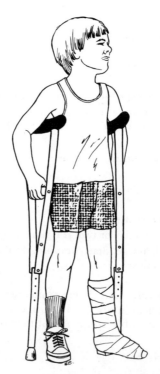

FIGURE 19   *When using crutches, bear your weight on your hands.*

Home Care of Casts

Prevent or reduce swelling by elevating the extremity and putting ice bags on the outside of the cast. Watch for poor circulation, noted by unrelieved pain, swelling, discoloration, numbness, burning sensations, tingling, an inability to move fingers or toes, or a change in the skin temperature. Check the circulation by gently pinching the nail beds and watching the pink pulsation when the color is almost out from under the nail. The color should return promptly when you let the nail go.

Plaster casts become soft and crumbly and often useless when wet. Spray the cast with some sort of clear varnish in order to help avoid getting it too wet. If the cast softens, notify you doctor. The more expensive plastic casts will tolerate water better than plaster casts and should not be sprayed.

FEVER

Fevers vary with the time of the day. Usually they are low in the morning and rise in the late afternoon and evening, only to go down again the next morning. The fact that a fever is gone in the morning doesn't mean that the child is better, and a higher evening temperature doesn't mean that the child is worse. Fevers themselves are usually not too important—it is the cause of the fever that is worrisome. There is not too great a correlation between the height of the fever and the degree of illness except in young infants, where high fever may mean significant illness. Parents often worry unduly about fevers of 104–105°, even if present for only a short time. However, for brain damage to occur from fever, a temperature above 107° rectally is required for a sustained length of time. Actually, fever is a friend—a method of defense against infection. A fever below 105° rectally is not a "high" fever. Aspirin or acetaminophen may be given if fever is elevated. Give one grain per year of life till age ten, when the dose is two adult (eight baby) aspirin. It takes aspirin at least thirty to forty minutes to work. If the temperature continues to rise, you can undress the child and sponge the skin with tepid water. Let the water dry by itself on the skin. Alcohol in the water speeds up the evaporation. As long as the skin is hot and flushed, you can cool the child by sponging. If the aspirin and sponging don't control the temperature, your doctor may need to give you some additional help (See page 97) .

Convulsions with Fever

Occasionally young children are unusually sensitive to abrupt rises in fever and develop convulsions. Febrile convulsions usually last only two to three minutes. Don't panic:

1. Place the child on his side with the head a little lower than the rest of the body. For a good airway, make certain that the tongue is forward.
2. Wrap a washcloth around a spoon. Feel along the outside of the teeth, and only *if* the tongue is caught by the teeth or if the child is blue or choking, pull open the jaw and insert the padded handle.
3. Remove excess clothes and sponge with tepid water while waiting.
4. Call the doctor and tell him what is happening.
5. As soon as the convulsion has ceased, take him to the doctor. (If it lasts over five minutes, take him anyway.) Febrile convulsions may occur in one child at 101° to 102° of fever, but in another not until the fever goes over 106°. Often, there is a family history of febrile convulsions. Most parents become quite adept at handling or preventing convulsions after the first hair-raising episode, and they have received education and medication from the doctor. Such convulsions are rarely very harmful unless they last over the usual time. One must keep in mind that the fever represents infection, and that the infection can be damaging. In febrile convulsions, convulsion is often the first sign; in meningitis, convulsions usually follow other signs of illness. Convulsions should never be treated lightly and should be reported each time they occur. Your physician may prescribe medicines to prevent recurrences.

Headache

If there are headache and fever, have the child lie on his side, curl up like a kitten, and touch his forehead to his knees. If he can do this, it rules out the stiff neck of meningitis (See also page 125 for headaches).

INSECT STINGS
(BEE, HORNET, WASP, AND YELLOW JACKET)

Insect stings are painful but they are dangerous only if the individual is hypersensitive. Most insect stings do not need to be seen or treated by a doctor. A little immediate redness and swelling at the point of the sting is normal. Often after a few hours there will be marked swelling at the site.

Routine Care

1. If the stinger is still in the skin, gently scrape it off with a knife edge or fingernail. Do not use tweezers, for they squeeze more of the toxin into the skin.
2. Immediate cold compresses are helpful. (One of our physicians believes that the old fashioned remedy of a moistened cigarette tobacco poultice on the sting will reduce swelling and pain. Another uses meat tenderizer.)
3. RX: Intermittently soak in warm epsom salts solution (one tablespoon/quart of water) for one or two days. Infection may occur. Look for: pus, red streaks going up from the sting, fever, or swollen glands.

Signs of Severe Hypersensitivity (With a Potential to Kill)
1. Shock, with pale, clammy skin and a feeling of faintness.
2. Hives, "welts," or a red rash in areas of the body away from the sting site.

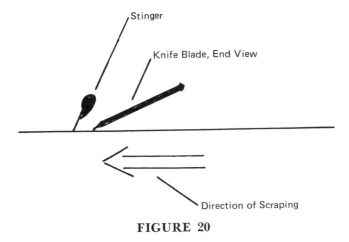

Stinger

Knife Blade, End View

Direction of Scraping

FIGURE 20

3. Swelling of the mouth, eyelids, or other areas.
4. Wheezing.

The *first thirty minutes* are the real danger. After that time has elapsed, there is not as much of a hurry. If the patient is known to be hypersensitive, he may have a kit of medications (See Chapter 20).

Care for Hypersensitivity Reactions

1. If you have an antihistamine on hand, give it at once.
2. Give the ephedrine tablet in the kit at once.
3. Put a mildly tight tourniquet between the sting and the heart. Loosen it every fifteen minutes. (See page 65.)
4. Use cold compresses on the entire limb at once, and continue this for the first half hour.
5. Give the adrenalin shot in the kit at once if the patient has severe symptoms, such as swelling around the mouth, wheezing, or unconsciousness.
6. If the adrenalin shot is not available and there is an adrenalin inhaler (used by asthmatics) around, have the patient inhale that.
7. If the color is poor, give oxygen. If respiration stops, give mouth to mouth resuscitation.

SPIDER BITES

1. Black Widow spider (black body with a red hourglass design on the abdomen) bites may cause painful abdominal cramps. The bites are rarely fatal, except in small children. See your doctor. Local cold packs may be helpful initially.
2. Brown Recluse spider (brown hairy body with violin mark on the back) bites may cause a large ulcer. See the doctor. (See pages 331 and 332.)

TICK BITES

Most tick bites are harmless, although some tick bites can cause paralysis (starting in the legs and working up) or cause serious infections such as Rocky Mountain Spotted Fever or Tick Bite Fever (with shaking chills). Sometimes the site of the bite can become a chronic sore whether or not the tick's head is left in. Secondary bacterial infection can also occur at the site of the bite.

To remove the tick, put some ether, gasoline, or kerosene on a cotton ball and tape it loosely over the tick for 15 or 20 minutes, or coat the tick heavily with vaseline or grease and wait 20 to 30 minutes. Sometimes they will loosen their attachment and back out themselves. If they don't, use a fine pair of tweezers or needlenose pliers and grasp the tick where his head enters the skin and slowly pull him straight out. Some advocate twisting counter-clockwise as you pull, but other experts tell us that this is an "old wives' tale." When the tick is out, examine him with a magnifying glass to see if the head is on the tick. It may be wise to report the bite to your doctor. If there is a black spot on the skin at the site of the bite, you should definitely call the doctor. Wash the area with soap and water, and dab with an antiseptic.

CHIGGER OR REDBUG BITES

These tiny insects, found mostly in the South, migrate to areas of the body bound closely by the clothes. They cluster around the ankles and about the belt line, and particularly on the genitalia, which frequently swell tremendously. RX: Sit in a basin of hot epsom salts water (one tablespoon/quart of water) for one-half hour three times a day for one or two days.

MOSQUITO, GNAT, FLEA, AND CHIGGER BITES

Use a soothing lotion, such as U.S.P. Calamine lotion, several times a day or an alcohol gel to cool the areas and to reduce the itch. Trim the fingernails. Watch the areas for infection. Antihistamines may help if there is swelling.

ANIMAL BITES

Most animal bites can be handled at home. There are four possible problems:

1. If it is a large bite or if the bite is on a cosmetically important area, it may have to be sutured, although animal bites are sometimes left open for better drainage.

2. A tetanus booster should be given if it is over five years since the last one.
3. The animal should be checked for possible rabies (See page 340).
4. Infection can occur from bacteria in the animal's mouth. Scrub the wound thoroughly with soap and water. Then apply a reliable antiseptic, such as betadine or Merthiolate.
5. Deep, penetrating dog bites should be cleaned out by a physician.
6. Report the bite to the police and make certain to locate the animal.

RATTLESNAKE BITES

1. Be sure the snake is venomous. Rattlesnakes have rattles. If marked swelling and pain starts at the site of the bite, and if there is discoloration, it is probably a venomous snake.
2. Remove rings, watches, and bracelets at once if the bite is on the hand or forearm.
3. Immediately place a tourniquet a few inches above the bite (between the bite and the heart). Use a belt, handkerchief, or a torn strip of cloth.
4. Tighten the tourniquet gently, enough to squeeze the skin firmly but not tight enough to block the pulse beyond the tourniquent:
   a. It should be tight enough that the veins beyond the tourniquet swell.
   b. It should be loose enough that the pulse beyond the tourniquet can be felt. The *wrist* pulse should be felt with the tip of your second and third fingers gently placed on the palm side, thumb hand edge, of the wrist. The *foot* pulse should be felt with firmer pressure of the fingertips behind the bone of the inner side of the ankle, big toe side.
   The amount of pressure applied should be equivalent to a moderately tight rubber band. Pulses are more difficult to feel in extreme cold or if the patient has gone into shock (pale, sweaty, faint).
   c. Loosen the tourniquet for thirty to sixty seconds every fifteen minutes.
5. Make a single cut one-half inch long, no more than $1/4$ inch deep (less on the wrist), through each fang puncture—parallel with the long axis of the arm—and cut down to the fatty tissue. The cut should be with a sterile or at least a moderately clean knife or blade if possible.
6. Suck the wound with a patented rubber suction cup, if you have one, or squeeze around the wound to milk out serum and venom. If you suck the wound with your mouth, there is danger of infecting the cut with mouth bacteria. For a large snake and a deep bite, however, there may be no choice if you don't have a suction bulb.
   a. Suck or milk continuously for the first twenty minutes.
   b. Suck for a few minutes every fifteen minutes thereafter.
7. Move the tourniquet upward as the swelling advances. Additional cuts can be made for suction near the bite if swelling is rapid.
8. Keep the site of the bite cool by immersing the entire extremity in cold water.
9. Keep the victim as quiet as possible, preferably lying down.
10. Transport the victim by stretcher to the nearest medical facility as soon as possible. A stretcher can be made with clothing and small tree branches. If it is not possible to move the patient, get him out of the sun, and keep him as comfortable and quiet as possible.

11. The use of snake antivenom is dangerous, even in professional hands. Its use in the field by laymen is questionable. The antivenom itself may cause severe allergic reactions, including immediate shock and swelling (anaphylaxis) or delayed serum sickness with swollen joints, fever, and hives. If it must be given, be certain to read the brochure that comes with the box, and do a sensitivity test for horse serum prior to administering the antivenom. It can be given into a vein or in the muscle. Do not give antivenom if the patient can be taken to a medical facility within three hours. The smaller the rattler, and the larger the individual, the less the need for antivenom. Some authorities believe that high doses of cortisone may be helpful—and this can be carried by a hiker in a ready-to-use syringe.

SUMMARY

There are other ways! Dr. Martin Smith, who did a good amount of the work on this section, points out that:

There are a number of ways to handle most emergencies and to give first and second aid. You may note differences between our advice and that of the Red Cross and others. Ours is a team approach which became acceptable to most of the physician authors and consultants, even though each of us might do it somewhat differently.

3

GOOD NUTRITION:
REQUIREMENTS,
PROBLEMS,
AND OBESITY

There is a lot of advice pushed on the public about nutrition. It includes both nutritional sense and nonsense. An exasperated mother was speaking for all parents when she said:

> We worry about the "too" fats, the "too" thins, the traumatic battle with acne, the snacks, the allergies, the additives, the vitamins, junk food—what is good nutrition? Most of us resolve these worries in a hit or miss fashion. What we'd all like to be told, once and for all, is precisely what foods to feed our children for a well-balanced diet. It would be good to know what preparation methods are healthiest, and which and how many (or if any) vitamins we should buy as supplements. We'd also want to hear about where to buy the freshest and best foods and how to tell when we have them. If some food wizard could swing yet another miracle, we'd even like to know how we could pay for this wonderful diet.

Despite the conflicting claims of various nutritional groups, the science of nutrition has made great strides since the discovery that eating limes would prevent scurvy among the sailors on the sailing ships of old. People are, in general, far better nourished now than at any time in history. Perhaps that is why people today are, on the average, taller and heavier than those in preceding generations. Nevertheless, many people today are challenging the nutritional "establishment." From "organic" food to the Zen macrobiotic diet, from Linus Pauling's pronouncements about vitamin C to the words of the American Medical Association Council of Foods and Nutrition—the public is bombarded with conflicting advice. All is well meant: Some is helpful and some harmful—but it certainly cannot all be right.

THE BEST ADVICE

Among all these sources, the most reliable advice comes from the Council on Foods and Nutrition of the American Medical Association. Theirs represents the professional scientific and clinical consensus that reflects our recent "proven" advances in nutritional knowledge. Yet I must profess that I don't like to rely on the advice of *any* single group or individual. Each may have proved his theory by studying a lot of people—but they didn't study *me*. To prove that any nutritional advice is sound for the norm may be fine, *if* I am in the norm. But each of us has a digestive, absorptive, metabolic, and excretory system that is probably as unique as our face or our finger prints; and I, for one, question how useful any advice based on a "norm" can be for *everyone*.

For example, take the basic four food groups put forth by the A.M.A. dieticians and nutritionists as a sound scientific foundation for a normal diet. A statement on "How to Map Out a Meal" from the Council on Foods and Nutrition of the A.M.A. advises: "You can hardly go wrong by following this plan."[1] For most of us, this is true, but I know many who can, and have, gone wrong on such a diet; and I know many who survive and thrive without eating all of the four basic foods. For example, milk foods are one group of the recommended four. But what if you are allergic to milk? I have seen infants develop bloody diarrhea from cow's milk. The second group is the vegetable–fruit group. Yet many people are allergic to citrus fruits. The sensitive bowels of some colitis sufferers may reject green or yellow vegetables as if they were poison to that particular individual. The third basic group is meat, yet many religious groups do not eat meat at all, and most of their members seem very well nourished. Fatty meat, in fact, is a source of unneeded cholesterol which may play a role in later heart attacks. The fourth group recommended is the bread-cereal group. Yet there are people who are allergic to corn, wheat, rye, and probably to oats. There are individuals who lack the enzyme to digest gluten, the cereal protein. So you don't have to have all of the "basic four" foods, even if they are part of "normal" scientific diet.

TABLE 1   *Sample diet using the basic four food groups.*

Milk–cheese group: Two to four glasses of milk a day, or substitute cheese, yogurt, ice cream, and so forth.

Meat–egg–nut group: Two or more servings of meat, fish, poultry, eggs, or cheese—or substitute dried beans, peas, and nuts.

Vegetable–fruit group: Four or more servings of a green or yellow vegetable; citrus fruit or tomatoes.

Bread–cereal group: Enriched or whole grain foods are advocated by many nutritionists. Servings as needed by the individual.

THE WORST ADVICE

After becoming aware of the exceptions to even the most scientifically and medically "valid" recommended diet, it should come as no surprise to learn that many of the fad diets we read about today are even more dangerous for even more people. At best, they are unscientific, unproven, and largely untrue. At worst, they are pure quackery. Some are nutritionally unsound for everyone. Yet each year brings new diets and new claims. There are two factors behind this phenomenon. First, there is the person who, having found a certain unique diet that seems to work for him, jumps to the assumption that it is good for everybody. He regards himself as the norm. Second, there is our primitive belief in magic and our penchant for wishful thinking. We *want* to eat a food which has magic good properties, or we *fear* to eat a food which may have magic bad properties. Considering our fond hope of finding *the* magic food, it can be difficult to remember that the best path towards good nutrition is to start from as scientific a base as possible, and then to modify this "recommended for the norm" diet in whatever way our own special needs dictate. The growing sophistication in the field of nutrition can help us in this task. As Dr. Thomas J. Conway notes:

Science is now distinguishing between those eating habits which are biologically important and those adopted for psychological and social reasons. Thanks to modern science, each of us has the information necessary to calculate our own energy needs and then to select food to provide that energy—food which would also contain the ingredients necessary for good health. In fact, such a possibility has existed for years; concerned nutritionists, dietitians, physicians, and parents have long been urging such mealtime wisdom, but to little avail.

IS YOUR WORRY OVER NUTRITION OR CUSTOM?

If we have this information, why, then, do so many of us worry about our children's eating habits? Part of the answer lies in the non-nutritional (i.e., psychological and social) reasons that people use to choose certain diets and modes of eating. Dr. Blackburn S. Joslin believes that many parental worries about nutrition are really over customs, not nutrition:

Offer a child a simple variety of good food several times a day with no fuss or comment, and he will maintain good nutrition. Consider the varieties of eating habits among different nationalities—Norwegian, South Pacific, Mexican, Chinese, Indian. Some eat on schedules, others on no schedule; some cook their food and some don't; some use utensils and some their fingers. It is all a matter of custom. Think of how many different ways a chicken can be prepared. Compare the type, and quantity of food served one hundred years ago with that of today. Then remember that, despite these variances, man survives. If you eat a moderate variety of good food, enough to satisfy hunger, the how, when, and how to prepare will take care of themselves. "Clean up your plate for mother" is really beside the point nutritionally, although it may represent an important battle cry in a parent–child power struggle.

VITAMINS

The attitude of many people towards vitamins seems to be, "If some is good, more is better." As a result, some physicians now see more examples of vitamin poisoning from overdosage than they do cases of vitamin deficiencies. With the easy availability of vitamins has come a great deal of misunderstanding on their proper use. Here are some simple facts about vitamins:

- Vitamins, in the proper amounts, are important parts of human nutrition, but either too much (of vitamin A and D) or too few of any can produce disease.
- In the United States, vitamin supplementation of foods is a widespread practice, by industrial design and/or governmental edict.
- Either natural or synthetic vitamins will serve to prevent deficiencies in normal persons.
- The dosage for treatment of an existing deficiency is much greater than that needed to *prevent* deficiency in a normal person.
- For children beyond the age of two, standard U.S. food supplements, plus the vitamins naturally contained in foods, will prevent deficiencies—for the normal child eating a normal diet. Before the age of two, the addition of vitamins A (5,000 IU/day), C (50 mgm.) and D (400 IU/day) is a wise practice.
- Other vitamin needs should be dealt with by the child's physicians. Such additions and dosages will depend on each child's needs.

TABLE 2   *Recommended daily dietary allowances of vitamins.*

	Infants	*Children*	*Adults*
Vitamin A (IU)	1,500	2,500 to 3,500	5,000
Vitamin D (IU)	400	400	400
Vitamin E (IU)	5	10 to 15	30
Vitamin C (mg)	35	40	60
Folacin (mg)	0.1	0.2 to 0.3	0.4
Niacin (mg)	8	9 to 15	20
Riboflavin (mg) (B_2)	0.6	0.8 to 1.2	1.7
B_1 (mg)	0.5	0.7 to 1.2	1.5
B_6 (mg)	0.4	0.7 to 1.2	2
B_{12} (mg)	0.2	3.5	6

TABLE 3 *Illness from lack of vitamins.*

Vitamin	Natural Sources	Early Signs of Deficiency Disease
A	Animal fats, fruits, and vegetables	Night blindness, susceptibility to infections, inflamed eyes, goose bumps
B_1	Whole grain cereals and cow's milk; beans	Lack of appetite, vomiting, puffy face, numbness, shortness of breath, mental disorientation
B_2	Meats, eggs, milk, cereals, and vegetables	Sores at the edge of the mouth, raw tongue
B_6	Meats, whole-grain cereals	Irritability, convulsions
C	Fruits and vegetables	Irritability, tender joints, weight loss, bleeding gums
D	Sunlight, fish, liver, and eggs	Lethargy, slow growth, bowed legs, rickets
Niacin	Milk, meat, fish	Rash-like sunburn, painful tongue, intestinal upset, weakness, anemia, weight loss.

Though uncommon now in the United States, deficiency diseases plagued our less fortunate ancestors, whose diets were frequently inadequate. Table 3 is a look at some vitamins, their sources, and what may result from a deficiency.

Dr. Thomas J. Conway expresses the views of many physicians on the need for vitamin supplements:

> Being aware of the importance of vitamins should impress us with the importance of a well-balanced diet, thoughtfully prepared. With such a diet, we need very few vitamin supplements. Without a well-balanced diet, even large doses of multiple vitamins cannot protect a child from problems. The child with a poor diet who snacks whenever he wants won't be helped much by vitamin supplements. His basic nutritional needs must be determined and properly provided. First, be sure your child is getting a balanced diet—then worry about whether or not he needs any extra vitamins. (See list of vitamin contents in foods, pages 390 to 395.)

Do We Need Extra Vitamin C?

One major vitamin controversy which still generates confusion is whether large doses of Vitamin C can stop colds. The issue is associated with Dr. Linus Pauling, a Nobel Prize winning biochemist (though his prize was not for his recommendations concerning Vitamin C). He claimed that thousand milligram doses of ascorbic acid prevent colds. Attempts by other scientists to verify this claim have been contradictory yet indicate that for some people there might be substance to the claim (see page 302). Other studies may indicate differences in growth with massive intake of vitamin C. We really don't know yet. I advise patients concerned about such "miracle cures" as huge doses of vitamin C not to forget the power of positive thinking.

For example, I was talking with the mother of a teenaged girl suffering with infectious mononucleosis, fever, and a strep throat. We were discussing how she could get enough fluids down to keep from dehydrating and becoming malnourished. The mother enthusiastically described a "milkshake" concoction of various health foods and vitamins, adding that the whole family took this mixture routinely, and that it really kept them in good health. I pointed out that her daughter's health was, at that time, hardly good, making her testimonial to the preventive powers of the vitamin mixture rather weak. The mother laughed, admitting that she hadn't thought about it "that way."

A Vitamin for the Teeth

A "vitamin" for the teeth is sodium fluoride, discussed in Chapter 8, which should be given from birth to at least the age of eight. Actually, it is a mineral and not a vitamin, but it acts almost like a vitamin for the teeth in preventing cavities.

THE WELL-BALANCED DIET

The scientific advice for a well-balanced diet is that you use foods from each of the four food categories: meat, cereal and grains, milk and dairy products, fruits and vegetables. We have partially debunked that advice, but, in fact, it is good advice for *most* people. We would like to be more precise and simplify dietary advice. However, the normal diet only works for the person with normal digestive, absorptive, and metabolic systems. Your child or you may not be completely normal as far as nutritional requirements go. We do know, of course, that there are essential ingredients in food that we all seem to need.

We can get by with 10% protein in our diet, although the quality of the protein used is important. Protein contains nine component amino acids required for human nutrition. Some proteins, like egg white, meat, milk, and fish, have an excellent balance of amino acids. Others, such as cereals, may lack some essential amino acids and therefore are of less value for growth and body repair. The American diet now averages about 14% protein.

Fat is primarily an energy food, but it often carries certain vitamins as well as essential fatty acids required for a healthy skin. Forty percent of the calories of the current average American diet come from fat.

Carbohydrate is an energy food. However, many starchy foods contain some protein. The current American diet contains 46% carbohydrate.

See Tables 1 and 4 for sources of protein, fat, and carbohydrates, and

TABLE 4   *Basic food sources.*

Sources of protein: Dried beans, breads, cereals, cheese, eggs, fish, meat, milk, nuts, peanut butter, peas, potatoes, and poultry. Use: Growth, healing, antibodies, and energy.

Sources of fat: Butter, cooking fats, meat, milk (whole or low fat), and salad oils. Use: Energy, helps keep skin smooth, carries vitamins A, D, E, K.

Sources of carbohydrates: Bread, cereals, corn, fruits, honey, jam, jelly, potatoes, sugar, and syrup. Use: Energy.

for a sample diet using the Basic Four Food Groups. See pages 385–396 in the Almanac Lists for the mineral, vitamin, and cholesterol contents of foods.

The key to a well-balanced diet is to eat a wide variety of foods—if they don't bother you. Make certain that some high quality proteins are included which contain all the essential amino acids. Check the Almanac food lists to find out if there is enough vitamin and iron content in your child's diet (see page 388). If you read the chapter on Basic Training in our companion volume, the Parent's Guide to Child Raising, you will remember that children are often streak eaters, and that the diet does not have to be balanced on a day to day basis. It should, however, hopefully be balanced on at least a weekly basis. If you are concerned, keep a list of all the foods your child eats and check their contents. Remember that there is a chance that your child (or you) may not be normal in your requirements or tolerance, so the average calorie requirements may not fit you, the average protein requirement may not be enough, and one or many "healthful" foods may cause illness in some. People *are* different. It follows that their diets must also be somewhat different, too. So start with a normal diet, but don't stop there: Make sure that it works for you or your child.

"NATURAL FOODS" AND FOOD ADDITIVES

"What is the truth about natural foods?" many parents ask. "We are terrified about everything we read about additives." Food additives do cause disease in some people. We discuss additives in Chapter 15 on allergy, because most of the known illness they cause occurs in allergic or sensitive individuals. After reading that section, you may well decide to eat only natural foods.

If you will check the lists of food additives starting on page 401, you will see that it isn't all that easy. Natural foods, however, are not all that safe, either. For instance, some faddists have claimed great things for unpasteurized milk, refusing to face the fact that such milk may contain very harmful bacteria. Prior to pasteurization of cow's milk, a baby had to be breastfed or he was not likely to survive. In those days, every year infants died by the thousands in every area of the world from "The Summer Complaint"—diarrhea from "naturally" contaminated milk. So, although it may be "unnatural" to protect our children by pasteurizing milk, it does work. Some nutritionists advise eating green and yellow vegetables raw so that their vitamins will not be destroyed. It should be pointed out, however, that moderate cooking does not deplete the basic vitamins in vegetables as much as many people think. A comparison of boiled and raw peas, for example, from the U.S. Agriculture Handbook (see the food lists on pages 385–396) shows only a minor loss of vitamins with cooking. No difference in vitamin content is found between raw and pasteurized milk. Canned carrots lose considerable vitamins, but retain their high content of vitamin A. Canned applesauce loses half its vitamin C and riboflavin, yet it still has reasonable amounts left. Of course, overcooking will increase the vitamin loss. On the other hand, raw vegetables, fruit, and grain must be thoroughly chewed if all their nourishment is to be absorbed and do us any good. Flours that are not finely ground may not be thoroughly digested and absorbed. Whole grain is so little digested by cattle that farmers let the pigs eat the cattle droppings as a source of grain.

Many of the vegetables we eat as a matter of routine have natural additives which are potentially dangerous. One of Mother Nature's "additives" is oxalic acid, which occurs naturally in plants such as spinach, beet tips, chard, and pokeweed. We must have an adequate calcium intake to balance the oxalic acid we take in when we eat these plants; laboratory animals fed these plants without enough calcium added to their diet actually died. Other foods contain a goiter-causing substance that blocks the uptake of iodine into the thyroid. These include broccoli, brussel sprouts, cabbage, chard, kale, rutabagas, and soybeans. Cyanide (in small amounts) is present in apples, green almonds, cherries, lima beans, and maize corn. Excessive nitrates and nitrites can be present in corn and other vegetables grown on some soils. This does not imply that you cannot or should not eat these foods; they are safe and nourishing. The point is that even "natural" foods often contain slightly toxic substances.

The ancient saying that "one man's meat is another man's poison" holds especially true for vegetables, fruit, and nuts. Poisoning by another man's fruit occurs through two basic mechanisms: allergy and digestion. A good percentage of humanity is allergic to many foods. I am well aware of this personally, because at the age of forty I began having hives, and then allergic swelling in the throat, which came close to suffocating me—from celery! I had patients who wheezed when they ate corn in any form. So allergy to Mother Nature's products is as real as allergy to man's additives. (And speaking of meat, before you experiment with eating raw meat, as some food faddists advise, read Chapter 19, on the various parasite infections you can contract by this practice—from tapeworms to trichinosis.)

Another way Mother Nature can "poison" us is through the individuality of our digestive, absorptive, metabolic and excretory systems. Most of these differences occur in the thousands of various enzyme systems which direct the biochemical actions of our cells; in each of us, some of these are genetically different from the norm. Some infants, for instance, are born without the enzymes to enable them to metabolize the milk sugar, galactose (after a milk feeding, forty percent of a baby's blood sugar is galactose). After severe diarrhea, something happens even in normal infants which prevents them from metabolizing galactose; as a result, they may be left with low usable blood sugar. With thousands of delicately balanced enzyme systems in our bodies, it is no wonder that we respond to foods in many different ways. So when you see nutritional advice, remember that it is usually designed for the "normal" person, whoever that is.

These facts should not frighten you away from good foods that are safely consumed by millions of people. They are presented to show that all that is natural is not necessarily good for many of us. Food additives have helped feed the hungry of the world better today than at any time in history, in spite of a massive population explosion. Yes, they harm some people: We should all be aware of this possibility, and be protected by adequate knowledge and labeling. At the same time, we should be aware that foods can be cooked, canned, ground, and even preserved in ways that may be more nourishing than the undigestible natural forms. More nourishing, that is, unless you happen to be allergic to the additive, allergic to the food, can't digest the food, or don't have the enzymes in your system to metabolize it properly.

Despite the "back-to-nature" movement hailed by the organic food enthusiasts as the true path to a nutritious and safe diet, I believe that the "establishment" food industry has done a fantastic job of producing, preparing, and preserving foods. The success of their efforts exceeds the wildest dreams of men and women at the turn of the century who had a hard time collecting enough food to get through the winter. Now we certainly have *enough* food, even if there are more pesticides used than we would like, or even if the food we eat contains hidden additives that are harmful to some of us. Yet we human beings have a penchant for surviving minor degrees of "poisoning." People are concerned, for example, about the effects of lead and arsenic in our systems—some of which comes from inhaling leaded gasoline fumes, smog, and garden sprays. But there is probably less arsenic in the average person today than a hundred years ago, when arsenicals were widely used in patent medicines—and less lead than two thousand years ago in Rome, which used lead-lined aqueducts for drinking water.

All food should certainly be clearly and accurately labeled, however. Without that protection, a rare, unfortunate person can be damaged by even "scientifically proven" safe products. Food additives may not be harmful to you or me, but they can be for some people—and for that reason we should know when we are eating them.

VEGETARIANISM

Vegetarianism, in various forms and for various reasons, is becoming more widespread. Some Seventh Day Adventists are vegetarians and seem quite nutritionally sound, so to find out how to maintain a vegetarian

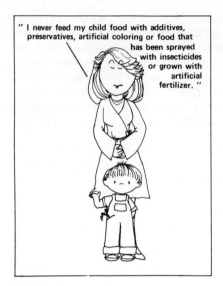
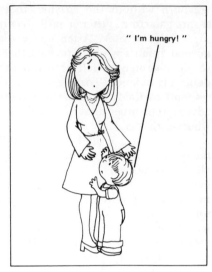

FIGURE 21

diet and still be assured of good nutrition, we asked **Dr. U. D. Register,** of the Seventh Day Adventist Medical School, Loma Linda University, to furnish nutritional guidelines (see also Table 5). Dr. Register pointed out that there are two types of vegetarian diets—the egg–milk vegetarian diet, and the no animal product, "pure" vegetarian diet. To follow either of these diets, you must modify the intake of the basic four food groups— meat, cereal and grains, milk and dairy products, and fruits and vegetables.

To change from a non-vegetarian diet to a milk-egg vegetarian diet:

1. Reduce substantially all "empty calorie" pure carbohydrate foods.
2. Increase the intake of all four food groups to supply adequate calories.
3. Delete meat from the protein-rich (meat) group; increase the intake of legumes, nuts, (especially peanuts, almonds, and cashews) ; use meat alternates such as soy bean cakes and so forth.
4. Increase the intake of breads and cereals, especially of whole grain products. This group supplies protein, B vitamins, and iron.
5. Increase the intake of nonfat and low-fat milk, and milk products such as cottage cheese. The milk group replaces part of the protein and Vitamin B_{12} which is reduced when you delete meat from your diet.

To maintain a "pure" vegetarian diet, follow the above steps, *and also* the following:

1. Maintain your calorie requirement. An adequate intake of calories is essential; when there is inadequate calorie intake, the body will burn up its protein for calories.

2. Increase foods which replace the nutrients in the milk groups, especially calcium and riboflavin.
3. Consider adding to your diet a fortified soybean milk preparation; more green leafy vegetables; and more legumes, particularly soybeans, nuts (especially almonds) , and dried fruits.
4. To get enough vitamin B_{12}, which is not present in plant products, add a supplement of B_{12} or fortified soybean milk to your diet.

TABLE 5   *Greens compared to cow's milk as sources of nutrients.*

Measure	Protein	Calcium	Riboflavin	Iron	Vitamin B_{12}
1 cup or 200 gm	gm	mg	mg	mg	mcg
Cow's milk	7.0	234	0.34	0.2	1.2
Soymilk	6.0	60	0.12	1.5	0.6
Broccoli	7.2	206	0.46	2.2	
Turnip greens	6.0	490	0.48	3.6	
Greens, average	6.7	305	0.39	3.0	
Soybeans, green	19.6	120	0.26	5.0	

THE ZEN DIETS

Far more care must be taken to eat the proper foods when you don't eat meat products. Even more care is needed if you eliminate all animal products. Greens can be used to replace the vital proteins, calcium, and vitamin B_{12}, although there are people unable to tolerate or absorb many nutrients from green vegetables. Nevertheless, the aforementioned diets will work for most people. The same cannot be said for the Zen macrobiotic diet, which has been popular among some people. Zen macrobiotic diets are an extreme example of the trend to natural and "organic" food. The series of diets varies from a mixed diet with many foods to an all-cereal diet. Fluids are restricted. Its inventor, Ohsawa, claims that his diet, along with exercise, cures diseases. Appendicitis, Ohsawa claims, will not occur in a "macrobiotic" person. Still, he does offer external plasters of ginger or albi for the treatment of appendicitis. The American Medical Association Council on Foods and Nutrition warns that there is great danger from the Zen macrobiotic diet fad, stating:

"The tragedy associated with application of this philosophy is well documented. . . . Cases of scurvy, anemia, hypoproteinemia, hypoglycemia, emaciation due to starvation, and other forms of malnutrition, in addition to loss of kidney function due to restricted fluid intake, have been reported, some of which have resulted in death." The A.M.A. statement notes the need for continuing dietary research and refuses to categorize all unusual diets as hazardous. However, it states that the Zen macrobiotic diet "should be roundly condemned as a threat to human health."[2]

WHAT ARE CALORIES?

Calories are the measure of the amount of energy in food. They are similar to the measure of energy in gasoline—the octane rating. High octane gas has more energy than low octane gas. Like gasoline, the energy of calories is used to supply energy for physical activity or heat. Unlike gasoline, calories can also be used to help build bone and muscle. If more calories than can be used are eaten and absorbed, they are converted to fat and stored for future energy use. Fat is burned when there is not enough sugar present in the blood to meet the body's physical energy requirements. The number of calories needed each day will vary with age and activity, but the following figures are accurate enough for most people.

Per Pound Per Day	Calories
Infants	40–50
Growing Children	30–40
Active Adults	20–25

Thus a child weighing 40 pounds may require (30 calories × 40 pounds) 1,200 to (40 calories × 40 pounds) to 1,600 calories a day.

"EMPTY CALORIE" FOODS

"Empty calorie" foods refer to foods containing large quantities of highly refined sugar, starch, and oils. These foods provide energy but few, if any, required minerals, vitamins, or other substances. Someone who is overweight or who must restrict his caloric intake should severely limit empty calorie foods—but an active child needs some of what they contain to give him the energy he needs. It is the large amount of highly refined sugar in these foods that receives a great deal of criticism today. Sugar is associated with hypoglycemia, diabetes, and dental cavities. A mother recently told me that sugar must not be any good because everything she read about it was bad. However, sugar in the form of glucose is a normal substance in the body and just as vital to our brain function and life as is oxygen. Without adequate levels of sugar in our blood, our brains cannot function; we could become unconscious and even die. Sugar is also necessary as the source of energy for muscles and many other body tissues.

Sugars (and starch) belong to a group of compounds called carbohydrates, made by plants with energy from the sun. Like logs in the fireplace, carbohydrates combine with oxygen to release heat, carbon dioxide, and water. This unseen "burning" of sugar within us provides energy for brain function and for other body uses.

There are different types of sugars. *Lactose* is a double sugar found in milk that splits during digestion to provide both *glucose* and *galactose*. Cane and beet sugars are also a double sugar, *sucrose*, which, in the intestinal tract, readily divides into *glucose* and *fructose*. Honey contains the same two simple sugars, glucose and fructose. Fructose is also found in fruits and fruit juices. Galactose, from milk sugar, and fructose are very similar to glucose, to which they are converted in the body after absorption from the intestinal tract.

Starches are found in grains and in other parts of plants. They are made up of complex chains of many glucose units which must be broken apart in the intestinal tract before absorption. Many people make an association between starch and potatoes, and then decide to cut out potatoes in order to keep their starch intake down. In fact, the lowly potato is one of the most healthful foods available.

The body normally stores sugar by combining glucose in a large, starch-like compound called glycogen which can be rapidly recalled to provide essential glucose. A limited reserve is normal and desirable. However, if we continually take in more calories than we need (whether carbohydrate, fat, or protein), our stores will become larger, and we will become fat.

Does Excess Sugar Cause Diabetes?

Diabetes is an inherited inability to utilize sugar. Obesity can bring out a tendency to diabetes, but overuse of sugar alone does not produce diabetes. Diabetics, like normal people, require sugar, but they do not

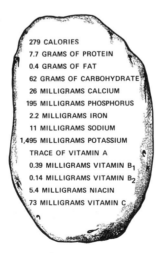

279 CALORIES
7.7 GRAMS OF PROTEIN
0.4 GRAMS OF FAT
62 GRAMS OF CARBOHYDRATE
26 MILLIGRAMS CALCIUM
195 MILLIGRAMS PHOSPHORUS
2.2 MILLIGRAMS IRON
11 MILLIGRAMS SODIUM
1,495 MILLIGRAMS POTASSIUM
TRACE OF VITAMIN A
0.39 MILLIGRAMS VITAMIN B_1
0.14 MILLIGRAMS VITAMIN B_2
5.4 MILLIGRAMS NIACIN
73 MILLIGRAMS VITAMIN C

FIGURE 22   *Nutrients contained in a potato.*

produce enough insulin to enable the sugar to get from the blood stream into the cells. The sugar piles up in the blood to such an extent that it spills into the urine, causing the diabetic to urinate more than most people. Because the cells are unable to get sugar, and are hungry, the diabetic eats and drinks a lot more than most people. This disease can be controlled with insulin shots. If too much insulin is given, all of the glucose goes out of the bloodstream into the cells. The problem is that the cells of the brain use up glucose very quickly and require a continuous supply. If glucose isn't available to the brain, it suffers from hypoglycemia. The treatment for overdose of insulin is sugar. Yet some doctors believe that too much sugar can cause hypoglycemia in some people.

Do Sugars Cause Hypoglycemia?

Dr. William Crook, a noted pediatric allergist, believes that many people suffer from hypoglycemia, or low blood sugar, which, peculiarly enough, may be caused by eating too much sugar. He also believes that some people are allergic to ordinary cane sugar. Some of the symptoms of hypoglycemia may also be caused by allergy: irritability, fatigue, restlessness, sleepiness, and impatience. Others, like being jittery or hungry, are more likely due only to hypoglycemia. The hypoglycemia from an overdose of insulin in a diabetic produces these same symptoms.

People with a tendency to hypoglycemia may have an oversensitive supply of insulin that responds to cane sugar by releasing a larger amount of insulin into the blood than is needed. The result is that the sugar is all absorbed by the cells, leaving a very low blood sugar, or hypoglycemia. The key factor here is that brain cells do not store glucose like many other body cells do, so brain cells require a continuous supply of glucose. If the brain cells don't get enough blood sugar, you become irritable; you want more sugar; and you become hungry, tired, sleepy, restless, and impatient. However, it is important to realize that people are different, and that not everyone is susceptible to hypoglycemia. Dr. Crook and other doctors who believe hypoglycemia is very prevalent point out that only 100 years ago people ate, on the average, only seven pounds of sugar a year and now we eat 115 pounds a year. Our bodies, they say, haven't adapted. Other doctors disagree and report very very few cases of hypoglycemia. Certainly, the symptoms of irritability, fatigue, hunger, and so forth can be due to many other causes, even including suppressed anger at your spouse or your child—or perhaps the symptoms arise from an illness, like a hidden kidney infection, or just from not enough sleep.

How do you tell if you are one of the rare ones with hypoglycemia? You can have a blood test, but doctors disagree as to their meaning, and as to what level of blood sugar is low enough to explain these symptoms. Another way of telling is to stop eating sugar and see if the symptoms vanish. Dr. Crook suggests a diet and a change in life style to prevent hypoglycemia:

- Stop eating sugar and other refined carbohydrates.
- Eat a good diet similar to that your ancestors ate.
- Eat six small meals a day.
- Exercise vigorously. This helps regulate your insulin.

If you do have a suspicion that your problem, or your child's, are due to something besides a bad disposition, you may want to try Dr. Crook's recommendation and his dietary changes (see Table 3–6).

It is fortunate that sugars are not "all bad," because it would be difficult, if not impossible, to survive on any kind of diet containing no source of sugar at all. Those parents who fear their children are sacrificing future health by maintaining a "junk food" diet can take heart from an analysis of the "typical" adolescent diet of hamburgers, french fries, and milk shakes which reveals that it is fairly well balanced. It can be completely balanced by a bit of liver, carrots or leafy vegetables given once a week.

OBESITY

Your proper body weight cannot be established by looking at a chart of so-called "normal" weights for people of various heights. Bone structure, muscle development, body build, and age all contribute to what your "best" weight should be. Obesity refers not to excess weight but to excess body fat. For older children and adults, the "pinch test" is probably the easiest way to measure body fat. Using the thumb and forefinger, simply grasp pinches of skin at the waist, upper arm, buttock, and calf. If

TABLE 6 *Foods you should and should not eat if you have hypoglycemia.*[7]

Foods You Should Eat	Foods You Should Avoid
All meats, fish, and shellfish (except lunchmeats) [a]	Potatoes, corn, macaroni, spaghetti, rice
Dairy products: milk, butter, and cheese; also margarine	Pie, cake, pastries, sugar, (white or brown),
All vegetables and fruits	candies, dates and
Salted nuts (excellent between meals)	raisins; limit honey.
Dietetic (no sugar) peanut butter	Colas and other soft drinks
Whole grain bread	Alcohol in all forms
Soybeans and soybean products	Coffee and strong tea
Decaffeinated coffee, weak tea (herb), and ice water	All hot and cold cereals, (except oatmeal,
Saccharin, as a substitute for sugar, in a limited quantity and frequency	occasionally).
Eat milk, fruit, or nuts between meals.	

[a] Lunch meats have carbohydrate extenders.

what you pinch is more than one-half inch thick in one or more of those places, then you are probably overweight.

The causes of obesity in children, as in adults, are a reduction in activity with no reduction in food intake; increased food intake without an increase in activity; a high carbohydrate diet; endocrine disorders; and brain damage. In over 95% of all cases of obesity, the cause is overeating—consuming more calories than your body burns up—although sudden changes in appetite or dietary habits are clues to metabolic changes which may, in turn, have their roots in emotional upsets or other disturbances. The first step in fighting obesity should be a thorough general physical examination to determine the actual cause.

Obesity Is Complicated

One of the major errors made in trying to solve obesity is in oversimplifying a very complex and somewhat poorly understood subject. Even programs of distinguished teaching hospitals often do not work as well as programs sponsored by lay organizations like T.O.P.S. (Take Off Pounds Sensibly) or commercial organizations like "Weight Watchers." Simplistic statements like "It's the calories that count!" don't explain why one person can eat 6,000 calories a day and stay thin while another eats 2,000 calories a day and stays fat. What we do know is that calories do count, but only if they are eaten, digested, absorbed, and metabolized. These functions vary to a degree with each individual. Then there is the recent scientific report that babies who are fed a lot develop a lot of fat cells and that the number of these fat cells evidently stays with us through life. Whether an individual's cells are full of fat or not is the significant factor in adult obesity. If, as is thought, overfeeding a baby increases fat cells and then the fat cells, when empty, somehow signal the baby (and later the adult) to eat enough to fill up the cells, then in theory we should simply avoid getting a large number of fat cells when we are babies. This may or may not be the case, but because few people successfully lose weight as adults, now some scientists are looking to the babies to solve the problem. So, there is a push to not overfeed infants. Unfortunately, some people get carried away, and, on occasions, end up underfeeding babies. Some fat is essential, and healthy babies put on a little before they start to walk and burn it off. Then there are just plain big babies, who are confused with fat babies. Large infants are sometimes brought to their doctors crying with hunger because they are denied some of the food they need by overconscientious parents, who, in their worry about preventing possible future obesity, are creating near starvation in the critical present.

How Much Food Do Babies Need?

How much food should your baby have? Newborns need two to three times more calories per pound than adults. An active, crying baby may need almost twice as many calories to thrive on as a placid baby. Only ten percent of the calories in food are utilized for growth. Different forms of calories are digested, absorbed, metabolized, and excreted differently. These processes also vary from individual to individual. Feeding, therefore, must be based on the specific individual infant's growth and contentment. Current popular concern about obesity may lead parents into underfeeding a baby, even though they follow all the expert advice—all the expert advice, that is, except the baby's. A good rule is to feed them when they are really hungry; but don't assume that all fussing is due to hunger: What they want may be holding and love, or dry pants and sleep.

Simple nutritional rules to avoid obesity in infants are:

1. Avoid whole milk in the first year of life, and limit it to a pint or less a day through the toddler years. Use formulas, which are better balanced nutritionally for human infants, but not over thirty-two ounces a day. However, don't let your baby become a "milk addict" even if you use formula. I offer the following rough guideline to my patients:

    Up to six months—*under* thirty-two ounces a day (one quart) .

    Up to twelve months—*under* twenty-four ounces a day (one and a half pints) .

    If too much milk is given, there isn't room for an adequate amount or variety of solids. Some babies will drink excessive amounts of milk and become obese. Don't let them!

2. Use vegetables and fruit as low calorie foods to supplement the breast or bottle. You can use meat as an extra source of growth protein and essential fatty acids although vegetarians believe this is not necessary.

3. Avoid high calorie foods, such as wet pack cereals, mixed breakfasts and dinners, and desserts.

4. Encourage physical exercise by limiting the use of play pens and including the baby in a physically active family life.

5. If a baby wants something he can't have, don't get into the habit of offering food first to stall him off; rather, play with him, hold him, and talk to him.

Should You Lose Weight?

Before you decide to lose weight, or especially before you decide your infant should lose weight or your adolescent daughter decides she should lose weight, check with your doctor. It is not uncommon to see beautifully shaped teenage girls who are not fat, who may even be thin, go on crash diets. They frequently have a fixation that skinny is beautiful. More often, the cause for their urge to diet is that they don't like themselves. A teenager with low self-esteem finds that dieting is one thing she can do to change her self-image. Whether her doctor says she needs to diet or not, you should make a serious effort to increase her self-esteem. This is especially true of large girls who have a heavy bone structure and simply do not fit the current fad for skinnyness. Don't let them confuse bigness with badness or fatness. Boys who are displeased with themselves usually want to grow bigger, although some of normal weight will also develop the urge to diet—spurred on by the constant public emphasis on obesity.

Treatment for Obesity

The number of "fat books" on the bestseller lists indicates our national concern with this problem—and the many "cures" that have been advanced over the years. There have been countless treatments for obesity: drugs, diets, hormones, hypnosis, psychotherapy, group therapy, mechanical and electrical devices, and exercise. None of these methods has been proved to be totally successful for all people; a determination to persevere is the key to the success of any weight control program.

Diets are the most popular method of losing weight. "Crash" diets can help, but only in the short run: As soon as the weight is lost, most dieters "go off" their diet, and promptly gain back the weight. The best dieting method is one that teaches the overweight person about nutrition, and helps him alter his eating habits, so that after he loses excess pounds, he can *maintain* his weight at the desired level without strenuous dieting and irrational self-denial. Such a program allows the person to eat those low calorie foods which also provide an intake of the basic vitamins and proteins.

Although people have lost weight by taking drugs that reduce the appetite and/or remove water from body tissues, most doctors discourage the use of these so-called "diet pills." Some don't help; some produce unwanted side effects—and, in any event, most people return to their normal eating habits as soon as they stop taking the drug. Some people can become almost addicted to diet pills—the amphetamines. Although there may be some justification in rare instances for the use of "diet pills" as an aid to getting started on a weight loss program, many doctors are against them on the grounds that they have no lasting effects—and that they may make the individual ill.

Dr. Blackburn S. Joslin lays out the hard truth for the millions of overweight Americans constantly on the lookout for the "quick and easy" diet that will cure their weight problems once and for all:

It is agreed by most authorities in medicine that being overweight is not healthy. Obesity increases the incidence of diabetes, heart trouble, high blood pressure, and vascular and bone malfunctions. No method of treating obesity is perfect. The truth is that each one of us must learn for ourselves just how many calories will keep our weight at a level that ensures good health, social acceptance, and a feeling of well-being. This means following good eating habits throughout our lives. To achieve this goal, we need nutritional knowledge and self-control.

What Is the Best Way to Lose Weight?

The long-term effects of most dieting are often poor. Although weight can be lost, as soon as the diet stops a lot of people gain right back to where they were. So weight goes up and down like a yo-yo, or more likely, down and up. There are many reasons why the long-run results of dieting are rather uninspiring: First, we should admit that the science of weight control is in its infancy—in fact, a lot remains to be discovered about nutrition. Second, human variability makes it almost impossible for even a "good" diet to work for everyone. Third, I believe that most mild obesity results from overeating caused by stress. An important type of stress is unhappiness. We rarely like to admit to being unhappy because bringing this emotional state into the open often seems to increase our suffering. Further, if we act unhappy, there is a tendency for other people to shun us, or to react with unhappiness themselves—and this leads to more unhappiness. So most of us "put on a happy face"—and go get something to eat. If we eat to satisfy our emotional needs rather than our physical needs—and most of us do—then we can get fat. Then, if we are fat, that makes us unhappy, for to say one is fat is to imply that one is "not good," is "ugly," and is therefore "not lovable." And when we diet to get thin, we are admitting to unhappiness. Then, to diet is to withdraw food; to withdraw food is to withdraw love. The result is more unhappiness, which underneath it all drives the individual to seek the comfort of eating. This vicious cycle is especially prevalent in children, although most of us who have tried to diet as adults have experienced these same feelings. It is especially bad if it is a child who is the only one in the family so criticized and the only one on a diet. Eating carries with it overtones of happiness, satisfaction, and love: To give love is to give food, in the minds of many parents. So it is little wonder that children equate receiving food with receiving love.

The vicious cycle of obesity then goes from unhappiness → overeating for comfort → overweight with a poorer self-image → unhappily trying to diet → driven to eat more for happiness. To break the cycle requires more emphasis on happiness than on diet. This is accomplished by establishing reward systems not involving food. All such systems should include:

- Faith in the person, whether he loses weight or not.
- Accepting and valuing the person, regardless of his weight.
- Love—given freely, not as a bribe for good behavior or dieting.
- Happiness, from doing things that are fun—from "kick the can" to bike rides to swimming parties.
- Contentment, from praise of the person and appreciation of the person's accomplishments.

Exercise Helps

Along with the reward system and building self-esteem, all of us need exercise. Exercise programs are helpful as aids to weight loss—and to one's general health, since they stimulate muscle tone, and improve circulation—but upon termination of the program, many people experience a rapid weight gain. (There is also the frequent reluctance of overweight people to go to a gym and expose their fat and clumsiness to other people.) Often a repetitive exercise with no purpose but losing weight or "keeping fit" becomes boring. In fact, it is a sort of admission that we are either fat or unfit (undesirable?), so it can actually increase unhappiness. Exercise should be rewarding in itself. It should accomplish something needed and of worth, or it should be fun for its own sake. Routine exercise includes walking to town rather than getting a ride, pushing a lawnmower rather than buying a power mower, or digging your garden. Episodic exercise includes after-school outdoor play and recreation, weekend ball games, or hikes in the country. Although team sport is excellent, it is harder to keep up when your children become adults. Try to get them interested in lifetime sports activities, such as swimming, tennis, golf, biking, and so forth, that they can continue as an integral part of their lives. Keep in mind that exercise outdoors tends to keep us away from the kitchen, where the temptation to snack is almost irresistible.

Don't expect rapid weight loss. There are approximately 4,000 calories in a pound of body fat; it is unrealistic and unhealthy to aim to lose more than two pounds a week. Keeping one's diet 700 calories *below* what is needed to maintain weight will produce a loss of approximately one and one-half pounds a week.

Final Cautionary Words on Dieting

Pre-adolescence is not the time to stress dieting. The best way to help the pre-adolescent child control his or her weight is by placing your emphasis on changing the eating habits that have led to obesity—not on weight loss per se. If you manage to slow down your child's excessive rate of weight gain, you've accomplished all that can be expected. During early puberty, rapid growth leads to such a striking increase in appetite that dieting is almost an impossibility. In fact, studies have shown that a prolonged low calorie diet during puberty can slow down growth and even interfere with sexual maturation. Consequently, it is not until the mid or late teens, when growth slows and appetites decrease, that an intensive weight loss program is a good idea. Also, by this age, most children have the motivation to look good; and without motivation (theirs, not yours), they will never manage to stay on a diet.

Finally—and perhaps most important—if you have an overweight child, support his efforts to control his weight by establishing good eating habits for the entire family—not a harsh regimen, just the kinds of general rules that will help the whole family form good eating habits. Some of these rules could include:

1. No between-meal eating, except for a small after-school snack.
2. If you are thirsty, drink water and low calorie drinks, not milk, juice, or soft drinks.
3. Prepare *limited amounts* of a favorite high calorie food, so that second portions are not available at meal time.

4. When shopping, buy limited amounts of snack foods, cookies, crackers, peanut butter, and ice cream. Establish a weekly family quota of "goodies" so that when they're gone, they stay gone until the next week.

5. Except for special occasions, serve low calorie desserts, such as fresh fruit, jello, and sherbet, rather than cake, pie, or ice cream.

6. Never tease or nag about overweight or overeating.

No rule need be so inflexible that it is never broken. Still, when reasonable rules are established and when the entire family makes an effort to stick to them, your overweight child—and the rest of you, for that matter—stand to achieve the best results.

4

UNDERSTANDING ILLNESS
AND ITS TREATMENT

Our aim in this section of *The Parents' Medical Manual* is to help you to understand the disease process, to recognize the complexity of human illness, and to learn how to avoid disease and doctors when possible. We don't aim to make doctors out of you. We do aim to increase your understanding of how and why medical decisions are made. This should help you make your own decisions on a more informed basis: What can you do at home; when should you call the doctor; and whether or not to follow your doctor's advice.

Our generation is the beneficiary of vastly improved scientific technology and health knowledge. Some of this you can use at home to keep your children and yourselves in better health. But medical advances don't necessarily mean good health. Today it is assumed that "health care" is the "right" of everyone, and many people feel that doctors should be able to cure almost everything. I once heard a woman berating an emergency room doctor because he wasn't able to bring her husband back to life after he had arrived at the emergency room not breathing and with no heart beat. It is because doctors sometimes can pull veritable miracles out of the hat and bring many heart attack victims back to life that some of the public seem to believe that they should *always* be successful, especially when dealing with "my family." This emotional misunderstanding is one of the causes for the high number of malpractice suits that raise the cost of medical care. Americans spend over a hundred and fifty billion dollars each year on hospitals, doctor's services, medicine, health insurance paperwork, and malpractice insurance. Our battle against sickness is so all-pervasive that we sometimes seem to forget that there is no such thing as lasting perfect health and that we *are* mortal.

Our life is a struggle from the moment of conception. The miracle of birth is that one out of ten conceptions actually survives to be born as a nearly perfect infant. The problems facing a fetus are phenomenal. First, it may be subject to its own inherited genetic weakness and thus, by faulty development, destroy itself by the first or second month. Of the survivors, those with the right combinations of genes, some face different hazards in the uterus. The fetus may become infected by viruses (such as German measles), protozoa (such as toxoplasmosis) or bacteria (such as syphilis). Others are damaged by drugs taken by the mother—cigarettes, alcohol, marihuana, and so forth. Some can be damaged because the blood supply from an abnormal placenta doesn't keep up with the growth of the fetus. Others may be damaged because their blood is destroyed by Rh antibodies in the mother's blood. Then comes birth, at best a traumatic procedure, that squeezes the infant through a narrow birth canal. And the umbilical cord can become twisted or knotted during the birth process, depriving the baby of oxygen. When born without damage, as most babies are, some may then suffer from chilling or may soon become infected by one of the universe of micro-organisms that now start growing on their skin, membranes, and intestinal tract. As the baby grows to adult life, he is subject to the attacks of organisms as small as viruses and as large as animals. And, of course, there are physical injuries (such as from sunshine), chemical poisons (like dishwasher detergent), and psychological stress (from worrying about all these hazards). Yet, God be praised, most infants are born healthy; and most of us survive and grow in good health, especially in our first half of life.

This book concentrates on the first half of life. Infants, children, and teenagers have some special medical problems, as do young adults. But you should be aware that children can get almost any disease that adults can. Pediatricians and family practitioners who are interested in pediatrics spend a lot of time studying the differences in disease between children and adults. We point out many of these. However, the information we learn about children is generally applicable to adults in the first half of life and beyond. I have seen appendicitis in a nine-day-old baby and a ninety-year-old man. To diagnose appendicitis in the baby, we had to be part veterinarian since, like an animal, he couldn't tell us anything except, by his actions, that he hurt. We had to depend on signs: vomiting, fever, abdominal swelling and hardness, diarrhea, and a high white blood count. The ninety-year-old had the same signs but could tell us the symptoms: loss of appetite and nausea, intestinal cramps, tenderness in the right lower abdomen, and that it hurt him to walk and to move. The significance of this is that the knowledge you learn in *The Parents' Medical Manual* may be useful to you as a parent for your children, or as a person for yourself. This is not a medical compendium that covers everything, and, specifically, we don't cover the ailments of middle and old age. Still, the information presented is useful in understanding illness at any age. To understand illness or disease requires a broad approach. The best definition of disease probably comes from archaic English (when they usually meant what they said), in which the word meant dis-ease—uneasiness or discomfort. This is what counts, regardless of more precise scientific definitions, which usually revolve around the fact that disease means there is damage, somehow, somewhere, to the body or to the mind. In order to understand the significance of this damage, we must look at many basic factors of disease: the cause, the location, the body's reactions, the symptoms, and the signs. But you first must realize that no one of these will stand alone.

A SINGLE "ENCYCLOPEDIA" APPROACH TO DISEASE WON'T WORK

Man is complicated, and so are his diseases. For example, a strep infection can cause symptoms in one part of the body (like headache), and signs in another (like a skin rash); it may be located in the tonsils, and caused by a germ called the beta-streptococcus. The same symptom, headache, can be caused by a host of things—from nervous tension to sinus infection to hangover. The same sign, skin rash, can be caused by other bacteria, some viruses, weeds in the lawn, or a detergent. The same location, the tonsils, may be diseased by many other bacteria, hundreds of viruses, allergy—or even by mechanical injury from ill-advised gargling with aspirin. Meanwhile, the same germ in the tonsils, beta-streptococcus, can cause damage to the heart (rheumatic fever), the kidneys (nephritis), the brain (chorea); or it can spread to the sinuses, causing sinusitis, and to the skin, causing impetigo. Then the body may respond to the same strep infection with a runny nose in an infant; a high fever and illness in a five-year-old; a sore throat, swollen glands, and fever in a teenager, and a scratchy throat with no illness in some adults; while in a few people, it may cause rheumatic fever or nephritis. Thus, one infection can produce many different diseases, in different locations, with different symptoms and signs, depending upon the age of the individual and the fact that different people react remarkably differently to disease.

Individual Differences

These differences between people represent one of the most important factors you can learn about illness and its treatment. Each of us, to one degree or another, reacts differently to infection, to disease, and to treatment. By measuring these differences, statisticians can define those whose differences are not enough to exclude them from the norm and those whose differences are enough to make them abnormal. The statistical result becomes our old friend, the bell-shaped curve we saw on page 3. Each of us is probably abnormal in some way. In fact, one of the characteristics that distinguishes man from animal is man's phenomenal variability and individuality. Of course, we can and do learn to act like the herd, and that is the basis of our social structure. But, in fact, we are all different. This is especially evident in our reaction to germs or other causes of disease. Thus one man's cold is another's viral meningitis. One man's medicine is another man's poison. Science seeks to make order out of this by classifying these reactions into the normal and the abnormal. Doctors armed with this knowledge seek to apply it to individuals. This is why doctors need to be sensitive to patients' reactions—for although we do the scientifically proper thing for the majority, we may inadvertently hurt a minority or a single "different" individual. Thus, what the doctor orders is usually good for you—but not necessarily all the time. Regardless, we have to have some place to start, and the statistical norm is a reasonable one. One of the first places we apply it is to the location of a disease. Thus we know that tonsillitis, for example, is statistically most often caused by a virus infection. But there are other causes of tonsillitis.

How to Sort Out Diseases

The various causes of disease are covered in separate chapters, as are the locations of disease—a handy way to start. In these, we concentrate on the type of information that will increase your decision making powers and that will help you do all that you yourself can do to prevent or relieve disease in your family. Keep in mind the complexity and diversity of illness resulting from a single cause, and the often abnormal response of differing people. It is this defensive response of the body to damage that causes most of the symptoms and signs of disease. An example of this response might be what happens when you get a sliver in your finger. As a start, it hurts.

Symptoms of Disease

As you have seen, symptoms are feelings of dis-ease. If you get a splinter in your finger, the damaged tissue sends a message to the brain, and you have the symptom of pain. Cellular chemicals released from the damaged tissue cause different responses. They attract white blood cells to the area, and cause specialized cells in the nearby tissue to release inflammatory chemicals. Some of these chemicals help the blood vessels in the area of the splinter open wide, bringing in more white blood cells and antibodies to fight the germs which came in with the splinter. The extra blood supply makes the finger hot and swollen. You feel these last two changes, but they are also seen as signs of infection of disease.

Signs of Disease

In the hot, swollen finger, the white cells accumulate around the splinter, engulfing any bacteria present. When a bacteria is "swallowed" by a white blood cell, the inside of the blood cell responds by releasing chemicals that form a germ-killing compound similar to the clorox that you buy in the store. This kills the germ, and, in the process, may kill the white blood cell. Thousands and thousands of these white blood cells surround the splinter, and as they die, they turn yellow. This yellow material causes another sign of infection, called pus.

We have discussed many other signs in this chapter. The baby with appendicitis had the signs of fever (measured with a thermometer) and a hard and swollen abdomen. Some of the people with strep throat had a foul breath, some a skin rash, and, in some, red urine from blood leaking into the kidney appeared, signaling nephritis. By discussing signs and symptoms, we discussed the body's reaction to disease. This comes under the complicated subject of immunity.

Immunity and Antibiotics

What you need to know most is will your own immunity, or your child's, handle most illnesses most of the time. Viral illness must either be handled by your own immune system or be prevented by building up your immunity beforehand with injections of killed or weakened viruses which stimulate a reaction but do not create a noticeable illness. But some very rare people have such a weak immune system that even a weakened virus is evidently able to make them quite sick, or, even more rarely, to kill them. These people would probably have soon died of something else anyway if they hadn't received the immunization.

Your immunity helps you fight bacterial and other types of infection. Antibiotics primarily fight bacterial infections. But neither immunity nor antibiotics are safe for everybody. Some people's immune systems overreact so much that their own antibodies seem to attack their own tissues—as well as bacteria. A common example of our own antibodies damaging us is hayfever. The pollen touches the membranes of the nose and the body mistakenly responds as if it is a four-alarm fire. Histamine, serotonin, and other potent chemicals are released, as if a bacterial infection is being fought—so the membranes in the nose swell and weep and itch. If severe enough, the same thing happens in the lungs, and, in addition to swelling, the muscles around the bronchial tubes go into spasm, causing the person to cough and wheeze with asthma. Antibiotics, which kill or damage bacteria, can be very helpful. However, if your body becomes allergic to the antibiotic, it may fight the antibiotic with its own antibodies as if the medicine were a bacteria. You can get hives, itching, swelling, and fever; in fact, a few can even get sick enough to die. So antibiotics have to be used with care. We discuss the relationship of antibodies to infections and fevers later.

Age Differences in Illness

An important factor in understanding illness and sorting out disease is the age of the individual. At times, the differences in response between newborns, toddlers, children, adults, and old people are so great that the same infection can cause markedly different diseases. Only recently, for example, has it been discovered that many small children seem to get infectious mononucleosis—and get over it without problems. It is certainly a different disease than teenagers have; in fact, we rarely recognize it in children even when they have it. And we often have to use a different set of criteria to determine when infants and toddlers are sick, whatever the cause.

How Can You Tell When Your Infant or Toddler Is Sick?

Symptoms of illness in infants include lethargy, excessive fussiness, poor fluid intake, sometimes fever, abnormal spitting, vomiting, diarrhea, cough, and the inability to suck. Still, your infant can be infected but not look ill and show none of these symptoms or signs. Because he reacts differently to infection than older children or adults do, it is sometimes hard to tell whether or not he is really sick. You should be suspicious if some member of the family or a visitor has "a cold." Infants can and do catch colds, skin infections, and bowel infections. It is reasonable to keep this sort of exposure to a minimum for the first several months of life. A mild adult infection can make an infant very ill; on the other hand, some severe adult infections bother infants very little. Because infant antibody production and reaction to infection is very limited in the first several months, an infant may not always have fever in response to infection. A rectal temperature around 100° F is normal; a fever is rarely significant unless it is over 101° F rectally. But a high fever in infants under nine months can indicate significant illness.

A high respiratory rate is a reliable sign of illness in infants. If a baby is bothered by infection, he usually breathes faster. An infant normally breathes less than thirty times a minute when quiet or asleep. If he gets a cold, the rate may go to forty to fifty a minute. If he breathes over sixty times a minute constantly, when quiet or asleep, it may be a sign of trouble. Sometimes it is just due to fever.

In order to count a baby's respiratory rate, it is best to use a watch or clock with a sweep second hand, or one with clearly marked minutes on the dial so that you can time a full minute accurately. Count the total number of breaths (one breath is breathing in and out) in a full minute when he is very quiet or asleep. A gas pain, a burp, or a dream may increase the rate temporarily, so a single count can be misleading. If the count is above sixty a minute, you should watch the baby closely for other signs of problems, or for a further increase in the rate above sixty.

Experienced pediatricians like Dr. A. S. Hashim rely on the general attitude of the infant to tell if he is sick: "If he is fussy for over two or three days, if his color is off, if he eats less or cries as if in pain, I would rather see him than wait." Experienced mothers like Bambi Scofield have their own ways: "It is hard to tell when your child is sick only for the first month or two. Then you learn what constitutes 'sick' for each individual child. It's a look—peculiar to each child."

Toddlers and Preschool Children

Around the time a baby starts to crawl and walk, there are some marked changes in the reaction to infection. The body responds with much higher fevers than it did in the first nine months of life. In fact, a minor infection can result in a very high fever. This tendency generally lasts until the age of three to four years, when the child begins to react more like an adult. Another change we mentioned earlier in this chapter is in a child's reaction to strep throats. Small children have little or no redness, while older children often have severe redness and pus.

Older Children

Although we make the point that there are differing reactions at different ages, symptoms and signs overlap enough that you should be aware that they can occur at any age. So, in addition to the above symptoms, parents should watch for earache, foul breath, swollen glands, croup, stomachache, headache, frequent or painful urination, red or purple spots on the skin, listlessness, or signs of pain. Be particularly suspicious of illness when an infant is unusually listless and refuses to suck, even if there is little or no fever. If these symptoms occur, or if there is fever over 101°–102° (rectally) and your child acts ill, you should call your child's physician. We will talk more about signs such as fever, and symptoms of illness a bit further on in this chapter.

What Is an Infection?

An infection is an invasion of germs that injure the body. The three most commonly known germs are viruses, bacteria, and fungi. Viruses live inside our living cells. Bacteria are single cell organisms that live in our body fluids outside the cells. Fungi live on or in our body, and are really a type of microscopic plant, like weeds in a garden. Ordinarily, a universe of micro-organisms lives on our skin and in our respiratory and intestinal tracts. Some of these organisms are friendly and aid our nutrition or protect our skin from "non-friendly" germs. But occasionally even "friendly" germs can cause trouble if they get into the wrong place. All of these are discussed in more detail in Chapters 16 and 17.

When a virus invades a part of the body, it creates what is called "primary infection." A "cold" is one example of a primary infection in which the throat, nasal, and respiratory tissues are affected. Depending on the particular virus and the particular individual, the affected tissue is damaged and therefore has less resistance to bacteria, which then invade and cause another infection in the same spot—a "secondary" infection. The toxic products excreted by the bacteria do more damage than most viruses. An ear abscess which follows a mild cold is an example of "secondary infection."

In either case, the body fights back. The tissues become red and swollen; white blood cells pour out to fight the germs; and antibodies seep into the area to neutralize the germs and their toxins. In some people, the body defenses kill germs with such ease that the victim doesn't know there is a fight. Others have a much harder time and have to fall back on defenses like fever to discourage the germs. Those who are not ill may carry the germs for a while and then destroy them with no apparent signs of disease.

Why Do Children Have So Many Infections?

The average preschool child in the United States has about one infection a month. Most infections are very mild and often are not even noticed; yet some children may get quite ill with an infection that doesn't bother other children. There are several reasons for this high incidence of infection in young children. First is the child's lack of immunity due to his body's lack of experience in fighting infections. Second is the individual child's basic resistance as he comes into contact with other children.

Infants are born with antibodies from the mother, but not all her antibodies pass through the placenta, so the immunity is incomplete. By three months of age, most of these maternal antibodies are gone. By three months, the infant's immune system has matured enough to start manufacturing antibodies; however, it isn't until around five years that a child's immunity level is the same as an adult's and there is enough immunity to protect against most common infections. Antibodies are produced in response to immunizing injections as D. P. T. (diphtheria, whooping cough, and tetanus) and in response to infections. Figure 23 shows the usual rise of antibody in children's blood, reaching an adult level by around five years of age.

Another reason for large numbers of infections is that nursery school is a bug factory! Preschool children's lack of immunity makes them very susceptible, so an infection starting in one child will spread rapidly to the others. The same thing happens in large famlies. The first baby rarely has infections before his first birthday, but succeeding babies have older brothers and sisters who bring germs home. This doesn't mean that children should not go to nursery school, although there are times when a very susceptible child should not.

Air travel is another reason for the increased incidence of infection. People and their germs are transported all over the world in a matter of

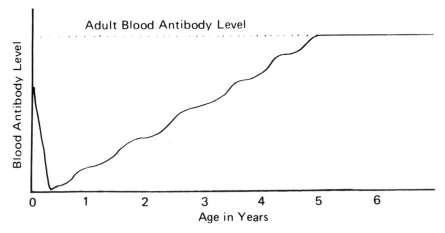

FIGURE 23   *The normal levels of antibodies in children.*

hours. Diarrhea from Tokyo and the "flu" from New York can be imported to California in one day. Multiplied by the phenomenal number of people who fly, travel becomes a major factor in explaining the increased incidence of viral diseases. There are certainly enough viruses to go around. Over 100 strains of the "common cold" virus are known, and at least 400 other viruses can infect humans.

Some children have real difficulty with common infections and require special help. People who handle colds or diarrhea easily have trouble recognizing that their minor illness can cause serious illness in a susceptible child. The world is full of "typhoid Marys." Mary was a healthy cook who carried the typhoid germ in her bowel. Unfortunately, she worked for families who had low resistance to her typhoid germs. Many of her employers died from the typhoid she carried. Mary couldn't believe that their typhoid and deaths were her fault, so she kept moving, cooking, and infecting people. There is little typhoid now; but many of our friends carry and occasionally infect us with an illness such as a virus, a cold, or a streptococcal throat. If your child keeps getting infections, check with your doctor—but suspect your friends.

Some colds are not colds at all but are allergies instead. It is difficult at times to distinguish an allergy from a viral infection. There is no question that at times allergy also lowers the body's resistance to infections. Often, there is a family history of allergy, even though neither parent is allergic. Your unique child may have granddad's unique gene which makes him more suceptible to allergy, and, therefore, to infection.

Do Your Children Give You Infections?

Preschool children bring home a lot of diseases. "Colds" alone occur six times a year in the "average" preschool child. But they occur from one to three times a year in most adults. Harmful bacteria such as the pneumococci exist in the noses and throats of about five percent of the general population. But it has been found that fifty percent of preschoolers and thirty percent of school age children carry this bacteria at times. Twenty percent of the parents of preschoolers carried pneumococcus, while parents of high schoolers had the average adult rate of five percent. It was noted that when the child became ill with a pneumococcal ear infection, it usually started with a viral cold. In adults, pneumococci are more likely to cause bacterial pneumonia than ear infections, although most adults are already fairly immune to the pneumococcus and simply carry it without problems. So, yes, your small children can definitely give you infections—but that's all right, you and they will survive from your own good resistance or with occasional help from modern medicine.

Colds and Allergy

We asked Florida pediatrician James Stem to explain the relationship of infection to allergy. He says:

> Allergy is often the culprit in some children who have more
> infections than others. As infants, these children frequently have

difficulty with milk and other foods: Weepy rashes occur behind the ears, in creases in the arm, or the back of the knees; or they vomited and had diarrhea from some food which could not be tolerated. Despite doctors' warnings, allergic children frequently continue to eat the offensive food. Such allergic reactions seem to make some individuals very susceptible to infections.

Infections are fought by our immune mechanism, which, in general terms, like a defensive army, swings into action when the body is invaded by virus or bacteria. In some people, allergens such as pollens or dust may cause the "defensive army" to react to them as if they were viruses or bacteria. This diverts the immune mechanism from the task of fighting infection and makes the allergic individual more susceptible. It is as simple as the age-old military strategy, "Divide and Conquer."

Parents who conscientiously and adequately reduce the allergens a child has to fight find a dramatic decrease in the incidence of infection. If the allergens cannot be avoided, allergy shots usually help. They produce a different sort of antibody that neutralizes the pollen or dust allergens and allows the body's usual immune mechanism to fight infection. (See also Chapter 15 on Allergy.)

TABLE 7 *Comparison of fahrenheit to centigrade temperature readings.*

°F = 98.6	100.4	102.1	103.9	105.6	107.6
°C = 37	38	39	40	41	42

FEVER

Fever is the body's way of letting us know that something is wrong—usually, that some kind of infection is present. One of the ways the body fights infection is by fever: Some types of bacteria do not grow well at temperatures we can stand. If bacteria or their toxins begin damaging tissues, the brain somehow decides to cause fever. It does this by sending messages telling your muscles to work very hard, creating heat. Messages are also sent to the blood vessels in the skin, causing them to narrow down in order to prevent the heat from being lost at the skin surface. The muscles, even those in the skin, contract or bunch up. This causes shaking and goose bumps on the skin. So, as a fever starts to build up, we often chill and feel cold and clammy. The body also may react with fever from toxins absorbed from the intestine or from some complicated types of delayed immune response. It appears that although fever was designed to fight bacterial and viral infections, it occasionally hurts some of us as much as the germs.

Fever in Children

Fever in an infant is always significant if it rises above 101° rectally, but a small child's fever can often be dramatic without being serious, especially in the one to three year age range. The height of the fever is not indicative of the severity of the infection. One mild child's illness, roseola infantum, may be accompanied by temperatures up to 105° or more. Occasionally, fever is caused from reactions to drugs—even to aspirin—or to dehydration, excessive sunshine, and the like.

Conversely, some very severe infections, such as meningitis, may not cause high fever in young babies. It should also be noted that wide swings in a fever do not necessarily indicate either a worsening or an improvement in the child's illness. It is natural for a youngster's fever to be lower in the morning and to rise in the evening. Much of this variance in temperature is due to the small child's heat regulating system. This system, which is a kind of thermostat located in the brain, has not had much "practice," and it is not as sophisticated as an adult's heat regulating system.

What Is a Normal Temperature?

The normal temperature in small children is usually below 100°, taken rectally, and any rise above this point is worthy of note. However, even high fevers rarely do harm in the range of 104°–105.5° orally, or 105°–106.5° rectally. The thermostat in the brain ordinarily helps protect the body temperature from going higher than that. The blood vessels dilate and the body perspires. If a child is uncomfortable and hot, he can be cooled artificially by wetting him with water and fanning him. Cooling sponge baths make him feel better, but it is doubtful if they are actually helpful in combating his illness. In fact, fever is beneficial in mobilizing the body's defenses against disease.

Body temperature is not stable—it is normally lower in the morning and higher in evening. So-called normal temperature, as recorded by the little red mark on the thermometer, is actually an *average* temperature. Some run a bit lower and some a bit higher; and in almost everybody, temperature fluctuates as much as one degree during the twenty-four hours of a day.

Fevers fluctuate even more. On a chart, many fevers follow a sawtooth pattern (see Figure 24). They rise in the evening and go down by the next morning. If your child had a fever last night and none this morning, that alone doesn't mean you can turn him loose. There is a fair chance that the fever will return tonight. If the fever is 101° F at noon, it will possibly be 104° F by ten P.M.

The minor variations in fever, say between 101° F and 105° F, are rarely significant. Parents waste a lot of time worrying about just how much fever a child has. Once you know there is a fever, you don't need to continue to take temperatures more than once a day. The morning temperature is often useless; for it may be normal but then rise that evening. The best time to take a temperature is once in the late afternoon. If you suspect the child is ill, or if you want to be sure he is over his recent illness, take his temperature at this time for a few days.

How Do You Check a Temperature?

You have to use a thermometer to check for a fever. Many times, the hand on the head technique doesn't work. That is why thermometers

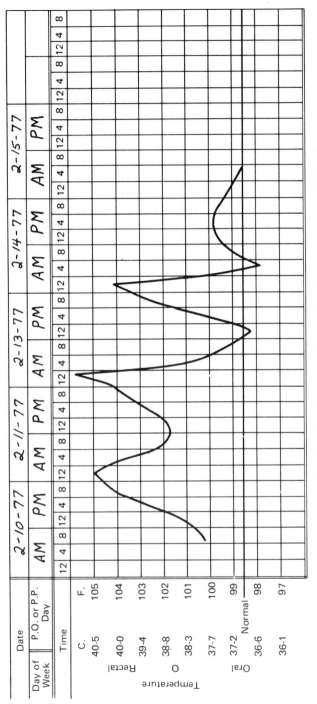

FIGURE 24 *An example of a five-day course of a spiking fever.*

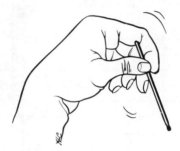

FIGURE 25　*Hold tightly to the thermometer as you snap your wrist to shake down the temperature reading to below 98°F or 36°C.*

were invented. The skin temperature is determined by how much blood is in the skin. Flushing and blushing and external warmth open the skin vessels up and warm the skin. Cold, shock, nervousness, and sweating will close the skin vessels down and cool the skin. I occasionally see children with cold skin and a 104° F fever. And I see children with hot skin and normal temperature. If you believe your child is sick—certainly if he is sick enough to call your doctor—then check the temperature with a thermometer and report these results when you make your call.

Before you take the temperature, read the thermometer to make sure it registers below the normal line. If it doesn't, shake the thermometer down until it reads under normal. Hold it like you would hold a pencil when writing but further out, not touching the hand—the bulb end would be where the lead of the pencil is. Hold tight with the thumb and first two fingers and shake it with a snapping wrist motion, as if you were trying to shake water off the thermometer. A rectal thermometer has a short bulb, while an oral thermometer has a longer bulb. Both register the same temperature, although the "normal" temperature arrow may be on the 99.7 mark for the rectal thermometer and on the 98.7 mark for the mouth thermometer.

How Do You Read a Thermometer?

Rotate the thermometer until you see the center clear line of mercury toward the bulb. Follow this line up until it becomes opaque. Sometimes you can see it better by changing the background from light to dark or by changing the direction of the light source.

Fahrenheit thermometers are marked off in degrees, with intermediate marks at two tenths of a degree. The "normal" mouth temperature is 98.7° F and the "normal" rectal temperature is 99.7° F. Since there is normal variation of around one degree, a temperature isn't considered a "fever" unless it is over 99° F by mouth or over 100° F by rectum.

Centigrade thermometer readings can be converted to fahrenheit readings with the following equations on the chart below:

°C to °F $°F = °C \ (9/5) + 32°$
°F to °C $°C = (°F - 32°) \times 5/9$

For easy conversion of centigrade to fahrenheit temperature readings, a "normal" mouth temperature is 37° C and 98.6° F. A temperature of 40° C is exactly 104° F and a fever is not "high" unless it is over 104° F.

How Do You Hold an Infant to Take a Temperature?

Lay him on his stomach on a firm surface. Spread the cheeks of the buttocks so you can see the rectum. Insert the greased metal end of the thermometer into the rectum about one inch. Place one hand on the buttocks, with the thermometer coming out between the fingers. Hold the buttocks of the child firmly and pinch the thermometer between your fingers firmly. If the child struggles, put the heel of the other hand in the small of the back with a stiff elbow and lean on him to hold him still. Leave the thermometer in for three minutes although sometimes it will register a fever more quickly. You may be able to watch the clear temperature line climb while the thermometer is still being held in the anus.

How Do You Get a Child to Hold a Thermometer Under the Tongue?

Have him open his mouth, gently put the bulb of the thermometer under the tongue, and instruct the child to kiss the thermometer with his lips only, not to bite on it. Tell him to hold it as though he were sucking on a straw. Hold the glass portion for him or let him hold it himself. Keep it at the proper angle, so that the bulb stays under the tongue. One minute will do if his mouth is closed and he has not just had a cold drink.

Treating Fever

Practicing pediatrician William Misbach gives the following advice: "The most important thing to do when your child has a fever is to keep

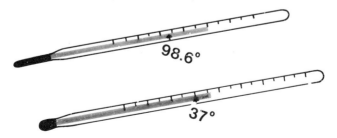

FIGURE 26 *Normal temperatures in oral (top) and rectal (bottom) thermometers in degrees fahrenheit and centigrade.*

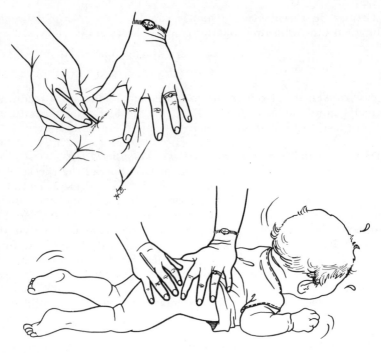

FIGURE 27   *The key to holding the thermometer in the rectum is to pinch it hard between your fingers while you press your hand firmly on the buttocks to hold the child still.*

him well hydrated with lots of fluids and to have him rest. It is permissible to give aspirin or other anti-fever drugs prescribed by the doctor to make the child more comfortable. However, aspirin is used far too often for the benefit of parents because it gives them the feeling that they have done something worthwhile, and that active treatment is under way. The dose is a grain for each year of age every four hours."

Sponging treats fever the same way that sweating does. In fact, sponging is actually artificial sweat. Undress the child, and wet the hot skin with tepid (warm) water. As the air dries the water, it cools the skin. As long as the skin is hot, you can bring the temperature down with continued spongings.

If the fever is above 105° F by mouth or 106° F by rectum, you may want to follow Dr. A. S. Hashim's advice:

1. Put the child in a cool water bath for up to half an hour.
2. Cover his skin with cloths wet with one half pint of rubbing alcohol mixed with a quart of water; keep changing cloths so they stay cool.
3. Give a cool water enema, with one teaspoon of salt in a pint of water.

TABLE 8   *Guidelines for fever medication.*

| | | *Every four hours give:* | |
| | | *Acetaminophen (Tylenol, Tempra, Liquipren, etc.)* | |
Age	*Baby Aspirin (1¼ grain)*	*Syrup*	*Drops*
6 months	½ tablet	¼th teaspoon	0.3 cc
1 year	1 tablet	½ teaspoon	0.6 cc
2 years	1½ to 2 tablets	¾ to 1 teaspoon	0.9 to 1.2 cc
3 years	2 to 3 tablets	1 to 1½ teaspoon	
5 years	4 tablets or one adult aspirin (5 grains)	2 teaspoons or 1 tablet	
10 years and up	2 adult aspirins	2 Tylenol tablets	

Medications for fever include aspirin and acetaminophen. They are both toxic if taken in excess, although aspirin is probably the most poisonous of the two. Because their poisonous effects are different, you can give both aspirin and acetophenetin at the same time if they really are needed.

Problems from Fever

When Is a Fever Dangerous?

Overall, fever is not dangerous; it is one of the body's ways of fighting infection. However, fever can be dangerous under several circumstances:

1. If it is above 106° F orally or 107° rectally.
2. If it lasts over two days without adequate intake of liquids and sugar.
3. If there is a possibility of a febrile convulsion.

Otherwise, fever is simply a general indication of infection or illness. A child with a 105° F oral temperature who doesn't act sick is far better off than a child with a 101° F temperature who looks and acts ill.

What Is a Febrile Convulsion?

For those who have never seen one, a convulsion can be a terrifying experience. The child stiffens, and becomes rigid and unconscious, often with an arched back. The eyes roll back and the saliva foams out of the mouth. Rhythmic contractions or movements of various muscles occur and cannot be stopped. Often, there is such muscle tightness that the child cannot breathe well, and he may become dusky. Once oxygen to the body is stopped, the muscles relax and the child's breathing resumes. So, of course, can yours! These spells are usually quite short—lasting only a few minutes—and then the child relaxes and sleeps.

Febrile convulsions usually occur at the onset of a fever when it first starts to rise. At times, a convulsion may be the first indication that a child is ill. It is rare for convulsions to occur when a fever has already reached a level around 105° F. Most febrile convulsions are self-limited and usually do little damage, although exceptions do occur. Convulsions with fever are not always simple febrile convulsions, and any convulsion always warrants a prompt call to the doctor.

Febrile convulsions are more likely to occur in a child where there is a family history of febrile convulsions. A child who has had one febrile convulsion is more likely to have others; and his physician may order medication to be taken routinely, or at the onset of any cold or infection. Most febrile convulsions occur between the ages of one to four years— beyond four they are rare, and if they occur in an older child, they deserve special consideration.

What Should You Do If Your Child Convulses?
Dr. A. S. Hashim notes that convulsions usually stop in a few minutes, although it seems longer:

Convulsions are more serious if they last much beyond five to ten minutes, if they recur frequently, or if the child is very sick. When your child does convulse:
1. Turn his face to the side to prevent him from choking on saliva. He will be better off on his stomach rather than on his back.
2. If his tongue is caught between his teeth or if he is blue, wrap a piece of cloth thickly around a spoon handle or small stick.
3. Force the jaw open and insert the cloth wrapped handle between the teeth.
4. Do not shake him, sit on him, scream at him, put your finger between his teeth, or push the spoon handle against the clenched teeth.
5. Have someone call the doctor.
6. Start cooling him if he is hot, as described on page 102.

Antibiotics

Antibiotics are chemicals produced in nature by fungi or produced artificially by man to act against bacteria. Antibiotics do not affect viruses because the virus lives inside our body as a part of the biochemical system of each cell. Thus, anything that will damage the virus will probably damage the cell. Bacteria live outside cells in body fluids, and can be bathed in antibiotics, which act on the bacteria cell wall. Antibiotics have successfully been used against so many illnesses that many parents become disturbed when they aren't prescribed, especially for colds. Parents often ask, "But why didn't Johnny get a penicillin shot?" "I don't see why the doctor didn't prescribe the same antibiotic Dr. X used to order for Susie." "I wish Mark had gotten a shot—he gets better so much quicker when he has one."

Dr. Glen Griffin explains why doctors often don't use antibiotics:

If a certain shot or red capsule or pink cinnamon syrup always "worked" and never caused problems, the practice of medicine would be simple. It isn't. There are no such all-purpose magic cures. There are simply more types of infection than any one medicine could possibly combat. Bacteria come as several kinds of cocci, bacilli, and spirillae. Then are are fungi, and parasites, and mycoplasma organisms, to say nothing of the rickettsiae, or the wide spectrum of viral agents.

Any one of many hundreds of infectious organisms may be responsible for a problem. Although sometimes a person may get repeated infections, it's rather foolish to think that "this medicine will always work for my child's fevers," or that this or that shot "never works for me."

It's true: Sometimes a shot doesn't work. Sometimes a medicine doesn't work. But that's because of the type of infection—not because of you. Certain organisms may become resistant to an antibiotic. People don't. (People may become allergic to an antibiotic and get a rash or other side effect—but they don't get resistant to it.)

How do doctors know what's going on? How do physicians make decisions about whether or not to give an antibiotic, and, if so, what kind? Experience helps. Knowing the pattern of current infections helps. A physical exam helps. Sometimes lab tests are needed. The main objective is to get you well—quickly. Other objectives are to do this as painlessly and as inexpensively as possible.

What we want to avoid is adding to your problem. Sometimes side effects happen—from every medicine—even aspirin. So good medicine is not always lots of medicine or lots of shots.

For this reason, sometimes you may not get a shot. Sometimes you may not even get a prescription. Many people become very unhappy when they don't get a certain prescription or when their child isn't given a shot. In fact, there are more dissatisfied patients who didn't get a shot, which they thought they needed, than there are complaints about getting a shot.

Why not an antibiotic? A virus infection wouldn't be helped by all the penicillin in the country. Some other infections are eradicated better with other medicines. There are many choices. You want the best choice for your particular problem. Why not an antibiotic? Because you don't need one this time.

Generally speaking, antibiotics are used in the following situations:

1. There is a beta hemolytic streptococcus infection.
2. There is a good likelihood of other types of bacterial infection such as the pneumococcus, hemophilus or staphylococcus germs.
3. The individual has a low immunity or a history of bacterial complications, such as pneumococcal ear infections, which start during viral infections.
4. There is suspicion of a possible highly contagious quick-acting infection, such as bacterial meningitis, which is "going around" in an area.

Antibiotics should usually not be used when:

1. The individual is allergic to the antibiotic.
2. The infection is probably caused by a virus.
3. The individual can fight off the infection himself without the help of antibiotics.

In spite of these generalities, there is a lot of criticism about the overuse of antibiotics, and doctors disagree with each other. Because we believe that parents are generally competent and can make rational decisions if they know the facts, we offer you not one opinion about antibiotics but several. When doctors disagree, it doesn't always mean that one is wrong. We hope the following "debate" will give you a better understanding of the complexities of the practice of medicine, and will also help you aid the doctor in finding the best means of treating you and your children.

Are Antibiotics Overused? Four Views

The editors of the *New England Journal of Medicine* believe that too many viral infections are treated unnecessarily with antibiotics:

> Among the commonest causes of acute illnesses with fever are the myriad respiratory viruses causing cold, cough, and signs of involvement of the upper and lower respiratory tract. It may be reasonable to assume that many of these illnesses are treated with antibiotics, at least when accompanied by significant fever. With the possible exception of some pleuro-pneumonia members [germs causing "viral" pneumonia], however, none of the viruses involved have been shown to be susceptible to currently available antibiotics, nor have prophylactic antibiotics [antibiotics used to prevent a secondary infection] been shown to be useful in decreasing bacterial complications: Indeed, complications appearing in patients already on antibiotic therapy may be even more difficult to treat.
>
> Although in the earlier stages minor viral respiratory illness may be difficult to distinguish from significant bacterial disease, its natural course is usually self-limited to a few days, often with spontaneous resolution becoming apparent by the second day, especially in younger patients. It therefore seems logical to withhold antibiotic therapy until unequivocal physical signs, culture reports, or lack of spontaneous improvement within a reasonable period form a more definite indication for its use. Since over ninety-five percent of acute respiratory disease is viral, there should be little risk in adhering to such a policy.
>
> It is nevertheless far easier for the harried physician to give all such patients antibiotics at the onset than to be faced with the task of explaining the germ theory of disease, the difference between viral and bacterial illness, and their response to antibiotics several times a day in the midst of a busy winter season. The tendency to buy time with antibiotics as sugar pills, however, carries with it the risks of the development of resistant bacterial strains, unnecessary sensitization to useful agents, and needless expense. Worse yet, the physician, when confronted with spontaneous resolution, may convince himself that he has actually administered specific therapy, thus encouraging the future neglect of adequate supportive therapy in similar cases.
>
> The public has, of course, come to believe over the last decades that anti-

biotics are truly miracle drugs devoid of limitations. The professional and lay press can share the credit for the creation of such a fantasy. The time seems at hand for a re-education to the fact that the need for antibiotics is relatively infrequent.[1]

On the other hand, as a practicing pediatrician, I believe that the editors of the *Journal* overstated their case. The debate on this topic can best be understood by the general public if people realize that most "authoritative medical opinions" are announced by the academic rather than the practicing physicians. For me, a practicing pediatrician, to debate with the respected *New England Journal of Medicine* is like trying to play tennis with Billie Jean King. Or is it? I respect the academic and research physicians who write such editorials, but they are often somewhat insulated from the day-to-day experience of the primary care of people. As a practitioner, I believe there are aspects of the "antibiotic debate" not clearly apparent to some of our learned academic colleagues.

In practice, many physicians find that there is less *total illness* if antibiotics are liberally used. Other practitioners don't report that experience. But remember, people are different. Many have good natural immunity. They dislike taking drugs; and, overall, they see physicians less often than the norm. When they do visit their doctors, they tend to have faith in their recuperative abilities: They are not likely to request antibiotics and are likely to reject a doctor's advice to use these drugs. On the other hand, there are persons whose every cold develops into an ear, sinus, or throat infection. These persons need antibiotics frequently. It would be unwise to withhold the drugs from them on the theory that antibiotics tend generally to be overused.

If, as it states in the *New England Journal of Medicine* article, ninety-five percent of acute respiratory disease is viral, then antibiotics are indeed overused. However, you may have noted, on page 96 that bacterial ear infections in children usually start with viral colds. In practice, the amount of secondary infection seen by physicians is far higher than five percent. This is an area where you should let your doctor make the decision—regardless of advice, pro or con, in books.

Doctors, as well as patients, can be different. Some remain conservative, while others who are more oriented to prevention tend to use antibiotics early. There is a certain amount of patient selection of a doctor, which helps to explain why physicians tend to continue their own way of practice. People who need (or want) antibiotics, or those who believe they suffered from an antibiotic being withheld, tend to seek "liberal" doctors. Those who found they didn't need the antibiotic prescribed, and who have excellent resistance, tend to seek "conservative" doctors. Thus the patients of both liberal and conservative doctors are generally content, leading each doctor to believe that he has done the best by that patient. And he probably has.

This does not mean that antibiotics are not overused. Some patients, remembering that penicillin cured a past "cold," demand more penicillin for other colds. And it is often easier for doctors to give a prescription rather than an explanation.

The key to avoiding an overuse of antibiotics is to let your physician know you and your medical background. First, have a complete history and physical done by your doctor. Allow him to get to know you well enough to know that he can trust you to follow his instructions and report potential complications to him—so he can *avoid* using antibiotics. If he doesn't know you, doesn't know your degree of immunity, or the likelihood of your following his instructions, he may have to assume the worst and treat you to cover all potentialities. Thus, it is important that you and your child establish a good relationship and mutual confidence with a personal physician. As Celsus of ancient Rome in the first century A.D. said: "Other things being equal, a friend makes a better physician than a stranger."

Pediatrician Merritt Low offers yet another view—perhaps we should replace antibiotics with a bit of faith.

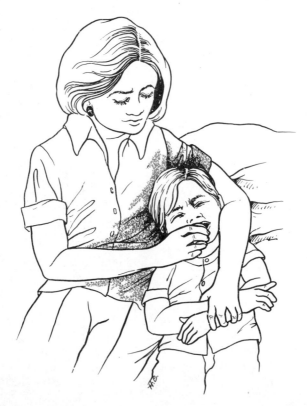

FIGURE 28   *Holding a child to force him to take medicine.*

With all our knowledge of miracle drugs, at times there is "nothing better than nothing!" I believe that overuse of antibiotics may interfere with naturally acquired immunity but I'm not sure yet. The best immunity —if it can be effected without danger—probably comes naturally through Mother Nature and Father Time. The wise physician is the one who knows when to step into the breach. A positive, optimistic attitude toward health seems to lessen illness. If Vitamin C engenders this attitude, why not use it?

Once I had a girl patient with bellyaches. Her mother shopped around and finally got her appendix out. I asked the girl several years later how her bellyaches were. She answered: "Just the same, but my mother doesn't worry about them any more!"

What Was Child Health Like Before Antibiotics?

In the reasonable effort to reduce the use of antibiotics, many of our academic researchers issue cautions about overuse of these life-saving drugs. It might help us all to look at what it was like to suffer an infection in the days before antibiotics. We have the opportunity to hear from a first hand witness, Dr. George R. Russell, who started practice back in the nineteen-twenties when, from a treatment standpoint, physicians had relatively little to offer. He recalls:

Our chief function as pediatricians before antibiotics were available was to recognize the type of disease and to give consolation and hope to our patients and parents as we followed the course of the disease process.

Oh, we could help by making the patient comfortable with aspirin and paregoric, but specific treatment for a given disease was for the most part lacking. In those summers, our hospitals were filled by "refugee-like" babies with sunken eyes due to dehydration, and in winter by victims of respiratory diseases, including chronic mastoid infections, pneumonia, and meningitis. A trip through the wards would show our primitive treatments—red noses from Mercurochrome, brown noses from argyrol, and purple noses from gentian violet—all with little or no apparent benefit.

During the twenties, contagious diseases were so common that there were special contagious disease hospitals, or "pest houses." In the winter of 1927, as a resident hospital physician, I saw more than 1,700 cases of diphtheria alone. At least twenty-five cases were in intensive care, with tubes in their windpipes to permit air passage.

The death rates in those days were high and much of the increased life expectancy of our time comes from the survival of children treated with antibiotics who would have died without them. Work with your doctor to decide whether you or any particular individual in your family may usually need treatment, or if the particular illness will respond as well to natural immunity.

FINDING AND USING MEDICAL CARE

In selecting and evaluating a doctor for you or your child you should take a lot of things into consideration. Is the doctor trained and skilled? Is he usually available? Can you communicate with him? Do you like or respect him? There are also less important considerations like how close you are to his offices, do you like his office help, and how much does he charge? One of the most important factors is: Will he serve as a primary physician?

The primary physician is the one you should turn to first when you have problems; he is the one you should go to for periodic checkups and preventive medicine; he is the one doctor who knows you best, and the one who keeps all your medical records and coordinates your care. As your primary source of health care, he is the one who will diagnose and treat you or send you on to the appropriate specialist in the medical care system for further care if it is needed. He is the doctor to whom all your medical reports should be sent by the various specialists. Usually, he is the one who will help you make the decision if there is conflicting advice or uncertainty about what path to follow in treating an illness. And he is the doctor you stay with over the years. This is especially important for children, because you are not just interested in their day to day care but also in having their health and growth supervised in a way that helps to avoid future problems and helps to encourage future growth and development.

If you are looking for a physician, you may want to check with friends and neighbors in the area to see if they have recommendations. If you are moving, your current doctor may be able to help with a referral. In any case, it is a good idea to check with the local County Medical Society to make certain that whichever doctor you choose is licensed and reputable. You should know, however, that county medical societies have little control over who practices in an area, although they do control who joins their society and who they recommend.

The first step in getting acquainted with a new doctor is to call his office and see what sort of staff and assistants he has. Are they helpful to *you?* Can the doctor take new patients? Then, when the opportunity arises, get in to see the doctor about something relatively minor. Be sure that he really listens to you, and that he cares about you. You have to feel that he is honest with you. And you have to feel that he is worth what he charges.

Time for the doctor and patient to spend together is vitally important. If a doctor is so busy that he doesn't have the time to try to know you, then you may want to change. In order to avoid future problems, there should be time to discuss them now. The best way to insure time for talk is to schedule each child for a complete initial history and physical, for annual checkups, and for consultations if necessary.

Value the doctor who suits you. Schedule complete history and physical examinations and get all the past medical records sent to the office. Open up and tell him of your problems and worries. Try to learn a little about him. Don't be hurt if he may not always remember your name. That is a knack that many people, including me, lack. Settle for the fact that he recognizes you in the office and knows your voice on the phone. Talk to his office nurse and receptionists; they can often help. Remember that primary physicians are personal physicians. They are usually at least as interested in people as in disease. Don't call him for frivolous things; but be certain to *insist* on talking to him personally if you really believe the problem is important.

Referrals to Specialists

If you need special help, let your personal primary physician lead you through the maze of specialists and institutions, and through the multitude of tests and procedures that will lead to the best result possible for your condition. This will save money, worry, disappointment, and suffering. It will reduce duplication of work and tests and increase the efficiency and ease with which you are treated. Insist that all specialists you see report back to your doctor, because someone has to keep *all* the pieces together.

Make certain that your primary physician is always available or always has a ready substitute when he is away. Avoid going to the hospital emergency rooms for treatment, and if you do, call your doctor first. Emergency room care requires much waiting and is more expensive then office care. If you do go to an emergency room, or if you see a strange doctor, request that the record be sent to *your* doctor. Ask your doctor how he wants you to proceed in case of emergency or night calls, and what hospital he uses. Find out who covers for him when he is on vacation, out of town, or off call.

If You Aren't Satisfied

If you aren't satisfied with the treatment you are getting from your physician, tell him! Ask for a referral. Let him know how you feel, what you want! You may be comforted in making your choices by the words of an experienced small town New England pediatrician, Dr. Merritt Low, a past president of the American Academy of Pediatrics, who offers sage advice about "doctoring."

There are 1,001 kinds of doctors and more kinds of people. Neither doctors themselves nor patients should look upon a physician as a god. People are human, and doctors are people. In these busy and frantic times, communicating, and understanding values and agreements are necessary. Usually this is achieved—wonder of wonders! This is because parents, by and large, are conscientious and flexible, and so are doctors. But if these things do not work out to everyone's satisfaction, a time for a change should be foreseen, discussed as openly as possible, and settled as amicably as possible —ahead of a crisis time.

Many physicians tend to cling to their patients, just as patients cling to them. Both sides should have choices. The patient is usually put in the position of having to make the choice, that is, the doctor will not precipitate a change, though his manner may almost force it. Perhaps under certain conditions—when he sees things are not going well—he should. Danger signs are: The patient is truly afraid to call the doctor (this can be dressed up and rationalized in various ways, like "I hate to bother you, but," "He's too busy for me," etc.); the doctor feels undue irritation when certain persons call; the patient cannot really air his problems but must "play games"; the doctor gives a patient the real brush-off or makes fun of him or takes away a child's or other person's dignity; there are certain little habits or mannerisms that are mutually aggravating; there are basic philosophic or intellectual differences or

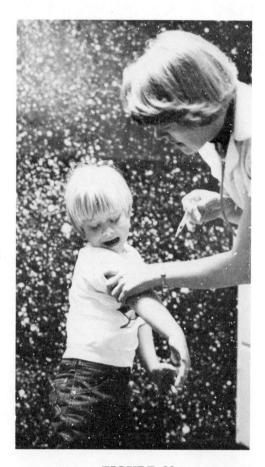

FIGURE 29

lack of feelings of trust in personality or knowledge, with an inability to adjust to them.

Complete agreement (usually on the doctor's terms!?) is neither necessary nor wise in the handling of problems. Open discussion *is* both necessary and wise. "Blow-ups" can be salutary and helpful in the long run, if we bear in mind they must not be deep, lasting, or severe —just as confrontations within a family can often have positive healthful results. Mutual empathy is a cornerstone of a good relationship. Often a doctor has an overriding concern for a particularly sick patient which may make others' complaints at the moment seem trivial. Good physicians can cope with this; good patients sense it or take no offense if it is voiced. Plain fatigue can also affect a doctor's personality temporarily (like a mother's!).

An unfortunate thing about "blow-ups" is that they are apt to occur at times of crisis, but good relationships shine at such times also. In conclusion, therefore, I speak for a preventive approach in patient–doctor relationships—prophylaxis, anticipatory examination, settling things at times when everyone is relatively calm and collected and when a serious problem is not of overriding, coloring concern. Every good doctor and every good patient should think these matters over. Though they should not always agree (life would be indeed dull if they did), they at least should feel comfortable, secure, mutually respectful, and empathetic. There may be 100,001 ways. The basic one is to talk things over, directly—this helps all present and future relationships. Personality conflicts must not be allowed to generate guilt and anxiety.

Health Supervision

When you get a doctor, and especially when you get a doctor for your child or teenager, then you must all get to know each other. One of the most efficient and economical ways is to have periodic health supervision examinations. These used to be called "well baby" or "well child" examinations. Those of us who do such examinations, and those of you who obtain them, know that wellness is a relative term. Many pediatricians find some sort of problem in 50 to 80 percent of periodic health supervision check ups. Parents learn to save minor problems for such thorough examinations, and doctors take the time to really look over the whole child, not just the throat or feet or whatever. Dr. David Sparling outlines guidelines for the frequency and content of health supervision examinations. How often should health supervision examinations occur?

Child's Age	Frequency of Exam
0 to 6 months	Every four to six weeks
6 months to 1 year	Every two to three months
1 to 2 years	Every three to six months
2 years to school age	One exam per year
During school years	Every one to three years

What Should You Expect in a Health Supervision Examination?

1. A discussion with the pediatrician about your child's physical and mental problems.
2. A complete physical examination.
3. Periodic checks of hearing, speech, and eyesight.
4. Periodic blood count, blood pressure, urine, and tuberculin skin tests.
5. Immunizations against contagious diseases, and booster shots when needed.
6. A discussion of the physician's findings, his comments about the child's developmental progress, and his recommendations for maintenance of health until the next examination.
7. Written instructions regarding any special health problems.
8. Pertinent pamphlet materials for home reading.
9. Updating of your child's office medical records.

Why Should Health Supervision Examinations Be Done?

1. Health supervision coordinates your medical care and increases its efficiency, economy, and results.
2. Health supervision allows the doctor and patient to get to know each other better, increasing mutual respect and appreciation.
3. By increasing the knowledge and improving the attitudes of those who deal with a child, health supervision may encourage the child's total character development in many ways including the emotional, intellectual, and social spheres.
4. Health supervision allows early discovery of minor problems that don't bother anyone very much which may become significant if allowed to progress. Examples include:
   a. Early diagnosis and treatment of hypothyroidism, which, in infants, may save them from becoming retarded.
   b. Finding a smoldering bladder infection which causes no symptoms but which may lead to future kidney and high blood pressure problems.
   c. Correction of dietary errors, such as hidden milk allergy, which may cause sluggishness and irritability.
   d. Early diagnosis of bone problems in the feet, legs, and hips—with exercises to prevent the need for later surgery.
   e. Early suspicion and investigation of learning or emotional problems which can lead to school failure and family tensions.
5. Health supervision includes the prevention of:
   a. Infectious diseases (e.g., tetanus), through immunization (See Table 10).
   b. Accidents, by early education and precautions.
   c. Dental cavities, by early prescriptions of fluoride.
   d. Emotional problems and family tension, by educating the parents about stages of growth and about possible problems which may occur with growing children and with parental attitudes.

Do You Avoid Doctors?

In spite of all of the good reasons to seek regular health supervision, many people avoid it for themselves and for their children. Some simply

TABLE 10   *One recommended schedule for immunizations.*

2 months	D.P.T., Polio
3 months	D.P.T.
4 months	D.P.T., Polio
12 months	Tuberculin test
15 months	Measles
1½ years	D.P.T., Polio, Mumps, Rubella (see Chapter 15)
4–6 years	D.P.T., Polio, Tuberculin test
14–16 years	D.T., Polio, Tuberculin test
Every 10 years	Tetanus and Tuberculin

haven't realized what it is or haven't seen any of its advantages and results. Others say they cannot afford it, even though the cost is small and the returns great. Usually, however, there is a deeper underlying emotional reason for avoiding doctors. Some people have great faith in their health or in the health of their children. Some avoid it because they may be ill, and if this is discovered, it will have to be faced. Others fear that something may be wrong and are afraid to find the truth. Some parents have fears so great that they have difficulty talking about them or even thinking about them: "Does my child have leukemia?" "Is my child doing poorly in school because I had venereal disease?"

Some people handle such fears by denying them. Others suppress the open fear and rush to the doctor with minor complaints, unable to voice their real concern. These anxieties should be relieved, because at least half of all human illness is probably based on anxiety and chronic stress. We create, through our emotions, many of our own headaches, ulcers, heart attacks, arthritis, and colitis. Anxiety and anger, hidden or open, are abrasive to our bodies as well as to our souls.

Faith

There are many people who have found that, through faith, they can reduce their anxieties—and therefore are not as ill. Others who are ill, but who are at peace with themselves because of their faith, seem to suffer far less from their illness. The value of faith is unchallengeable. Faith in family, science, doctors, religion, or self—it is an effective gift to health. However, faith should not blind us to the human qualities of intelligence and to the practical abilities of doctors to help. Nor should people be so desperate for faith that they invest their doctor with powers far beyond what he has. Of course doctors don't scorn, and do use, the therapeutic value of faith. The problem is that some people attach to whatever fad or charlatan catches their fancy. This is self-deception, even if it is faith. It may protect against the inner trauma of psychosomatic stress, but it will not protect against the law of gravity, the measles virus, or the tuberculosis bacteria.

HOW TO GET THE MOST OUT OF
YOUR DOCTOR BY TELEPHONE

Before you call the doctor, what should you do, what should you know, and what is the best way to make certain you get the most out of your call? Your doctor may be able to avoid having you come in for an office visit, may be able to treat some conditions over the phone, and will have far better grounds for decisions he must make on whether or not you must be seen if you have your story clearly summarized. This, of course, assumes that he knows you well enough to assess your complaint accurately. If he doesn't know you, he may have to see you anyway.

To decide when you should or shouldn't call the doctor can be difficult. You can learn many key reasons why you should call as you read *The Parents' Medical Manual.* You learn others from your doctor and through experience. No list we can offer will replace your good judgment. And no list we can offer will replace your consideration for your doctors.

Most doctors would rather be called early in the day than late at night. It isn't just that late calls interrupt rest—there are the problems of no help in the office, of the drug stores being closed, and of the increased cost of night visits. Children don't get sick only at night, but it is often at night that the parents finally get around to checking a child. With many infections, fever is usually low or absent in the morning and goes higher in the evenings. It is rarely reasonable to call in the evening or night for an illness that has persisted unchanged for several days.

It is certainly unreasonable to call in the evening or night for routine type questions about feeding, vitamins, or immunizations. Regardless, it is reasonable to call at any time if a child is exceptionally sick, if he has problems breathing or urinating, or if he looks shocky (pale, cold, sweaty, rapid pulse). Some patients complain that there should be some good old-fashioned doctors around who will pay more attention to midnight telephone calls. An "old-fashioned" doctor himself, Merritt Low replies:

> There may not be any "good old-fashioned doctors" left, but there aren't many "good old-fashioned patients" around either. Life has become too complicated. To uncomplicate it, it helps to communicate with meaningful and mutually understood words in a pleasant manner.

Dr. Low suggests some basic principles for using the telephone. The telephone is many things to many people.

Before You Call the Doctor

1. Have a pencil and paper by the telephone.
2. Have the telephone number of your drug store by the telephone, and, if possible, know if the drugstore is open and if you wish delivery service.
3. Avoid meaningless phrases such as: "awful sick," or "burning up"; "very bad runs," or "a pink liquid that Doctor X gave me. . . ." Instead, use words

with more meaning: "Temperature of 102 degrees by rectum"; "he can't even sit up"; "he won't even watch his favorite television show"; "ten large watery green mucus-containing stools in the last six hours."

4. Have clearly in mind all information you can obtain. If it helps you, jot down an outline of the points you wish to make. Use the outline below on how to describe problems over the telephone to help you determine what information is needed.

5. Summarize the major problem:
   a. The main reason you are calling: for example, injury, earache, cough, stomachache, rash, and so forth.
   b. In your opinion, how *sick* is the child?
   c. Why are you calling at this time?
   d. When did the illness or injury start and how many hours or days has he been sick?

How to Describe Problems Over the Telephone

For respiratory illnesses, have the following information:

A. What is the major problem: cough, sore throat, earache, headache, swollen glands, stuffy nose?

B. Other symptoms of the illness, such as: stomachache, nausea, diarrhea, skin rash, muscle aches, pains.

C. Before you call, check the following:
   1. Take the temperature with a thermometer.
   2. Smell around the mouth, nose, and ears for foul odor.
   3. Look at his mouth with a good light over your shoulder.
      a. Are there sores, ulcers, or red spots on his tongue, gums, cheeks, or palate?
      b. Are the tonsils big or red; do they have grey, white, or yellow pus spots? With a good light over your shoulder, have him look up at you, open his mouth wide, and yawn.
   4. Feel gently under the ears and jaws and the back of the neck and head for swollen or tender lymph glands. Have him look at the ceiling, and you can usually see the swollen "tonsillar" lymph glands on each side and a little above the "Adam's apple."
   5. Have the child curl up and kiss his knee. If he can do this, the neck is not stiff.
   6. Watch him breathe without clothing covering the chest.
      a. Does he sink in between the ribs with each breath?
      b. Count the respiratory rate.
   7. Note the type of cough: hoarse or barky? Loose (do you hear mucus rattling) or dry? Throat clearing or hacky? Constant, every few minutes, steadily, or occasional spasms?
   8. Look at the skin for rash.

For stomach and intestinal upsets, have the following information:

A. The primary problem: vomiting, pain, diarrhea, lack of appetite, or nausea.

B. Was he exposed to an illness or has he had an injury?

C. Other symptoms, including:
   1. Are there respiratory symptoms?
   2. How long ago (days, hours) did the illness start?
   3. How much and what kind of liquid has he kept down over the past twenty-four hours?
   4. How often and how many times has he vomited? Is it only with a cough?
   5. When did he urinate last?
   6. When was the last bowel movement? How many stools in the last twenty-four hours, and what color and amount?
   7. Does it hurt the child to walk? Where? Does he walk bent over as if it hurts him to straighten up?
   8. Was he hit in the abdomen recently?
   9. Does it hurt when he urinates? Does he urinate more frequently than usual?
   10. Is there pain in the back, groin, testicles, or penis?
D. Before you call:
   1. Check the temperature, rectally or orally.
   2. See how sick he looks.
   3. Is his mouth dry?
   4. Is his stomach noisy (put your ear on it) ?
   5. Does it hurt when you press the flat of your hand on the stomach? Any special area?
   6. Are there any bruises on the abdomen?

For small infants, have the following information:

A. What is the primary problem: vomiting, crying, lethargy or dopiness, refusal to eat, diarrhea.
B. Know the following general information:
   1. How old is the baby?
   2. What is the weight?
   3. Breast or type of formula?
   4. Is he eating well?
   5. Did the problem start after a new food?
   6. Has he been exposed to any colds, intestinal infections, or viruses?
   7. Is the baby happy, fussy, or quiet?
   8. Does he seem to be in pain?
   9. Is there a change in the type of bowel movements?
C. What other symptoms and signs are there?
   1. Does the baby cry when urinating?
   2. Does he vomit? How far does the vomitus shoot out?
   3. Does he pull at an ear?
   4. Is it hard to breathe through the nose?
   5. Is there a wheeze or chest rattle?
D. Before you call:
   1. Listen to the stomach; is it noisy?
   2. Press the stomach around the belly button; does it seem to hurt?
   3. Count the respiratory rate (see page 93) .

For possible poison ingestion, have the following information:

A. If it is a cleaning agent—Drāno, lye and so forth—first give a glass of milk, soup, or at least water *immediately* (see page 26) .
B. For most other things, give two tablespoons (or six teaspoons) of syrup of ipecac at once. If you are not certain, wait till you have talked to your doctor. If your doctor is not immediately available, call the poison control center or the emergency ward at the hospital.
C. Tell the doctor:
   1. How long ago did the child take the possible poison?
   2. How much did he take (count or estimate the number of pills or quantity of liquid in teaspoons) ?
   3. What is the product? Have the label handy to read the ingredients.
   4. Any symptoms yet?

HOSPITALIZATION, DOCTORS, AND KIDS

Should you force your child to go to the doctor? Should you stay with him in the hospital? How do you help your child handle fear? These questions are often a real bother to parents. As a start, you have to get your child to the doctor. Family practitioner Raymond Kahn counsels:

You do what you know is in the child's best interest. When the preschooler is brought to the physician's office for an examination and shot, neither the parent or doctor inquires, 'Do you want your shot?' We know the answer well before hearing the frenzied cry of 'No-o-o.' Parents should make every attempt to explain to the child, calmly, the necessity for medical treatment and 'shots,' the fear inspiring element of medicine. Regardless of his response, the treatment, of course, must go on.

Should You Stay With Your Child in the Hospital?

Not too long ago, parents were not allowed to stay long in the hospital with their children. Rules with very limited visiting hours are still prevalent in many areas. On the other hand, there has been a movement to have parents stay with their children during the entire hospitalization. Some pediatricians believe that if it is a toddler who isn't seriously ill, then mother need only stay for the first day or two. They advise, "The child doesn't need her around. If the child is very sick, it is best for the parents not to stay. The mother who wants to stay all the time is more attached to the child than the child is to her."

This angers many parents. One mother reviewing this chapter said:

As a parent, I resent being shunted aside. We can help our children in the hospital in many ways: bathing, feeding, diapering, walking, reading to sleep, recording food and fluid intake, helping with physical therapy, answering questions, bringing allowed snacks from the kitchen, helping the child to the bathroom and recording the results or even collecting the urine or stool if required. A parent may stay with the child for neurotic reasons, but there can also be excellent reasons. There may not be enough nursing help, and overworked nurses can be short-tempered with children. In some cases, a parent may be able to get a child to take a medicine when the nurse has trouble. Sometimes doctors don't know what goes on in these rooms all day!

My opinion about parents staying with the child have changed. In my residency training, we found that the children generally did very well and we were able to get work done more efficiently and were often able to get along with the children better if the parents were not there. Personally, I have not seen significant lasting emotional trauma from the parents leaving a child in the hospital. Some experts, however, claim it is the parents' "duty" to stay with the child, and that the child will feel abandoned if you don't. That I believe, is an oversimplification. It depends on whether or not you can be of real help to the child. *My best advice is to try it and see.* Parents are not all the same. An apprehensive parent who communicates fear to the child may make a bad situation worse. Anyway, children *may* get the idea that things must be really bad if a parent stays in the same room with them twenty-four hours a day since this ordinarily never happens. I have seen parents who were close to exhaustion, a bundle of nerves with a bladder about to burst! There is no justification for a parent physically and emotionally running himself down by sleepless anxiety in an uncomfortable cot. One of the things a child needs the most is a healthy happy parent. Several days at the bedside achieves neither of these.

The worst thing you can do for your child is stay in the room while someone "tortures him" and scares him, while he cries his heart out for you to make them stop. And you don't make them stop, because what they do is essential for your child's recovery. If you leave while the doctor, nurse, and technician do their work, it represents a display of trust the child will not miss. It also is likely that the child will not cry as much or hurt as much, for your presence in the room may exaggerate his problem. Furthermore, it allows the professionals to relate directly with the child, who isn't so busy trying to escape to mother. More often than not, their words and attitude make the procedure far less traumatic and result in the child's trust. With you in the room they have less of a chance.

I had an amusing and instructive experience which shows how a child can think about hospital trauma. He was a three-year-old boy who had diarrhea with dehydration, and he required intravenous feedings. The parents were panicky and refused to leave. So the child continued to struggle and thrash, crying, "Mommy, Mommy, Mommy," while I tried to get the needle into the jumping arm. It was difficult. The child switched his crying, but not his struggling, to "Daddy, Daddy, Daddy." Dad did nothing more than Mom; both were crying and telling the boy how sorry they were. So was I, but it did no good to say so. After a minute or so more of wriggling and screaming "Daddy," making the insertion of the needle almost impossible, the little guy suddenly stopped quite still for a short pause, and then in a quiet but intense voice demanded, "Somebody call the cops!" After a good laugh, I was able to get the needle in, but it could have been quicker and easier on the child *and* me had the parents stayed out of the room. On the other hand, some hospital pediatric wards have completely open visiting hours, and even allow other children to visit. Parents can be very helpful. I have often asked parents to stay with the child to make certain that enough fluids were offered, to help watch the breathing, or to help feed. This may be especially helpful when the nursing staff is overworked.

PART TWO

ILLNESS: THE LOCATION

There are many ways of looking at illness; the first one is usually the location. Whatever the symptom, it usually is located somewhere—an ache in the head, a pain in a joint, or itchy skin. As we have seen, location alone is not an adequate way to understand disease, but it certainly helps. Even though there are probably hundreds of causes of sore throat, it helps to know that sore throats usually involve the tonsils and adenoids. You should appreciate that the openings to the middle ears are located next to the adenoids so that such an infection can easily spread to the middle ear. And infections that involve the throat and the nose may easily spread into the sinuses. In this section, we discuss some common diseases in each area of the body. We concentrate on those we believe you should know about because you may be able to prevent a problem or treat it at home. Knowledge is also included about some diseases you can do little about; understanding, here, may either alert you to the necessity for treatment by your doctor or relieve your mind from unnecessary concern. After you have looked up the disease by location, you may then want to check the next part, on causes of disease, in order to improve your understanding and your abilities to help yourself and your family avoid or minimize the effects of illness.

5

THE HEAD

HEADACHES

When a child complains of headache, it is often associated with the onset of fever or infection. Headaches that appear as an isolated symptom and recur over a period of several days or weeks can offer a real challenge to the physician. Even when it is certain that the headache is not due to a serious disease, the symptom can be a source of real distress to both the child and his parents.

Preschool children rarely complain of headaches, probably because they just don't know how to describe how they feel. As the pre-teen years approach, headache becomes a relatively common complaint, often due to fatigue and the increasing stress of "growing up." Although better able to describe where and how the head hurts, older children can be very vague in their description, while insistent that the headache is "really bad." In general, one can be relatively unconcerned about a headache that does not interfere with the child's play or prevent the teenager from taking part in activities that are interesting or fun. Also, a headache that is relieved quickly by a short period of rest or a single dose of aspirin is usually of little consequence, even when the complaint is mentioned by the child every few days. Sometimes headache is a symptom of serious disease, and for this reason parents should seek medical advice when simple measures fail to give relief or when headaches recur at frequent intervals.

Types of Headaches

Two of the more common headaches in children, writes pediatrician Jack G. Shiller, in his common sense book, *Childhood Illness,* are febrile headaches and muscle tension headaches.

Febrile Headaches

Toddlers are usually incapable of localizing pain to the head (except in the case of earache), but children four years old or older will often complain of headache during the course of a febrile illness. Frequently the headache will precede the onset of fever by a few hours. This headache is mild and disappears after the first dose of aspirin. It usually does not recur, even though the fever may wax and wane. No further treatment is necessary unless the headache persists, gets worse, or is associated with vomiting or unusual sleepiness. These symptoms require a call to the doctor.[1]

Muscle Tension Headaches

Muscle-spasm tension of the back of the head, neck, and shoulders sets up headache patterns after varying periods of time. The underlying reason for the headache may indeed be emotional, but the actual pain is caused by muscular tension. Children, like adults, get this kind of headache after exams or any kind of concentrated activity, in school or out, at any time of day or night. Any unpleasurable situation can make children and the muscles tense, and can therefore set up a headache.

These headaches may be frequent or recurrent, usually depending on what's really causing them. It is obvious that if a child is unhappy about something on a long-term basis (for example, a teacher–student problem), this may be the basis for recurrent tension headaches.

Tension headaches respond to aspirin and rest. Your child should have his full dosage of aspirin. Don't give a smaller dose for a small headache. The full dose will give him faster and better relief, thus cutting down on the necessity for repetitive doses. Encourage him to lie down for a while. Read him a story. But don't let him watch television—the eyes have to work too hard.

What about prevention, especially in the recurrent cases? Is there a problem at school? Perhaps on the school bus? Is there a neighborhood bully? Too many extracurricular activities? You can't take the child's word for this. I've known kids involved in scouting, music lessons, swimming at the Y, religious instruction, varsity sports or intramurals, getting straight A's, and having headaches! Yet they don't want to give anything up. In this situation, you have to be firm.

The more specifically emotional causes of headache may be harder to spot. Many problems upset children, and anything that upsets them can cause headaches. If your child's mood, behavior, and enjoyment of activities are frequently impaired because of headaches, then it's time to seek the doctor's help. He will try to rule out some of the other causes of headaches but he will first want to know if there are any emotional situations that may be contributing to the problem. Go through the mental gymnastics beforehand and try to figure out what's bugging the child. Your responses will be more thoroughly thought out, and the doctor will have a better chance of accurately assessing what's behind the headache.[2]

Dr. Merritt Low adds a pearl about headaches in pre-adolescents and adolescents: "These are not infrequently due to masked depression. Don't expect the child to tell you 'what's bothering' him. It's not as simple as that, and he usually can't give an answer. And don't accuse him of 'faking.' He truly doesn't know."

Treatment for Tension Headaches

I have found that a good treatment for tension headaches is heat. Tense or tight muscles relax with a heating pad or hot water bottle on the back of the neck, the scalp, or the face. A hot shower frequently cures a tension headache. Massage is also helpful. Use the tips of the fingers to move—deeply—the muscles of the shoulders, the back of the neck, and the scalp itself. If your child (or you) complains that the scalp is sore to touch, you can be certain that you are on the right track—just rub and massage more gently. A mechanical vibrator is a good substitute.

Some children will visibly relax after eating, and their headaches will vanish. Eating should be a relaxing experience anyway, a signal that the trials and tribulations of the day have ceased, at least for a while. Children whose headaches are caused by low blood sugar will find relief from the increase in blood sugar. Sleep cures most tension headaches. If it doesn't, you should suspect that the headache might be due to other causes and check with your physician.

Recurrent Headaches

Recurrent headaches in children are not uncommon. A Canadian study revealed that five percent of children between ten and twelve years of age had migraine, and that thirteen percent more had frequent headaches of other types: One school age child in five has frequent recurring headaches.

Sinus Headaches

A true sinus headache comes from a vacuum, infection, or pressure in the sinuses. Sinuses don't exist at birth and are very small in infants. They gradually grow as the baby grows, but they cannot be seen by x-ray until age three. There are several pairs of sinuses, all with small openings into the nasal cavity. They are lined with the same type of mucosal surface as the rest of the nose and throat. Irritation and swelling of this mucosa may plug the openings, as will swollen adenoidal tissue or swollen nasal turbinates. (The turbinates are spongy masses of blood vessel tissue which warm the breathed-in air and trap dust, germs, and smog in their mucus coat.) This spongy tissue will swell with irritation from smog, infection, allergy, nervous tension, and, in some people, even from cold air. Infection in the turbinates can cause headaches, whether the sinuses are plugged or not.

Many people feel that a headache with a stuffy nose is a "sinus headache," but true sinus headaches aren't common. Headaches and stuffy nose can occur with virus infections or even with tension. True sinus headaches result from a plugging of the sinus openings. The air in the sinus is absorbed by the mucosal lining, resulting in a vacuum. This hurts. The membranes excrete mucus and serum, and the sinus fills. Then germs grow in the mucus and create pressure. This hurts.

Preventing and Treating Sinus Headaches

There are several techniques which help to open blocked sinus openings. The first is to sleep propped up, with the head of the bed elevated by blocks, or with a wedge between the mattress and box springs. This allows the sinuses to drain better during the night. It also reduces the shift in body fluids from the feet, which are swollen during the day. That fluid moves to the head when you are flat. Another help in preventing sinusitis is the use of a humidifier at night to keep the mucus thin and the membranes damp and healthy. Reducing dust and other allergens in the bedroom reduces another source of sinus blockage.

Once the sinuses are blocked, it may help to use antihistamines, decongestants, or nose drops. To open all the sinuses with drops requires special positioning when you use the drops (see page 159). Once the membranes are washed off and the swelling reduced, the normal outlets open. If there is a vacuum present, air rushes in, causing temporary pain. If there is mucus, it usually drains down the back of the throat and into the stomach, where it does no harm.

Migraine Headache

Migraines occur in children as well as adults. They are vascular headaches caused by spasm or dilation of the arteries in the brain. Pain starts when the muscles in the arteries constrict, depriving that portion of the blood vessels and the brain beyond the point of constriction of blood and oxygen. In the early stage of migraines, there may be disturbances in vision, numbness, or vomiting because of the lack of oxygen to certain parts of the brain. Finally, the muscles in the arteries, like all muscles, tire. When they relax completely, they cause the artery to dilate and swell, and that causes even more pain.

The muscles of the arteries are controlled by nerves. Nervous tension may be the cause of many migraines. Yet these headaches frequently come on when there should be no tension. In some individuals, allergy may be the cause. In any case, the pain is intense, often one-sided, and causes nausea. Usually, this type of headache is unaffected by aspirin. Many people with vascular headaches have attacks repeatedly, and should beware of addiction to strong pain killers such as codeine or demerol.

Treatment of Migraine Headaches

Sometimes, relief from migraines can be obtained from head massage or heat, which may relax the spasm of the vessels as well as the neck muscles. Conversely, cold may give relief by constricting dilated vessels. A heating pad or hot shower, followed with a cold rag or a cold shower on the back of the neck and head, may help. Your doctor can help you with good prescription medications. Research by electronic bio-feedback points to self-control of the blood vessel spasm as a method of preventing headaches. Many people with migraines have discovered for themselves that they can control some of their headaches by a change in attitude toward life and toward themselves.

Critical Headaches

All headaches are significant to those who have them, but some are of far more importance than others. Luckily, critical headaches are very rare. The following symptoms may help you to decide which headaches might be critical.

- Stiff neck: If a person with a headache has a stiff neck, it may indicate infection or irritation of the membrane covering the brain. This is not the type of stiff neck that hurts to move from side to side; it is a neck that hurts when the head is flexed upon the chest. However, if a child can either curl up and touch his forehead to his knees, or, with the mouth closed, touch the chin to the chest, then the neck is not stiff. The ability to do either of these procedures makes it very unlikely that there is a meningitis.
- Swollen face or legs or red, tea, or coffee colored urine: Headaches from high blood pressure in children is most often associated with kidney problems, such as nephritis.
- Headaches on awakening in the morning: Waking up with a headache that goes away when you are up and about is most often due to sinus blockage or allergy. Continual morning headache, however, can possibly be due to a brain tumor or a swelling of the brain. In any case, a visit to the physician is indicated.
- Persistent vomiting: This may be the result of a concussion from a blow on the head, a brain tumor, or swelling of the brain due to an infection. However, most episodes of headache with vomiting, especially with fever, are due to a flu-like viral infection with an upset stomach that passes in from a few hours to a day or so. Be sure to check for a stiff neck as described above.
- Concussion: Headache after being hit on the head is reasonable to expect, and if there is only a headache, it usually goes away overnight. However, if there is vomiting more than twice, and especially if there is marked sleepiness, unsteadiness of gait, unequal pupils, peculiar eye movements, amnesia, or disorientation, you should talk with the doctor.

Headaches in children due to serious diseases are unusual. These usually require extensive evaluation and diagnostic tests by a physician. They are mentioned here so that you will remain alert to the possibility that headache can be a sign of a serious disease.

Other Headaches

Other causes of headache, says Dr. Shiller in his book are:

- Ear Pain: Most children can identify localized ear pain. However, the younger the child and the *less* acute the problem, the more likely he is to respond with irritability and/or headache, rather than with a specific ear complaint.
- A Tooth: Most people who experience tooth pain, either from spontaneous toothache or from a rough experience in the dentist's office, get a headache. But a child with a mild toothache frequently complains about a headache first. Sometimes this starts as face pain, or jaw pain, usually one-sided, which may then spread to the whole side of the head. Obviously, fix the cause and you fix the headache.
- Eye Strain: Eye strain may cause headache. Farsightedness and astigmatism

are the most common causes, with nearsightedness and muscle balance problems running a close second.[3]

Eye specialist Dr. Frank Berry assures us, however, that only a small percentage of headaches are caused by eyestrain or poor vision, or are corrected by glasses.

Allergic Headache
Dr. William G. Crook believes that

Many children's headaches are caused by allergy. Allergens, especially foods, rather than producing a rash or causing sneezing or wheezing, may cause an allergic reaction inside the head. As part of this reaction, spasm and other changes take place in some of the blood vessels; extra fluid may leak out, and the brain may swell—all leading to pain and throbbing.

However, Dr. Merritt Low comments: "Some people are allergic to people, including themselves, and get headaches."

When Should You See The Doctor?
Pediatrician Sid Rosin advises:

Any child's headache deserves at least a telephone check with his physician. If a headache lasts, recurs, doesn't respond to aspirin and rest, or is chronic, see a physician to rule out serious disease. Most headaches in children, however, come from two sources: infection and the people around them.

6

THE EYES
AND VISION

The eye is a marvel of mechanical, optical, and biological engineering. Usually, its recording of the outside world is accurate but not always. There are significant signs to be looked for to detect visual problems, and steps to be taken to preserve and improve vision. Where possible, we emphasize those things you can do at home.

THE ANATOMY AND FUNCTION OF THE EYE

1. At the base of the eyelashes, along the edge of the eyelids, there are a series of small oil glands. These may become infected in various ways from mites to small abscesses which lead to sties.
2. Most foreign bodies lodge underneath the upper eyelid, which has a hard piece of cartilage in it called the *tarsal plate.*
3. The best protection for the eyes is nature's method—blinking.
4. Tears are constantly formed in order to keep the eye moist. These are removed to the back of the nose through the lachrymal ducts, which have small openings on the inner edges of the eyelids.
5. The sclera or white of the eye is the tough outer covering that encloses the entire eyeball except the cornea.
6. The cornea is the window-clear curved membrane that overlies the colored portion of the eye, the doughnut shaped iris, which expands or contracts to control the amount of light admitted through the pupil, which is the hole in the doughnut that contains the lens.
7. This lens is flexible and changes shape so we may focus on near or distant objects.
8. The chamber between the cornea and the lens and iris is filled with a crystal clear fluid.

9. Behind the lens and iris, inside the eyeball, there is a clear heavy gelatin substance which fills the interior of the eyeball. Light rays are bent by the cornea and lens to focus and pass through this gelatin to the retina, the lining of the inside of the back of the eyeball.

10. The shape and length of the eyeball varies in different people and at different ages. It may be too short, causing farsightedness, or too long, causing nearsightedness.

11. The image hitting the retina is instantaneously transmitted by very complex nerve pathways to an even more complex visual area in the back of the brain which integrates and sorts out the images, transmitting information to the rest of the brain. In the immature brains of some children, these images are poorly handled, making reading quite difficult, a condition called dyslexia.

What Signals Visual Problems?

Only one child in four with faulty vision complains about it—they don't know that their blurred vision isn't normal. It is up to you to look for clues of faulty vision at home or at school, as well as to take your child to a doctor who periodically checks the vision, writes pediatrician Isaac Reid. The following signs should alert you:

- Abnormal watering
- Blurred or double vision
- Swollen or encrusted eyelids
- Tilting or thrusting head forward
- Squinting at distant objects
- Tripping over small objects
- Frequent appearance of styes
- Excessive blinking
- Frequent rubbing
- Inflamed red eyes
- Red-rimmed or chronically swollen eyelids
- Shutting one eye to read
- Excessive scowling or squinting while reading
- Crossed eyes
- Holding books and objects very close
- Pain in or around eyes
- Habitually avoiding close work
- Seeing halos or rainbow colors at night

Does Your Baby See?

Parents frequently ask, "When can my baby see?" This question bothers pediatrician David Sparling who complains that:

It is a pity that we have been told that babies don't see during their early months. There *are* babies who at first do nothing but eat and sleep. However, you have only to watch a more alert newborn to realize that from the beginning he stares at and studies everything in his environment. Vision is one of our most valuable resources, and is very important in the process of learning, even for the small infant.

Children born at term may start following large objects with their eyes at anywhere from two to six weeks of age. At first, they cannot follow up and down or side to side motion, past the midline. I recommend that a mobile be hung right over the baby's head; it is both pleasurable and stimulating for the infant.

By six weeks, the baby will study the motion of a speaker's lips and recognize mother by sight. Even before two months of age, a child may be attracted to certain colors and patterns or "turned off" by others.

Soon he will recognize a bottle, a spoon, his bathtub, and other objects in his environment. By four or five months, he will differentiate strangers from family and friends. During the first six months, an infant's eyes occasionally fail to focus together. Persistent crossing or turning-out of the eyes is abnormal. This or any other concerns regarding the development of vision deserves careful and prompt evaluation by the child's physician, who may then recommend an ophthalmologist (medical eye specialist).

What Is Lazy Eye?

In some children under age six, one eye, for a variety of reasons, is not being used to the fullest. This condition is called "lazy eye" or amblyopia. One common cause is crossed eyes. In this instance, the brain blocks out the image of one eye in order to prevent double vision, which is disabling to the child. The eye that is not used progressively loses more sight and may become blind.

Amblyopia is preventable, but must be treated as early as possible. Treatment involves patching the good eye for the proper length of time, forcing the brain to use the lazy eye. Parents should watch for a crossed eye; if noticed, the eyes should be checked by the doctor. Sometimes, eyes only cross when fatigued; if so, bring the child to the doctor late in the day. However, crossed eyes are not the only cause of amblyopia; so be certain that your young child has an eye examination on one of his checkups even if there is no crossing.

What Are "False" Crossed Eyes?

A misleading sign of crossing often occurs where the bridge of the infant's nose is broad, and the inner folds of the eyelids drop down sharply, cutting across the colored iris. These are not crossed eyes. Eyes will "cross" when you look at something really close. If they cross when looking at a distant object, it is very significant. Sometimes, eyes cross only when fatigued and are normal when examined by the physician.

Test Your Children's Eyes at Home

Home eye tests are especially valuable in the preschool years. They may enable you to pick up a lazy eye or other problems. Also, home eye

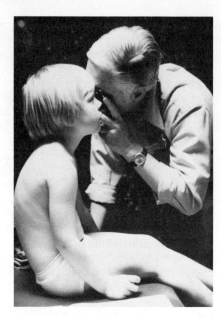

FIGURE 30   *Look for the reflection of a light in the pupils. If the reflection is in the same place in each pupil, the eyes are not crossed.*

tests train the child so that he may respond better to the doctor's examination. Unfortunately, few children are able to cooperate well enough for adequate eye testing before the age of three or four years. Observant parents, however, can detect poor vision in many ways just by being alert.

One early home test is to patch one eye and have a toddler pick up small objects such as candy parfait (cake decorating) beads. Note his accuracy in spotting the candies with each eye. Often it is reward enough to keep the child going if he is allowed to eat each one he picks up. A more sophisticated free home eye test kit for preschoolers is available from the National Society for the Prevention of Blindness, Inc. in both English and Spanish. A kit will be sent without charge in the United States. Write: Home Eye Test Program, 79 Madison Ave., New York, N.Y. 10016.

The "E" test, used to determine if the vision is the same in both eyes, can be done successfully at home with most three-year-olds. It helps if the parent has some patience and humor. Three-year-olds are motivated by instant reward, so make a fun "game" out of the test. Hang the "E" chart on the wall, and put easily recognized pictures on each side, above and below. Then you "point" the "E" to a picture of a rabbit or a car or a flower, and so forth. Vary the pattern you use so that the child will not memorize your route. Start with the largest "E" and work down to the smallest one he can see. Your aim is to know that he sees equally

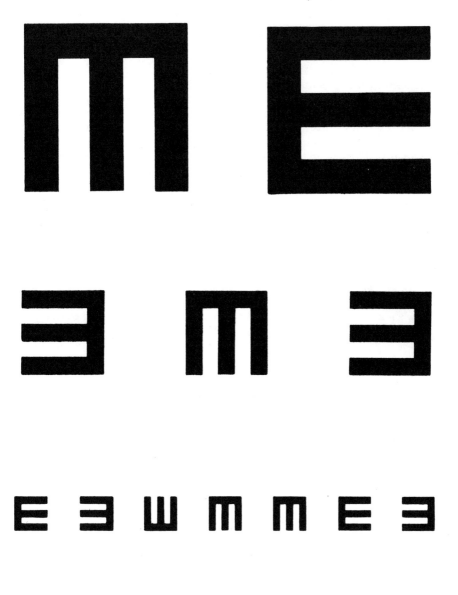

FIGURE 31   *E chart for home eye test.*

with each eye. So cover one eye while you test the other. Remember that in order to get a reward, a child with a bad eye may peek with his good eye. To prevent "cheating," hold a card over the eye across the bridge of the nose. Don't press the card against the covered eye, as this might blur the vision when it is uncovered.

If the child doesn't see equally well with each eye, the weak eye may get progressively weaker, leading to further visual loss. If you are unable to get reliable results, put the test away and repeat it in a month. (Don't forget to mark the date on the calendar.) Keep trying until you have a valid test. If there is a possibility that a lazy eye is present, check with your child's doctor for a referral to an ophthalmologist.

Many cases of amblyopia are treated by patching one eye or by glasses or eye exercises. If the cause is a crossed eye, surgical correction is sometimes needed—this is one reason we suggest an ophthalomologist for the initial evaluation. People occasionally become confused with the differences between ophthalomologists and optometrists. The Federal government has defined them as follows:

1. An *ophthalmologist* or *oculist* is a physician—an M.D.—who specializes in diagnosis and treatment of defects and diseases of the eye, performing surgery when necessary or prescribing other types of treatment, including glasses.
2. An *optometrist,* a licensed, nonmedical practitioner, measures refractive errors —that is, irregularities in the size or shape of the eyeball or surface of the cornea—and eye muscle disturbances. In this treatment, the optometrist uses glasses, prisms, and exercises only.
3. An *optician* grinds lenses, fits them into frames, and adjusts the frames to the wearer.

How Do You Protect Eyes?
An unfortunately large number of people are blind because of accidents. Much of this is preventable, contends pediatrician Sparling:

> Babies and small children should not be in a position where they can stare for long at the sun. Cover the eyes while children are sunbathing. They should never have sharp pointed pencils, toys, scissors, or knives. Older children must be taught always to point sharp objects away from their faces, and never to run with a sharp tool. Toys need to be checked periodically for safety. Teach your child never to rub his eyes with dirty hands. If he wears glasses and is in sports, consult your eye specialist about hardened or plastic lenses. Supervise the use of sharp tools, B-B guns, sling shots, bows and arrows, and fireworks. Do not look directly at eclipses of the sun.

Ophthalmologist Frank Berry agrees, pointing out that:

> At least half of all blindness is probably preventable. The most important signs are:
> 1. Persistent strabismus or crossing which might indicate a congenital cataract, congenital glaucoma, or a retinal tumor.

2. A white reflection in the pupil of the eye (like a cat's eye), in place of the usual black or red reflection, can indicate a tumor.
3. Extreme sensitivity to light or excessive tearing can indicate glaucoma.

    Other preventable causes of blindness include injuires, which are responsible for three percent of blindness. The use of safety glasses will reduce blindness from this cause. Diabetes is a major cause of blindness. Adequate dietary and insulin control may reduce this problem.

Other causes of visual loss, adds Dr. Lendon Smith, include some less common conditions:

1. Corneal inflammation from virus infection, congenital syphilis, or gonorrhea.
2. Cataracts, an opaque lens which blocks rather than transmits light, may be due to genetics, maternal rubella infection when the baby's eyes are forming, galactosuria (a genetic disorder of the blood sugar), hypocalcemia (low blood calcium), or injury to the lens.
3. Retinal inflammation or chorioretinitis, from infections such as tuberculosis, histoplasmosis, syphilis, and toxoplasmosis.
4. Optic nerve damage, or atrophy from glaucoma, encephalitis, optic neuritis, and degenerative diseases.
5. Night blindness due to inadequate vitamin A is rare nowadays.
6. Color blindness—usually red-green—occurs in five percent of males.

Tumors in the Eye

Martin H. Smith, M.D., says:

    There are several different types of tumors or cancers that may originate in other portions of the body and spread secondarily to the eye. However, the most important tumor, a retinoblastoma, begins in the eye. This cancer is often fatal. If the retinoblastoma is discovered *early* enough it can be treated surgically.

    This particular type of cancer may occur in several members of the same family, so it is particularly important for all members of the family to be closely followed for any evidence of the development of this type of growth. Even without such a family history, the possible occurrence of this type of cancer is one reason that your pediatrician will probably periodically examine your child with an instrument called the opththalmoscope. This enables him to see the interior of the eye, including the surface of the retina, so that evidence of the development of this type of growth or of other abnormality of the retina can be detected.

What Is Nearsightedness?

Nearsightedness, or simple myopia, explains Dr. Lendon Smith, is due to an eyeball growing slightly longer than it should.

Because of the extra length, the lens brings distant light rays to a focus at a point in front of the retina, rather than right on the retina. Near objects are very clear, even with a long eyeball, but distant objects are a fuzzy blur. Nearsightedness can be inherited. It may be responsible for poor classroom performance.

A more extreme form of myopia, also more rare, is that in which the eyeball is extra deep or long. The retina in these long eyeballs is so stretched out that it is more easily jarred loose or detached. People with severe myopia should avoid contact sports such as boxing, football, or high diving.

What Is Farsightedness?

Farsightedness, or hyperopia, is due to an inability of the cornea to bend nearby light rays sufficiently to focus the image on the retina because the eyeball is shorter or shallower than it should be. One can see better at a distance than near. A child may see the words on the blackboard, or on the eye chart at twenty feet, but have trouble reading the letters in his book. Fatigue, headache, and disinterest in reading may result. It could also be one cause of hyperactivity. This condition tends to improve with age, while myopia may get worse.

Farsightedness problems are rarer in children than in adults. Most children see close things very well; in fact, they tend to put their nose almost on top of what they are reading or watching. This usually does not mean poor vision.

Do You Have Astigmatism?

Astigmatism is a defect in the curvature of the cornea or lens. It may give you blurred or distorted vision. Your ophthalmologist, of course, is the one to test for this defect. Glasses may be in order to correct this defect.

Will It Harm Your Child's Eyes to Read Excessively?

No. Fatigue may create eyestrain or headaches, but, like fatigued muscles elsewhere, they recover. More pertinent is the question of the child's general inactivity. Excessive reading may preclude adequate exercise or may mean that the child is escaping from his world. He may need success and happiness in the real world rather than new glasses or the substitute of reading.

Types of Eye Irritation

If you have a rash that is similar to chicken pox on the face near the eye, and the eye becomes irritated, this may be caused by a Herpes infection which can cause serious visual loss. We discussed foreign bodies in the eye in chapter 2 under emergency care. Foreign bodies, minor cuts or scratches on the cornea, or sunburn of the cornea can be very painful; often the pain isn't too severe until the middle of the night. Other types of eye irritation are less threatening to the vision but nonetheless deserve treatment writes Dr. Lendon Smith:

1. *Gelatinous swelling of the white of the eye:* This allergic reaction to pollen is alarming but innocuous. It looks like gelatin has been stuck on the eye. The condition responds rapidly to cortisone eye drops, but recurs until the airborne irritant is removed. To help, get the animals outside if possible. You can't do much about the grass pollen until a good rainfall comes, but staying indoors as much as possible may help.

2. *Watery, clear, or milky fluid flowing from the eye, or excessive tearing:* Another allergic response, usually to "something in the air" —such as pollens in the spring. The lids are often swollen and itch. An antihistamine should control the allergy temporarily. The mucus in the tears is a good culture medium; if green or yellow matter appears, local antibiotic drops or ointment may be required. Check with your doctor.

3. *Pink eye:* Redness of the white of the eye, or pink eye. An inflamed eye, or eyes with pus, may be due to several types of bacterial infection. Many viral infections can cause pink eye, and there is less likelihood of pus. Redness can be due to sand or other foreign bodies in the eye.

4. *Crusty, red-edged eyelids:* These are a sign of seborrhea, a trait of excessive oil production which is inherited. Victims of this are usually blue-eyed blondes and have dandruff and adolescent acne. They do better if they limit the amount of dairy products and chocolate. [Dr. Richards (and probably Dr. Jacobs) questions this statement. I don't know. Some foods might affect a few sensitive individuals in this manner.] Cortisone and antibiotic ointments may have to be used for flare-ups.

5. *Red, tender swelling at the lid edge:* Usually, this is a sty. Although the eye may become swollen shut and be painful, it is safe to let it progress until the small boil bursts. Hot packs will help a little. Recurrences of sties are found in families with skin infections (boils, fingernail runarounds, impetigo, etc.). A whole family may have to be treated with an antibiotic that works against the staphylococcus. Some doctors will give a series of injections, hoping to improve the patient's immunity against this tough staph germ. Incidentally, eating chocolate may be enough to bring on a sty.

6. *Tender, swollen, red lids without itchiness:* This type of eyelid infection usually follows a cold or purulent drainage from the eyes or nose. The infection gets into the tissue around the eyes or into sinus tissue behind the bridge of the nose. This is serious and demands the doctor's attention and heavy antibiotic therapy.

Eye Infections

Pus in the eyes of newborns ordinarily doesn't indicate infection explains Lendon Smith:

Every new baby born in the hospital has had his eyes treated with a silver nitrate solution that is supposed to prevent *ophthalmia neonatorum,* a severe eye infection due to the gonorrhea germ. A few babies will develop irritation and a mucus discharge because of this chemical. This clears in a few days, and nothing need be done. Tears will wash it out in time. If a profuse yellow discharge appears, a conjunctivitis has developed. Your doctor should see this. He may want to take a culture to find out what germ is responsible. Antibiotics, taken locally or injected into the muscle, will usually clear this rapidly.

If a *purulent discharge* (green or yellow) develops in one or both eyes after a week or so, it suggests that the baby has a plugged tear duct—the tube that carries the tears from the inner corner of the lids down into the nasal cavity. Each newborn comes equipped with a thin membrane at the end of the duct, which usually breaks with the first tears. If it does not break, and tears do not drain, germs grow, and pus appears. The opththalmologist will probably pass a probe through the tube to open the duct. Generally, this will come up before the baby is eight months old. The trouble generally clears after this has been done. On rare occasions, the problem is more complicated, as there may be a bony or tissue obstruction which will need surgery.

Pus in the eye may frighten mother and child, because the lids are stuck shut after a night's sleep. A warm, wet wash cloth will soon unglue the lids, and an antibiotic ointment or drops can be placed in the pocket between the pulled-down lower lid and the eyeball. (Three people are needed to help hold the child.)

This conjunctivitis may result from one of many conditions: The germ causing it may be airborne; someone may have coughed near the child's eye; the child may have picked his nose and then touched his eye; he may have been swimming in a contaminated pool; and so forth. If the child also has a cold with purulent matter in the nose, the local eye antibiotics may have to be supplemented with oral antibiotics.

To treat an eye infection:

1. Hot compresses usually help, and are more effective if a dry towel is held over them in order to keep the heat in. Usually, the greater the amount of time the heat is applied, the better the results. Hot packs to treat eye infection are easy to prepare: Fold a clean, hot, wash cloth and wring it dry. Hold it on the eye with a dry towel over it for several minutes several times a day. Cold compresses may temporarily relieve the irritation and swelling.
2. Avoid rubbing.
3. If the infection, redness, and pain do not promptly subside, or if there is accompanying nausea or vomiting, glaucoma or iritis may be present. See your doctor at once.
4. If the eye infection is associated with other respiratory symptoms, especially hearing loss or earache, see the doctor.

DO THE EYES CAUSE DYSLEXIA?

Reading disability, or dyslexia, is unrelated to visual acuity of the eyes themselves. Occasionally early symptoms such as mirror writing, reversals in printing and right-left confusion are noted. The condition is usually found by the first grade teacher who tries to teach the child to read. As to the role of the eyes, ophthalmologist Frank Berry advises that the most important aspect of dyslexia is recognition of the problem by teachers and parents so educational help may be given. For a more in-depth discussion of dyslexia and other learning problems see Chapter 8 of our companion volume, *The Parents' Guide to Child Raising.*

SUMMARY: THE EYE

1. A painful eye should be seen by a physician.
2. Emergency treatment for chemical burns in the eye is flushing with water or milk.
3. A foreign body may be removed at home by everting the tarsal plate and brushing it with cotton, but often a doctor is required.
4. Burns in the eye may be relieved with cold compresses.
5. Double vision after an injury around the eye requires prompt attention.
6. Treat eye infections with hot compresses, avoiding rubbing, and be alert for signs of infection in the ears or nose. If response is not prompt, see your doctor at once.
7. There are many types of eye irritations:
   a. Allergic gelatinous swelling of the white of the eye.
   b. Watery or milky discharge from itchy eyes of hayfever.
   c. Pus-like green or yellow discharge of infection.
   d. Inflamed white of the eye or "pink eye" from many bacterial and viral infections, occasionally from a foreign body.
   e. Crusty red eyelids from oil gland irritation.
   f. Red swollen spots on the eyelid from abscesses.
   g. Tender red swollen eyelids from sinus infection.
8. Pus in a baby's eye is usually from the irritating silver nitrate put in the eye at birth. Pus in the eye of a newborn who did not get silver nitrate at birth may be due to gonorrhea and result in blindness.
9. Chronic tearing in a baby's eye is usually due to an obstructed tear duct.
10. Babies see earlier than most imagine, and should be given visual stimulation.
11. Children's eyes should be protected from sharp toys, dirty hands, B-B guns, sling shots, and so forth.
12. Lazy eye, or amblyopia, is a common preventable cause of blindness in one eye. Home eye testing should be started before the age of two, and crossing of the eyes should be reported early to prevent such visual loss.
13. False crossed eyes occur in infants when the bridge of the nose is broad.
14. Half of all blindness is preventable: Look for crossing of the eyes, a white reflection in the pupil, and excessive tearing.
15. Nearsightedness, farsightedness, and astigmatism tests can be done at home; but for definitive testing, an ophthalmologist is recommended.
16. It does not hurt the eyes to read excessively or to read with poor light, even though it may tire them.
17. Cancer of the eye can occur, and often there is a family history of such disease; health supervision checks frequently include ophthalmoscopic examinations of the inside of the eyes in order to pick up such tumors early.
18. Dyslexia has nothing to do with vision or with eye muscle balance.

7

EARS, NOSE,
AND THROAT

Each day we breathe over 2,000 gallons of air. The nose is the first to receive this onslaught of allergens, smog, dry air, or chemical irritants. The mouth and throat have the dubious distinction of being the first to experience bacterial, viral, and allergic attacks as well as chemical contents of our food and drink. All these factors make the ears, nose, and throat susceptible to a variety of problems and diseases. Fortunately, many of these can be prevented by sensible and simple precautions, and many existing conditions can be helped by the proper home treatment.

Figure 32 shows the anatomy and diseases of the ears, nose, and throat. The numbers 1 through 8 in the front of the figure refer to the anatomy, and the numbers 9 through 14 at the back of the figure refer to diseases, as follows: (1) Frontal and spenoid sinuses, air filled cavities in the bone lined with mucus membranes and having small openings into the nasal cavity. The ethmoid sinuses behind the eyes are too small to show. (2) The nasal turbinates, spongy masses of tissue on each side of the nasal cavity, partially visible through the nostrils. They lap over the openings of the maxillary sinuses in the cheekbones. They warm inspired air, excrete antibodies to fight germs and pollens, and trap inhaled dirt and germs. (3) The opening of the eustachian tubes which allows air to fill the middle ear behind the ear drum. (4) The adenoids are tonsillar tissue which can infect and swell, making breathing through the nose difficult: They can plug off the openings of the eustachian tubes. (5) The uvula, a finger of tissue that hangs from the soft palate in the back of the mouth. (6) The tonsils, on each side of the throat just behind the soft palate. They trap germs and start the process that causes white blood cells and antibodies to fight the germs. (7) The epiglottis, a stiff cartilage valve that covers the windpipe when you swallow so food and liquid will

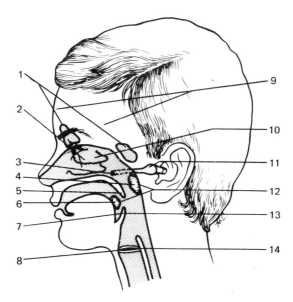

FIGURE 32 *Anatomy and diseases of ears, nose, and throat.*

not get into the lungs. (8) The vocal cords, paper thin membranes covered with mucus excreting cells that keep the cords moist in spite of the continual drying effect of breathed air. (9) Sinusitis from infected membranes or plugged off openings in the sinuses. May cause headache, swollen eyelids, aching cheeks, and fever. (10) Infected turbinates from colds or bacteria, or swollen weeping turbinates from hayfever or smog. The source of nasal discharge, stuffy nose, itching nose and sneezing. (11) The middle ear becomes full of mucus from a plugged eustachian tube causing hearing loss. Bacteria easily grow in mucus, causing infection (otitis media) and pressure on the ear drum which causes pain. (12) Tonsillitis infections usually also includes the adenoids. They may be red, they usually swell with infection (and can with allergy), and they may be covered with white blood cells (pus) fighting the germs. (13) Epiglotitis is an infection of the membrane covering the cartilage. It can cause swelling which, if severe, can interfere with breathing. (14) Infection of the vocal cords (laryngitis) can cause them to swell and go into spasm with hoarseness, a dry croupy cough, or trouble breathing air in, causing a croupy wheeze (stridor).

What If You Wake Up with a Dry Nose and Throat?

I believe that one reason for the increase in "colds" is the dry air in homes in the winter. Heating air dries it out, especially air recirculated through blower furnaces. The same problem undoubtedly existed with pot bellied stoves, but one of our forebearers handled it elegantly. Many Franklin stoves from the 1776 era had an iron basin fixed on the top of the stove for water to humidify the air. Our current heaters are not always that well thought out, but humidifiers which attach to furnaces are available.

In any case, the dry air dries out the nasal membranes, which are covered with a protective coating of moist mucus. This constantly replenished mucus contains antibodies to fight virus and bacteria. The mucus, with all of the debris, is swept away by little microscopic moving whiplike projections of our cells called cilia. If the air is too dry (and I have heard that some suburban houses have air at night with less humidity than the Sahara Desert), then the mucus dries and ceases to function. You waken in the morning with a dry nose and throat, and are probably much more susceptible to colds and infection.

Another major factor in night nasal irritation is allergy. The furnace blows not only the air but also dust, fragments of feather pillows, wool rugs, hair rug pads, and other irritating and allergic substances.

A third important factor is gravity. When you stand up all day, your feet and ankles may swell some from edema, the fluid that leaks out of the blood and lymph vessels. When you lie flat all night, this edema fluid may end up in your face and cause swelling under the eyes and in the nasal cavity. This complicates nasal stuffiness. It is interesting that man is about the only creature who lies flat to sleep. The rest of Mother Nature's mammals seem to have better instinctive sense. Primates, such as monkeys and gorillas, generally sleep sitting up. Cattle, horses, and most dogs sleep with the head in its daytime position. I have a crazy collie who sleeps on her back—but she thinks she is human anyway. What can you do about all this?

1. Keep the heat low at night. Use more night clothes or blankets to keep warm.
2. Keep the house as dust free as possible. Some people should avoid feather pillows.
3. Use some source of water to increase humidity.
4. Sleep with your head higher than your feet.
5. Prop the bed up with blocks under the legs at the head of the bed or with a wedge or bolster between the mattress and box springs, in hospital bed fashion.

What Causes Tonsillitis and "Sore Throats"?

Sore throats are caused by viral and/or bacterial infections, allergies, and such irritants as smog. Along with soreness, the membranes are usually red, swollen, or ulcerated, and in some cases they are covered with pus. The same germ may cause a severe sore throat in one person and not cause much reaction at all in the next. Some of the soreness is from the membranes, and some from an inflammation of deeper muscle and lymph gland tissue.

The throat can be sore whether or not tonsils are present. The process of inflammation of the throat is both complicated and interesting. Noxious agents, including germs, land on the mucosal surfaces of the nose and throat. These surfaces are covered with microscopic hair-like cilia that continually sweep off the tender membranes with an antibody-containing mucus which runs into the tonsillar tissue. Together, the adenoids and tonsils (including the tonsils on the back of the tongue) literally form a ring around the posterior area of the mouth and nose. Almost all incoming agents are trapped or sampled.

The tonsils are made of a lymphoid tissue that has deep crypts or folds in which germs are trapped. This tissue contains a high concentration of white blood cells and immune bodies. When an offending germ lodges in the tissue, white cells migrate to the area and sample the germ. These white cells go to the lymph glands in the neck, and give them a sample of the germ. The lymph glands use this sample as a pattern and manufacture antibodies to fight the germ. White cells and antibodies migrate out of the tonsil, surround the germ and, if possible, destroy it. All of this requires a lot of traffic through the blood and lymph vessels in the tonsils. The increased supply of blood, lymph, and white cells causes the tonsils to become swollen, red, pussy, and inflamed. This condition is called tonsillitis. If the tonsils are not present, the same germ may lodge on the membranes of the throat and cause infection anyway.

You do not treat tonsillitis directly with antibiotics. Antibiotics act on bacteria. If the tonsils are infected with a certain bacteria, and a specific antibiotic will kill that bacteria, then *that* antibiotic is treatment for *that* particular infection. If the tonsils are infected with a virus, antibiotics will not cure the infection. People are often misled, and say: "Penicillin really works well on my tonsils." Tonsillitis is often associated with other symptoms such as headaches, fever, stomachache, vomiting, and fatigue. Sometimes this is from the local infection in the tonsils, other times it is from a generalized infection that also includes the tonsils. Let your doctor decide what antibiotic, if any, will probably work best under the circumstances.

Sore throats and tonsillitis can be caused by:

* Several hundred viruses, including:
    Adenovirus
    Chicken pox
    Coxsackie
    Herpes
    Influenza
    Para influenza virus
    Infectious mononucleosis
    Measles
* Many bacteria, including:
    Betahemolytic streptococcus
    Diphtheria
    Gonorrhea
    Hemophilus
    Pneumococcus
    Syphilis

- In-between germs, including:
  Chalymidia
  Mycoplasma
  Psittacosis
  Yeast
  Irritants
  Drano
  Smog
  Aspirin gargles
  Allergy

Should Tonsils and Adenoids Come Out?

Not many years ago, recalls pediatrician Sid Rosin, it was fashionable to have tonsils removed automatically at around the age of five years.

It was not uncommon to see newspaper stories of all the children in a family having their tonsils and adenoids removed at one sitting. Now the pendulum has swung to the other extreme of "no tonsillectomy," except in cases of suspected cancer of the organ. To do a tonsillo-adenoidectomy without indication is bad, but to retain a diseased organ is equally harmful. I believe that tonsil surgery is indicated when:

1. The tonsils have become diseased by repeated severe infections, especially beta-streptococcal infections. At this stage, tonsils are simply filled with "pus pockets." To retain the tonsils is to invite serious problems.
2. Abscesses develop under the tonsil (quinsy). Today, these abscesses may be cured by antibiotics alone without lancing. However, the damage is there and recurrences are possible, so the best cure is to remove the diseased organ.
3. Significant swollen lymph glands in the neck persist after repeated tonsillar infections. This happens when the infection has left the tonsils and moved to the nearby lymph glands. It means that the tonsils are usually deeply and severely infected, and are best removed.
4. There is obstruction of the nose and throat passages from large tonsils or adenoids. Generally, this is the child who walks around or sleeps with his mouth constantly open. He is uncomfortable and cannot function at his best. Orthodontia may be required later, for the jaw cannot develop normally while the child's mouth remains constantly open.
5. Your child has repeated earaches or hearing loss caused by inflammation of the middle ear (otitis media). Swollen adenoids may plug the opening of the Eustachian tube that drain the middle ear. As a result, hearing is decreased. Medication may help *some* children, but it has no chance against the glue-like mucus which often builds up behind the eardrum. In such cases, an

adenoidectomy, in conjunction with drainage of the ear, relieves the problem. Under most circumstances, it is wise to do a tonsillectomy if an adenoidectomy is planned.

Good health supervision allows a doctor to follow the child over the years and permits him to conclude more efficiently what is best for his patient. Fragmentary care can be most harmful, especially if snap judgments are made.

In the pre-antibiotic days, tonsillectomy almost always did more good than harm. Chronic streptococcal infections and abscesses in the tonsils effectively "poisoned" many children. The toll of resulting ear infections was high, and hospitals were full of patients with severe mastoid infections. Large numbers of draftees for World War II were turned down because of such ear problems. Chronic draining ears were commonplace; many adults still have chronic draining mastoid and ear infections left over from childhood. Today, children who receive adequate health supervision and early illness care have fewer such major problems.

If the tonsils and adenoids are taken out very early in life, they usually grow back. "Mother nature" wants them there. In fact, the tonsils and adenoids grow faster than the rest of the body between the ages of one to five. Usually, they peak in size at around five years; after that the body grows faster than the tonsils, which begin to shrink in size. At about this time, the measurable antibodies in the body reach an adult level. Tonsils and adenoids aren't all bad and shouldn't come out just because "they are there." They are like two soldiers guarding the entrance to the body, and are important in immunity.

Physicians argue in the scientific journals over the proper indications for tonsillectomy. But there is no question that many children are better off without the tonsils and adenoids. Large tonsils, however, do not necessarily mean bad tonsils.

A tonsillectomy is not without psychological trauma and some risk, usually bleeding and the anesthetic risk tied to any surgical procedure. If there is a family history of bleeders (especially if they bled from tooth extraction or a tonsillectomy), be sure to tell your doctor. Pediatricians also point to other factors that can affect the decision about a T. and A. Nature causes adenoids to shrink spontaneously. By the age of fourteen years no significant adenoids are left. There can also be a need for adenoidectomy from obstruction or a need for tonsillectomy from infection. Separate procedures are sometimes recommended. Pediatric allergist Dr. William Crook adds another viewpoint:

Many mouth-breathing children appear to have a continuous "cold" due to enlarged tonsils and adenoids. So the tonsils and adenoids may be removed. However, if allergy has led to the enlargement of the tonsils and adenoids, such surgery, although it may relieve some of the breathing obstruction, does nothing to help the underlying allergic swelling of the nose and other respiratory membranes. Many of these children continue to have breathing difficulties until the underlying allergy is identified and treated. Unless such allergies are identified and treated, adenoid tissue will regrow and the adenoidectomy might have to be repeated. Allergy, the great masquerader, may block your child's breathing and cause you, mistakenly, to blame your child's trouble on enlarged tonsils and adenoids.

Beta-streptococcal Sore Throats

The bacteria beta-streptococcus is such an important cause of human misery that we asked pediatrician William Misback to explain about it here, somewhat out of turn, even though this section is about where disease occurs rather than the causes of disease.

Strep infections are common in children and adults, can occur with or without tonsils being present, and can occur in other places, especially the skin. The versatile strep is highly contagious and somewhat sneaky. It can cause disease of different severity in different individuals. Some infections may be so mild as to go unrecognized, while others cause severe sore throat, swollen glands in the neck, scarlet fever, and even blood stream infections.

The strep germ is especially contagious among children in the same family or in the same school room. In some families, one child has scarlet fever, another sore throat, and a third a runny nose—yet all have the same strep germ. To make it even more difficult, one or both parents may be infected and have no symptoms. Those who have the germ but who are not sick are called carriers. Such carriers can re-infect their children or others. When a child in the family has strep throat, it may be necessary to culture the other members or to treat them, because they may have strep infections without showing it. Some physicians do not believe in culturing the family or contacts, feeling that carriers are rarely harmed. Others believe that strep infections recur so often in some children that it is less expensive in the long run to culture and treat the carriers. Some pediatricians culture routinely not only for strep infections but for another bacteria such as the pneumococcus.

It is important to get rid of the streptococcus, not only to cure the sick child but also to prevent the development of rheumatic fever or acute nephritis (kidney disease). Although not common, these complications occur in three percent of the children, two to three weeks after an inadequately treated strep infection.

Treatment: Fortunately, the strep germ responds to most of the antibiotic drugs, especially penicillin. To kill the germ completely, penicillin must be given as follows:

1. By mouth, in dosage prescribed, for *ten full days,* or:
2. By one or two injections of a long-acting penicillin. This is absorbed slowly from the muscles and gives a high blood level of penicillin for ten days. (A disadvantage is that it may cause a sore hip for a few days.)

3. It is advisable to reculture the throat about two weeks or so after an injection of long-acting penicillin, or four to five days after completion of oral therapy. The urine should be watched for a change in color, such as cloudy, brown, or red. After twenty-four hours on penicillin, the child is not contagious.

   The child will feel better after a few days or even a few hours on the penicillin, and it may be tempting to discontinue the medication. To be effective, it must be given for a full ten days.

What Is a Good Gargle?

A gargle can work in several ways: to clean the mouth, tonsils and pharynx, kill a few germs, and bring heat and relaxation to the throat. Hot salt water is an excellent gargle. It cleans and soothes. The heat relaxes tense inflamed throat muscles and reduces soreness. It increases the blood supply to the area of infection. Gargle as often and as long as you can with half a teaspoon of salt in eight ounces of hot water. Avoid aspirin gargles and Aspergum, as they burn the tissue and make the inflammation worse.

Some commercial gargles contain a cleansing detergent that helps by washing pus and germs out of the crypts of the tonsils. It is doubtful if their germ-killing properties are of significant value, because the germs are usually imbedded out of reach in the mucosa and in the deep tonsil and adenoidal crypts, which are not reached by the gargle. Occasional individuals may become allergic to the gargle and be worse after gargling because of a local reaction, but this is rare.

For small children unable to gargle, the medication can be sprayed onto the back of the throat—if you are lucky.

Much of the soreness in throats results from swollen tender lymph glands which put surrounding muscles into spasm. A warm towel wrapped around the neck gives some temporary relief.

What Should You Do for Sores in the Mouth?

There are many causes of sores in the mouth:

1. Canker sores—small ulcers with a grey or yellow base—are the most common mouth sores. They often occur in series, lasting four to five days each (See page 304).
2. Herpetic stomatitis is a herpes virus infection that lasts up to two weeks, with fever and ulcers throughout the mouth (See page 303).
3. Herpangina, from a coxsackie virus, which causes fever and painful ulcers on the back of the mouth, and lasts around five days (See page 304).
4. Allergy to drugs.
5. Damage from aspirin gargles.
6. Burns from lye or spicy foods.

Any of these can become secondarily infected, causing "trench mouth." Before you call your doctor to report, check several things:

1. What is the temperature?
2. Is the breath foul?
3. Are the sores on the outer lips, the inner lips and inside the cheeks, on the gums, the tongue, near the tonsils, or on the roof of the mouth?
4. Are there swollen lymph glands under the jaw, under the ears, or elsewhere in the neck?
5. Is the child sick or just uncomfortable?

Giving the nurse this information will help the doctor to decide whether your child needs to be seen or treated. While you are waiting for an answer, it won't hurt to use a mouth wash. Pediatrician Charles Hoffman suggests that some relief can be obtained from half-strength peroxide mouth wash and a solution of glyoxide painted on the sores after meals. The various throat and cough lozenges are of questionable medical value but are at least of psychological value. Aspirin may be swallowed for relief of pain if needed. Encourage fluids, ice chips, popsicles, and so forth. Some of us feel that it is best to avoid milk and ice cream, as in some individuals they thicken the nose and mouth secretions, increasing the congestion. Other physicians ignore this aspect of milk. Yogurt is acceptable to all.

What Causes Foul Breath?
Foul breath (not stomach-sour or the sickly sweet fever breath) frequently means the presence of a bacterial infection. Don't have the child breathe on you to check. You will be smelling lung air rather than mouth and nose air, and you may catch the infection yourself. Have him open his mouth, then smell around it. Foulness can mean many things aside from unwashed teeth. With bleeding gums, it can mean trench mouth or gingivitis (infection of the gums). With fever and swollen glands, it can indicate a streptococcal infection, an abscess in the tonsils, or even "a bean up the nose." These deserve a call—and probably a visit—to the doctor.

Pediatrician R. Wendell Coffelt notes that a foreign body up one nostril is more common than many suspect. He adds that gasses from the intestinal tract are another cause of foul breath and believes that eating yogurt daily helps reduce this odor. Dr. Thomas Conway believes that a common site of infection is around obstructing adenoids and that this is often better appreciated by the parents because they hear the child and smell his breath at night. Sometimes this is secondary to allergy, which causes the adenoids to enlarge.

How Should You Treat Croup?
Croup is an infection of the respiratory passages that causes noisy breathing and a bark-like cough. If the trouble is in the larynx, at the vocal cords, there is also hoarseness. Laryngeal croup often comes at night with frightening and puzzling suddenness, reports pediatrician David Sparling.

One reason for the night time onset of croup is that the hot dry air, blowing out of the furnace, causes spasms of the vocal cords. Symptoms may improve greatly by day, but may return for three or four consecutive nights. In mild cases, a vaporizer and an increased intake of clear liquids is all that is necessary. Expectorant or loosening cough syrups help. If the breathing is hard, the child may rest better propped up to a near-sitting position.

It is important to cough up the increased mucus in the chest. In order to help a child to do this, take him to the bathroom two or three times during the night, close the door, turn on all the hot water to create steam, and turn him over your knee, face hanging down. Pat him on the back, or even gag him with your finger, to encourage him to cough up the mucus. Tell him why you do this so that he won't be frightened. The results will allow you both to sleep better.

If the child's croup is moderately bad, a tent may be constructed over his crib. Cover the crib about three-quarters of the way with a blanket, and also drape the blanket over a chair beside the crib. Place the vaporizer under the tent between the chair and crib, but do not turn the vaporizer directly on the child. If a warm vaporizer is used, dress the child lightly enough to avoid overheating. If a cold mist is used, dress him a bit warmer than usual because of the chilled air. Use only water in the vaporizer; smelly medications do no good and can ruin the vaporizer. Though croup is frightening, particularly the way it comes on, it is seldom dangerous. Emergency attention is required on the rare occasions when croup may rapidly cause such severe breathing difficulties that the child cannot lie down or sleep or starts to turn blue.

Dr. Thomas Conway cautions: "If you have a steam vaporizer make certain the child cannot reach through the crib rail and be burned by the hot steam. Have the cord to the vaporizer out of the child's reach so he can't tip it over on himself." Other suggestions for both emergency and routine treatment of croup are covered on page 48.

Signs of Dangerous Croup

There are several ways in which you can determine if croup is becoming serious:

1. An increasing rate of breathing is an early sign. The normal respiratory rate is twenty breaths a minute when quiet or asleep. Children with croup and colds often breathe above forty times per minute. If the rate increases steadily above fifty when the child is quiet, it may indicate problems.

2. Retracting, or "sinking in" between the ribs, below the ribs, and in the neck with each inspired breath is another signal. Mild retractions are not unusual, but if severe, they should be reported. To experience retraction, pinch your nostrils shut, close your lips tightly and attempt to breathe in; no air can get in. You will sink in between the ribs as described. Doing this, you understand the restlessness and panic that can occur in a child with severe croup.

3. Fever above 102–104° F with croup may occasionally indicate the presence of a bacterial infection requiring antibiotic treatment.
4. Episodes of choking unrelieved by vomiting should be reported to the doctor.
5. Extremely pale, dusky, or bluish skin color can indicate lack of oxygen.
6. Croup so severe that the child can't lie down or sleep requires treatment.
7. Uncontrollable cough and labored breathing deserve a call to the doctor.

LARYNGITIS

Laryngitis is an inflammation of the vocal cords. It is almost the same disease as croup. Occasionally an adult or older child in a family will have a viral laryngitis, and the smaller brother and sister will develop croup from the same virus. It can also be caused by screaming and hollering a lot—or even singing and talking too much. Sometimes the voice goes completely or only a whisper is left. Often there is a dry, croupy, barky cough. Treat it like croup—where the first and usually unwelcome rule is *stop talking*. If there is high fever, a general illness, or choking, you should see the doctor.

WHY DO CHILDREN GET EARACHES?

In order to understand ear problems it helps to know about the three main parts of the ear:

1. The external ear includes the visible part and the canal that leads to the ear drum.
2. The middle ear is a cavity behind the eardrum. It is filled with air from the short but narrow Eustachian tube, which opens at the back of the nasal cavity near the adenoids. A series of small movable bones carry the sound waves from the eardrum to the inner ear.
3. The inner ear is a fluid-filled cavity containing the delicate nerves of hearing and the organs of balance.

The external ear canal can hurt from "swimmer's" ear and can become plugged with ear wax, beans, cotton—or whatever a toddler can put into it.

Pain in the middle ear usually results from pressure on, or inflammation of, the paper-thin membrane of the eardrum. Inward pressure results from a vacuum in the middle ear. This occurs when the Eustachian tube is plugged and the mucus membranes in the middle ear absorb the air, creating a vacuum. A vacuum can also result from going down quickly from high altitude to low altitude in an airplane or auto. The sudden pressure change collapses the opening of the Eustachian tube. The pressure also holds the eardrum tight and reduces its ability to transmit sound. Mucus secreted by the membranes of the middle ear replaces the vacuum. This mucus reduces hearing by suppressing the transmission of sound via the small moveable ear bones from the eardrum to the inner ear. The ear may or may not hurt during the time it is filled with mucus,

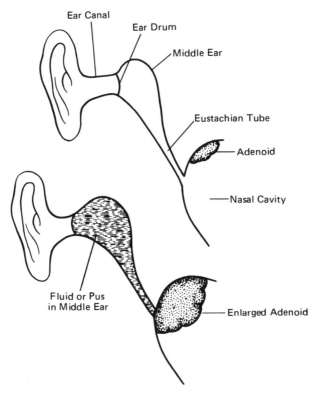

FIGURE 33   *Top: Normal air filled middle ear. Mucus drains out the eustachian tube. Bottom: Swollen adenoid tissue blocks the eustachian tube. Mucus or pus cannot drain out and presses on ear drum.*

although older children and adults complain of a stuffy feeling. If the pressure of the mucus builds up, it will push the eardrum out, causing some pain. If the mucus remains in the ear too long, it thickens to a glue-like substance which further reduces hearing, and if it stays long enough it is replaced by scar material that can cause permanent hearing loss.

Pain from cold air reaching the eardrum occurs only if the eardrum already hurts or is inflamed. Aside from the discomfort, it does not make the ear problem worse. Middle ear problems start in the back of the nasal cavity. This is the reason that hats or ear muffs do not prevent ear infections.

Mucus in the middle ear is a dandy place for bacteria to grow. Their growth brings white cells into the mucus to fight the bacteria. The resulting pus greatly increases the pressure, causing the eardrum to bulge out and hurt. Both bacteria and viruses can cause an inflamed red eardrum; if the process is severe enough, the thin eardrum may pop and pus will drain from the ear canal, relieving most of the pain. If a baby cries a lot at night, it might be due to an ear infection, and should be checked.

Most middle ear problems result from mucus in the middle ear, due to an obstruction of the Eustachian tube. This may be caused mechanically by mucus in the nasal cavity, or from swollen adenoids. The Eustachian tube membranes themselves may become inflamed and swollen, plugging off the opening. Such swelling may be triggered by many things, including: smog, chemical irritation (chlorine in swimming pools), allergy, viral infection (various "colds"), or bacterial infection. It can also be started by blowing the nose hard and forcing mucus or pus into the Eustachian tube.

How do you remove a foreign body from the ear? See emergency care, Chapter 2. What can you do for an insect in the ear? See emergency care, Chapter 2. How about altitude ear aches? See emergency care, Chapter 2.

What Can One Do to Prevent "Swimmer's Ear?"

"Swimmer's ear" (external otitis), an infection in the ear canal, occurs when the ear canal gets wet and stays wet for a long time. It often shows up in children engaged in competitive swimming. The soggy skin reacts like "dishpan hands." The victim finds it painful to wiggle the outer ear. This is one infection that can be diagnosed by telephone. It usually requires medical attention and can last a long time.

"Swimmer's ear" can be prevented. Have your child take along a dropper bottle containing 90% to 99% isopropyl or ethyl alcohol, and instruct him to fill his ear canals with the alcohol when he leaves the water, then turn the head down, letting the solution drain out. This treatment leaves a sterile, clean, dry ear canal and prevents soggy skin and resulting infection. Do not use alcohol in the ear if it is painful. Remember that isopropyl alcohol—rubbing alcohol—is a poison if taken internally. Dr. Misbach uses a mixture of equal parts alcohol and white vinegar.

How to Use Ear Drops

Ear drops are used for:

1. Relief of local external ear infections (swimmer's ear).
2. *Temporary* relief of earache from a middle ear infection.

Pediatrician Marvin McClellan points out that the materials used for the treatment of external otitis are medications designed to reduce swelling or infection whereas:

> The material used for middle ear pain is some type of oil or glycerin that contains a local pain reliever, conducts warmth to the drum, and possibly attracts some moisture by osmosis through the eardrum.

To apply ear drops, have the child lie down on his side with the affected ear up. Put the prescribed number of drops in that ear. Then put a cotton wick, twisted to a shape similar to a golf tee, in the ear. This helps keep the drops in contact with the eardrum. If both ears hurt, turn the child to the other side and repeat the same process. Leave the cotton wick in the ear until the next application of drops; then use new wicks. Remember to remove the wick after the pain has gone.

Except in the case of a local skin infection such as swimmer's ear, ear drops have a very limited curative power. The use of drops for pain is only justified on a temporary basis. If you use them to stop pain, and then ignore the underlying cause, the child could end up with some hearing loss due to ear-drum damage. Check with your physician when earaches occur.

What Do You Do About Dirty Ears?

Family practitioner Ben McGann, like the rest of us, frequently sees a worried mother with a child who has a painful ear. This, he contends, is frequently caused by mother!

All too often the physician finds impacted wax with a smooth surface in the ear canal. This is caused by injudicious use of cotton-tipped applicators. Mothers become very concerned about wax building up in the ear—or just about "dirty ears." Television and magazine advertising contribute to the problem—encouraging the use of cotton tipped applicators in every possible human orifice.

Do not use cotton-tipped applicators. The ear canal is very sensitive. It is a bony canal, lined with a thin layer of tissue containing small glands that secrete an oily waxy material to protect and lubricate the ear canal. The lubricant acts as a protective lining for the canal to remove dust, dirt, and debris. If the flow of wax is not impaired—by toothpicks, hairpins, or cotton tipped applicators—the ear canal will take care of itself. So leave the ear canal alone and don't worry about a little wax. The old adage holds—what you can't get out with a washcloth—don't worry about!

Most of the trouble comes from trying to clean the absolutely normal dark wax out of the ear canal. No matter how much is pulled out by the cotton tipped applicator, some is pushed farther back. It dries; wax then piles up behind it; and the ear canal becomes plugged. Hearing is diminished, and at times, infection occurs under the old dry wax.

If the wax piles up and doesn't come out, it can be softened by pouring a thin baby oil into the ear canal. Don't try this if the ear hurts at all or if there is already some drainage from the canal. Let the excess oil run out by itself. A few days of such treatment often clears out the wax. Follow this treatment with the treatment recommended for swimmer's ear to remove the oil. Your physician can prescribe more sophisticated medications if needed. If it hurts when you wiggle the external ear, or if hearing is still diminished, a visit to your physician may be in order.

What Causes "Glue Ear"?

Serous otitis is caused by a thin fluid that gradually becomes thick or "glue-like" and fills the normally air filled middle ear. It causes a feeling of fullness in the ear and hearing loss, or a popping sensation with chewing or swallowing. Small children are rarely able to tell the parent they have a stuffy ear.

Pediatric allergist William Crook notes that of a group of 512 allergic children with ear trouble, 97% had good results from careful allergic study and management. However, I still believe that most cases are due to incompletely treated ear infections that often end up in glue ears or that they just develop after repeated colds. Pediatrician James Stem sides in with Dr. Crook:

> Most physicians now agree with the allergists that most "glue ears" are caused by nasal allergy. This may be obvious when there is sneezing, itchy eyes, and nose—but more often, though, it is sneaky, accompanied only by a low grade nasal obstruction which plugs the opening of the Eustachian tube. There are, of course, other causes of Eustachian tube obstruction, such as large adenoids or a deviated nasal septum. However, studies of the fluid withdrawn from "glue ears" show an amazingly high concentration of antibodies against ragweed, house dust, or other common allergens.
>
> Aside from such scientific indications, there is more practical proof. Allergy treatment frequently results in the disappearance of the fluid from the middle ear. The Eustachian tube opens and air bubbles appear, heralding the beginning of the end of "Sneaky Serous Otitis." The treatment may be as simple as avoiding a feather pillow or giving away the family cat. Conscientious administration of an antihistamine nasal decongestant combination often controls serous otitis. If these do not work, a tailor-made allergy vaccine can be made on the basis of skin tests and given as allergy shots to desensitize the individual and open the Eustachian tube.

What is Sinusitis?

The sinuses are air-filled cavities in the bones of the face with openings into the nasal passage. When the openings are plugged off by swollen membranes, the mucosa absorbs the air in the sinuses, creating a vacuum. This is one cause of sinus headache. The vacuum draws mucus into the sinus and bacteria can grow in the mucus, creating infection. Another cause of infection is from contaminated mucus or pus being forced into the sinus openings when one "blows the nose."

Most sinus infections are just an extension of a nasal infection. Because the openings seal off with swelling, a sinus infection can be more severe than a nasal infection or a simple "cold." One contributing factor to many sinus infections is allergy, as the pollens cause the membranes to swell, blocking sinus openings.

The spongy tissues lining the nasal passage are called the nasal turbinates. They serve to warm and humidify inspired air, and their large mucus surface traps dust, pollens, and germs. The turbinates lie over the openings of some of the sinuses and are the culprits in blockage. The swelling may become so severe that polyps or grape-like growths are formed on these membranes.

How Do You Teach Your Child to Blow His Nose?

Don't, please! To blow the nose and clean it of mucus or pus requires considerable air pressure, which may push the mucus or pus into the Eustachian tube or into the sinuses. It is a common way of starting middle ear and sinus infections. Sniffing the mucus pulls it away from the openings of the Eustachian tubes and sinuses. It may not sound attractive, but it *is* healthier. True, it runs down the back of the throat and is swallowed, but the stomach acid kills the germs and no harm is done. Mothers and grandmothers, contain yourselves: Remember that a sniff sounds no worse than a blow to some, and that it serves a better purpose.

What Causes Nose Bleeds?

There is a network of blood vessels on the wall of the lower part of the central septum of the nose, covered by a thin layer of mucus membrane. If this dries out, or if the nose is picked or bumped, the fragile vessels may break or bleed. Don't worry about a few minor nose bleeds a year. See your doctor if the nose bleeds are frequent, if the bleeding is quite severe, or if it refuses to stop. Your doctor may cauterize the area, or he may do a complete physical and laboratory examination to rule out rare blood diseases.

How Do You Stop a Nose Bleed?

Have your child sit up and lean forward. With your thumb and forefinger, pinch the soft part of the nostrils into the septum in the center and hold it that way firmly for five minutes without letting go. (See Figure 10 on page 42.) Don't press on the bony part of the nose, as that does no good. Put a cold wet rag on the back of the neck or cheeks. After the bleeding stops, don't let him blow or pick his nose, and don't let him lie down for an hour or so without propping him up or the nosebleed may start again. Put a small amount of lotion or cream in each nostril twice a day for several days. If the nose continues to bleed when you release the pressure, or if it bleeds again later, call your doctor. There are other techniques. Dr. William Misbach advises:

> Press the nose on the side that is bleeding. If it doesn't stop immediately, roll up a small piece of cotton and put it up the nostril on the bleeding side. Now press again or pinch as shown and hold for some time. Remove the cotton a few hours later. If it is removed too soon, bleeding may restart. If it recurs, call the doctor.

Other pediatricians caution that small children may get a type of pneumonia from grease dripping into the lungs if too much ointment is used in the nostrils. Some recommend an A and D vitamin *cream*. The amount of cream used should be smaller than a match head for each nostril.

Another Cause of Sinus and Ear Infections and Nose Bleeds

If the cartilage in the septum in the center of the nose is broken and heals out of position, the septum is deviated to one side or the other. This changes the air currents breathed in through the nose, which may result in one area being dried out from excessive air, or in another being plugged easily from too little space. Such drying or plugging causes irritated membranes, plugged off sinuses and ears, and, occasionally, nosebleeds. If it is a severe enough problem, the septum can be straightened surgically. We usually wait until the child has stopped growing before performing surgery.

Should You Use Nose Drops?

Doctors vigorously disagree about recommending nose drops, because nose drops are so easily *misused*. But first the good news. The drops function in two ways. First, they wash and flush off the membranes. Second, they cause the blood vessels in the nasal membranes to constrict. This opens the nose so you are able to breath better. More important, the drops shrink the swollen membranes around the openings of the sinuses and the Eustachian tubes to the middle ear. This allows the ears and sinuses to drain and makes it less likely that these organs will become infected.

Now for the bad news. After continued use of nose drops, the muscles in the walls of the blood vessels get fatigued; then the vessels open and the membranes swell. This happens most often with strong nose drops, but it can happen with "weak" ones if they are used too long. Your particular nose might overreact to *any* nose drops, or conversely, react to none.

Avoid strong nose drops unless they are prescribed by your doctor. And don't use *any* nose drops for too long a period of time. A good rule of thumb is to use the common, non-prescription nose drops (Neosynephrine $\frac{1}{4}$%, Alconefrin 25, Isofrin $\frac{1}{4}$%) four times a day for five days. Then stop for at least three days, even if your nose is stuffy. Give those poor tired blood vessel muscles a rest. For infants, check with your doctor. Baby nose drops are available (Alconefrin 12, Neosynephrin $\frac{1}{8}$%).

If you do use nose drops, use them correctly. They have to reach the membranes, flush off the mucus, and then shrink the tissue. It is especially important that they reach the openings of the sinuses and middle ears (Eustachian tubes) and stay there long enough to work. Sprays are handy, but they are wasteful as the drops run quickly down the back of the throat.

I advise lying with the shoulders off the bed and the head upside down as if you were going to stand on your head. Put in the drops, hold your nostrils together with your thumb and finger, and say slowly, out loud, once with each breath, "K," "K," "K," fifty times. *Then,* still holding the nose and keeping your head down, roll over onto your

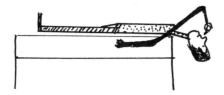

FIGURE 34   *Get your head upside down (as if you were standing on your head) so that when you put the nose drops in they won't just run down your throat.*

stomach so you are face down and say another fifty "K"'s. Then sit up and allow the sinuses to drain. Sometimes you can open up ears and sinuses this way and prevent infections and mucus accumulating in the ear.

Infants and toddlers rarely think well of this fine advice. But remember that you *are* bigger than they are. You can usually achieve some relief for them if you have the will, the muscle, and the following technique. Put the baby across your lap with his head clamped between your knees. Hold his hands with your left hand. With the right hand, squirt the drops quickly in each nostril. Don't put the dropper in the nostril. For the nose drops mentioned above, use about a quarter of an inch in the dropper for each nostril.

If your back is up to it, you can make a game of swinging the baby around like a centrifuge (but don't bump his head on things!), which puts the drops right up where they belong. If you make this a "fun game" before using the drops, it often makes the whole procedure less traumatic.

If your maxillary sinuses—in the cheek bones under the eyes—are full and aching, there is a better way to get at their openings. Lie on the bed on your side and let your head angle down. Put the drops in the lower nostril and wait a few minutes. Then roll over and repeat this for the other side.

If you are trying to do this to your child and he screams so much that he gets more congested, you may want to chuck the whole idea. If, after temporary relief, you find that the nose is worse than before, you may be suffering from nasal membranes swollen from the action of the nose drops—beware the "nose drop nose."

Pediatrician Marvin McClellan suggests that you get the best results if you use the nose drops before meals so that you can eat and breath at the same time. He cautions about bedtime use because they may make some susceptible individuals more wakeful. Dr. Merritt Low suggests that you gently use nasal suction bulbs or one ounce rubber ear syringes for babies under two years of age to suck the mucus from the nose. I have found this to be of value only when there is a very heavy nasal discharge.

How Do You Know Your Decongestant or Allergy Medicines are Working?

Antihistamines help reduce swelling caused by an allergy, whether it is in the nose or skin. If you have hives and itch, the results of antihistamine treatment are as plain as the bumps on your skin. If you have a stuffy or runny nose and the antihistamine works for you, then within an hour after taking the medicine the running and/or the nasal stuffiness will decrease.

The problem is that there are hundreds of antihistamines and millions of people. The same drug does not react the same way on everybody. In some it works, and on some it doesn't—or it doesn't work well. If it does work, is it worth suffering the possible side effects? The same drug will make some people sleepy, some irritable, some nervous and hyperactive, and will leave most unaffected in any way. Using an antihistamine is an experiment on everyone. If it works, fine. If it doesn't work, ask your doctor for a different one. Sooner or later, you may find one that works and is worth it. Dr. Thomas Conway cautions:

> In some people, decongestants may produce side actions, such as speeding up the heart rate or causing nervousness. Antihistamines have a helpful drying effect in nasal allergy, but this dryness can, in turn, make an asthmatic episode worse. Therefore, I don't recommend antihistamines when there is wheezing or chest cough. Above all, don't take "cold medicines" just to be taking medicines. Don't force them on your children unless their symptoms are severe enough to require chemical relief.

SUMMARY

Our facial organs are both simple and complex. At least there are relatively simple things to remember which will help you to avoid complex problems and which will not necessitate a visit to the doctor each time. You can stop most nose bleeds, kill and remove most insects in the ear canal, and blow most foreign bodies out of the nose. Simple effective home treatments for croup, laryngitis, and mild sore throats may prevent serious problems.

Prevention is the name of the game. Sleeping propped up with adequate humidity in the air may prevent many earaches and infections. Check Chapter 15 on allergies to learn how to keep dust out of the bedroom, and, therefore, irritation out of the nose. Keep the ears and sinuses less full of mucus by the simple rule: "Sniff—don't blow." Get early diagnosis of streptococcal infections and treat your allergy before it harms you. Keep hearing acute by putting nothing in the ear smaller than your elbow. Don't let acute hearing loss become chronic. Make certain that your child can hear.

8

THE MOUTH
AND ITS CONTENTS:
TEETH AND BRACES,
THUMB OR PACIFIER!

Ah, the mouth! A source of pleasure with almost as many nerves per square centimeter as the genitalia. The conduit of nutrients to our body and of our thoughts to our society. Among its organs are the teeth, without which either of the above functions is distorted. Among its vices are sucking on a thumb or pacifier. Yes, teeth are important. Throughout life they serve us, plague us, and demand constant care and expense.

THE PREVENTION OF DENTAL BILLS

I asked my dentist, Dr. Frank McDaniel, D.D.S., "How can you prevent dental bills?" He responded with the following advice:

The prevention of dental disease is a goal of the entire dental profession, for what we cannot prevent we must restore. The backlog for restorative dentistry is enormous. Our only alternative is prevention —to solve dental problems before they occur. The concepts involved in preventive dentistry have been taught, preached, and practiced for many years. Dental publications from the last hundred years suggest many ways to prevent dental problems before they become serious.

Good dental hygiene starts with proper instruction of both parent and child. Some of this can be done by pediatricians and family practitioners who see dental problems begin, and who refer the child for periodic preventive visits to the dentists. Once the child reaches the dentist, our first step is careful visual examination of the oral cavity. The second step is to take dental x-rays. The number of x-rays taken will depend upon the dentist's visual evaluation of the child's problems: the number of caries (cavities) detected, the age of the child, and the number of teeth present. If there is no visual decay, then two to four x-rays should suffice *to reveal possible decay between the teeth.* When the patient has many carious areas, the dentist will need more x-rays for adequate diagnosis. With the use of the latest fast films, a lead apron, improved developing techniques, and good x-ray machines, the minimal exposure to radiation is not dangerous to the patient.

The dentist or dental hygienist will clean the teeth when necessary, and show the patient how to care for the teeth adequately at home in order to prevent tooth decay or gum disease. This requires an understanding of plaque on the teeth—the first step in the events leading to tooth decay. Plaques are small colonies of bacteria in a gel-like membrane which sticks to the surface of your teeth. Bacteria in plaque metabolize sugar from food in the diet—the second big factor in the formation of cavities—producing acid in the plaque which can dissolve tooth enamel. The degree of dissolving depends upon the third factor in cavity formation, the inherited softness or hardness of the enamel. Another factor besides genetics affecting the hardness of enamel is the amount of fluoride in the drinking water. Still another factor is mechanical crowding of teeth, making plaque difficult to remove. Cavities, as well as gum irritation caused by the acid, may be dramatically reduced by removing plaque or by reducing sugar intake.

How to Control Plaque

Plaque can be controlled. First, find out how much plaque you have by using a disclosing solution or tablets which makes plaque visible. Your dentist can show you how best to use the kit and the disclosing solution, a harmless temporary dye.

How to Use Disclosure Solution to See Your Plaque
1. Chew a tablet or swish a solution around in your mouth.
2. Spit it out or swallow—it is harmless.
3. Examine your teeth with a mirror and a good light. The color on the teeth is plaque that you must remove by flossing or brushing. When the color has gone, the plaque has gone.
4. Once you become more experienced in cleaning your teeth of plaques, you will only have to spot check occasionally.

Dental tape or floss should be used between the teeth, especially to remove plaque near the gum line and debris from areas where a toothbrush can't reach. Dental caries and gum disease will be reduced by brushing and flossing.

Sugar Causes Cavities

Reduction of sugar intake is the other major method of preventing cavities arising from plaques. Plaque bacteria are dependent on the nutrients received in the mouth. If they do not have sugar, they will not form acid. If they do not form acid, there will be far less enamel dissolved and far fewer cavities. If you are careful about what you eat, if you reduce sugar content, and if you brush after eating, you can prevent cavities.

Dentists have a responsibility to make their patients aware of every possibility available to improve dental care and to prevent tooth disease. Each patient is an individual, so use of any or all preventive techniques should be based on accurate personal diagnosis. The only certain method at this time is the regular professional care provided by your dentist, combined with your home dental care, a balanced diet, and the use of fluorides.

FLUORIDE: FACT AND FICTION

Dentists tell us that a fluoridated water supply is the easiest method of reducing cavities. If fluoridated water is not available, then children up to twelve years of age should take fluoride tablets daily. Those whose teeth are more subject to decay should have their dentist apply fluoride one to four times a year, depending on need. Fluoride toothpaste is also helpful in hardening and making the tooth enamel more decay resistant. Fluoride achieves this by entering the chemical structure of the enamel, making it harder and more acid resistant. Yet in spite of this knowledge, which is accepted by the American Dental Association, the American Medical Association, the American Academy of Pediatrics, and all responsible scientific bodies, some people persist in criticizing fluoride and making rather wild claims about all the harm it does.

The use of fluorides to harden teeth was accepted when Mother Nature put it in the water. Once man tried to imitate Mother Nature, other men became suspicious. Its safety wasn't challenged when it was found that people had fewer cavities when their drinking water naturally contained ten parts per million of fluoride. People had lived well in these areas for generations. Ten parts per million of fluoride has the disadvantage of causing a slight mottled stain of the teeth—and the advantage of around 80% fewer cavities. In infants and children, dietary fluoride enters growing teeth forming under the gums and becomes part of the harder enamel. You can look at fluoride as a vitamin for the teeth. In old folks, it hardens the bones.

Most drinking water contains some fluoride. In many communities, however, the amount of fluoride in the public water supply is not enough to protect teeth against decay. The amount should be increased to one part per million—the equivalent of one drop of fluoride in a bathtub one-third full of water. No mottling occurs at this level, but the decay resistance is greatly increased.

Like many other substances aside from fluoride—salt and vitamins, for example, an excess is dangerous. Some opponents of fluoridation have used the argument that fluoride is used as a rat poison. But the amount used in rat poison is huge compared to the amount used to fluoridate water. An equivalent amount of overdose of table salt or vitamin D would probably kill a child. Too much of anything is dangerous. There is no evidence of danger from fluoride when taken properly. The amount added to public water supplies is safe and far below any potentially dangerous concentration. Check with your dentist or doctor to see if fluoride has been added to your water; if not, he can prescribe fluoride drops or chewable tablets with or without vitamins. Your dentist or dental hygienist may apply fluoride directly once the teeth have erupted, and fluoride toothpaste is helpful locally.

A few dentists believe that fluoride tablets, even in the accepted dose, will cause a small amount of mottling or color change in the teeth. Most of us do not see these changes, even after decades of following children on fluoride. Even if mottling occurs, the trade-off of reducing cavities by 80% would overbalance any minimal color changes in the teeth.

Isn't Fluoride Toothpaste Enough?

The television advertising about fluoride toothpaste might lead one to think that using fluoride toothpaste and seeing your dentist twice a year is enough. However, brushing with fluoride toothpaste does nothing for the teeth that have not come in. As long as teeth are growing, they need a supply of fluoride absorbed from the water—or a fluoride pill or drops. Some 90% of tooth growth is complete by eight years, and 100% is usually complete by twelve years.

Before the Teeth Erupt

Teeth assume importance well before they erupt through the gums. They can be damaged by high fever, possibly by infections, by poor diet, by lack of fluoride, and by tetracycline antibiotics. Excessive amounts of

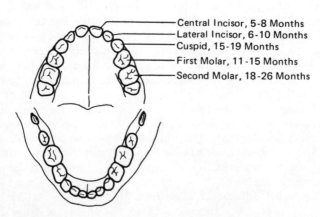

Central Incisor, 5-8 Months
Lateral Incisor, 6-10 Months
Cuspid, 15-19 Months
First Molar, 11-15 Months
Second Molar, 18-26 Months

FIGURE 35   *Usual times of eruption of primary teeth.*

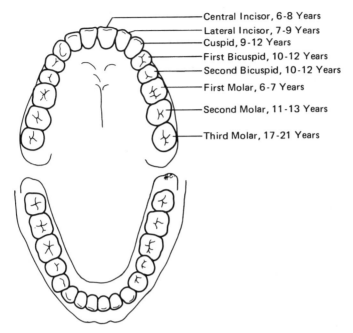

Central Incisor, 6-8 Years
Lateral Incisor, 7-9 Years
Cuspid, 9-12 Years
First Bicuspid, 10-12 Years
Second Bicuspid, 10-12 Years
First Molar, 6-7 Years
Second Molar, 11-13 Years
Third Molar, 17-21 Years

FIGURE 36 *Usual time of eruption of permanent teeth.*

tetracyclines given to infants and young children for various infections may cause stain in the tooth enamel. However, the most important and common problem with teeth at this stage is teething.

The Teething Myths

"How bad is teething?" we asked experienced pediatrician A. S. Hashim. "Not bad at all," he replied.

> Teething is a natural process. We all go through it. Grandma and the public have scary ideas about teething. Fortunately, those ideas are wrong. Will teething give your child any high temperature? The answer is *no*. Any bad cough? The answer is *no*. Any vomiting? The answer is *no*. Any diarrhea? The answer is *no*. Any important degree of fussing? The answer is *no*.
>
> What the heck is causing all those problems? Certainly not the teething process. It is something else, often infection. It so happens that during the teething age (six months to two and one-half years) the child is extremely susceptible to infections. When he gets the infection, the poor teeth get the blame. My fear is that you may miss noticing a good deal of trouble the infection is giving you. It is infection—teething should not be blamed for these symptoms.

Won't teething give any trouble whatsoever? Perhaps some tenderness of the gums. The baby may try to bite on his finger or a teething ring. Actually, it is better not to use any medicine whatsoever, but if you want to busy yourself, you may use a medicine that you rub on the gums.

When you stop to consider that we are teething from birth until all our permanent teeth erupt, we could blame all of our actions on teething. Even professionals sometimes use the teething ploy, because it is an easier way to reassure parents than to explain about the latest viral cold. The urge for pat explanations will probably keep the teething myth alive a long time. However, when we observe the fact that most teeth, including the six year molars and wisdom teeth, erupt without fever, we are hard put to logically blame fever, colds, or whatever onto teething, comforting though it might be.

When Do The Teeth Erupt?

When do the first teeth come in? At almost any time from birth to eighteen months. It depends on the individual. The average or "normal" time of eruption is given in Figures 36 and 37. Don't let such statistical norms bother you; it is of no great consequence (except perhaps to you and the baby) when the teeth come in.

Clean Your Teeth Three Ways

Teeth should be cleaned by all three basic methods: brushing, flossing, and rinsing. These should become habits engrained early in life, when the teeth are most susceptible to decay. To do this requires commitment and self-discipline on the part of the parents to see that adequate tooth cleaning is done. It also requires a knowledge of the proper techniques. There have been changes in recommended techniques in the past, but over the recent years there has been more consistency in advice from dentists. Apparently, a consensus has been reached. We suggest you check this advice out with your own dentist.

Brushing Baby Teeth

When the teeth do erupt, when do you start brushing them? The American Dental Association recommends that parents should start cleaning their baby's teeth as soon as they first come in. However, for the first few months, teeth are usually coated with a yellowish protective membrane. Since children are prone to tooth decay, the teeth should be cleaned right after eating and every night before bedtime.

Preschool children can learn to brush and floss effectively, but parental help and supervision are necessary for several more years. Make the use of the toothbrush an opportunity for the child to "be big." Patience and persistence are required.

Basic Brushing

The toothbrush should be small enough to reach every tooth, so small children need small brushes. The brush handle should be straight, the bristle edges soft and rounded, and the bristle surface flat. If the fibers are too soft or worn out, they are ineffective—so replace your brush often.

Angle the brush so that it points at 45 degrees against the gum line. You should feel the bristles on the gum as you gently brush back and forth over one to two teeth at a time, while slightly wiggling or rotating the brush. This scrubbing motion is also applied to the chewing surfaces and to the inside tooth surfaces.

Children's six year molars deserve special attention. These permanent molars are the sixth teeth back from the center front of the mouth. They are difficult to reach, and have pits and fissures on the chewing surfaces which can develop decay-producing plaque. The dentist should check these six year molars soon after they erupt. Some dentists recommend sealing the pits and fissures with a protective coating.

Electric Toothbrushes

Electric toothbrushes, like handbrushes, are effective for both teeth and gums. Electric toothbrushes can be very useful for some of the handicapped, and they often appeal to children who otherwise resent the time taken from play to hand brush their teeth adequately.

Using Floss

Most plaque cannot be removed from between the teeth by brushing, so dental floss should be used. For children, tie the ends of a twenty inch piece of floss together and hold the circle in both hands. Slide the floss gently between two teeth, curve it around the sides of the teeth, and scrape away from the gums. For adults, wind the ends of a shorter piece around a middle finger and guide the floss with your thumb and index finger. Scrape away from the gum. Using floss the first few times may cause some bleeding and soreness. This ceases as the plaque is broken up and the gums heal. If it persists, see your dentist.

Rinsing the Mouth

Mouthwashes may feel good and may freshen the breath, but they do not prevent decay or gum disease. A good rinsing with water is worthwhile after brushing and after meals, snacks, sweet drinks, or candy.

Stained Teeth

Teeth can be stained or mottled from many causes. Sometimes it is genetic—the teeth are just made that way. Sometimes it is from infections, especially if the infant is still in the uterus. A very high excess of fluoride taken over a period of time may cause mottling.

A not uncommon stain is from iron supplements, points out pediatrician David Sparling:

Iron medications for anemia are frequently prescribed. Unfortunately, some liquid iron preparations and some iron tablets, if they are chewed, may cause a stubborn black stain on the teeth. Swallowing the iron from the back of the mouth and brushing the teeth with baking soda immediately after taking the medicine generally prevent this stain. As an aside, constipation or diarrhea may be caused by some iron preparations, but often this can be relieved by a change of prescription. Keep iron medications safely away from curious children, since taking a three to five days' supply or more all at once may cause dangerous poisoning.

It is encouraging that there is treatment for stained teeth. The dentist can bleach them, depending on the severity of the stain, or cap or crown the teeth at an appropriate age in order to hide the stain.

Cavities in Toddlers

Once the teeth are in, they are susceptible to the "nursing bottle mouth." Children who run around during the day, or who go to bed at night, with bottles of sugar-containing fluids, especially acid juices (orange juice, apple juice, or "pop"), may develop severe caries. The older your child is when he is put down with a bottle, the worse the damage. Pediatrician Hashim has, in his practice, seen "the teeth become 'chewed up' down to the gum line, even as early as the age of two years." He believes that it's "really sinful" to see such a thing happen and recommends that the bottle should be stopped by the age of seventeen months at the latest, and brushing the teeth before going to bed should be observed rigorously. No food should be given *after* the teeth have been brushed at bed time.

Bad Breath

Teeth are one of the causes of bad breath, so they should be checked if the breath is offensive to see if there is accumulated caries, cavities, or pyorrhea. There are other causes of bad breath, including infection in the tonsils, or the sinuses, or indigestion with constipation (especially if there is too much fat intake). Don't forget the possibility of a foreign body in the nose, such as a lollipop stick, kleenex, and so forth. Some of the stuff removed from the noses of these little stinkers is amazing.

Gum Boil

Frequently, a tender swelling will appear on the gum adjacent to the root of an abscessed tooth. Dr. Hashim explains:

Usually, there is a cavity in the tooth, a chip on the enamel, or the tooth may be non-vital and gradually darkening. Germs multiply in the diseased tooth, burrowing a tunnel through the root of the tooth into the jawbone, causing infection. The pus may come to a point or drain at the gums. The infection can even go into the soft tissue of the cheek and can be quite dangerous. This is especially true for the area of the upper lip and the base of the nose, because there is a network of veins in that vicinity that can pick up the infection and transfer it to certain areas of the brain. It is a scary thing to think about, so we should try to prevent it. If you see signs of infection from the teeth, get the child to the dentist at once.

Toothache

Gum boils usually don't hurt much, but cavities and infection do cause toothache. Aspirin helps, but Nebraska pediatrician Hobart Wallace cautions: "My dentist friends report seeing severe mouth burns caused by applying aspirin over or into the decayed teeth. Aspirin benefits only after absorption into the system. When applied locally, aspirin burns the mucosa of the mouth."

Of course, the best course is to repair cavities early so that they don't progress to abscesses. In children, however, the primary teeth all fall out and are replaced, so some have questioned the practical need to fill cavities in children's teeth. Rather than ask a dentist, we asked pediatrician. Hashim his opinion on fixing cavities in primary teeth. He replied:

Don't say, 'Since these are primary teeth they will fall out anyway and the cavity will go away with them.' If it is not fixed, the cavity in a primary tooth can act as a focus of infection for the permanent teeth, or it can become so big that it destroys the whole tooth, may lead to a tooth abscess, or give trouble with toothache and bad breath. The primary teeth are needed for chewing, speaking, and appearance; and they hold the space for the permanent teeth.

SAVING BAD TEETH

How Teeth Get Bad

A tooth has the crown protected by a hard outer enamel coat and roots bound to the socket with fibers. Most of the tooth is made up of a moderately hard substance called dentin. In the center, there is a channel of pulp which carries the nerves and blood supply to the tooth, although some blood supply goes from the socket to the outside of the roots. If the pulp is injured by decay, it often becomes infected by germs which may spread through the pulp to the jawbone in the socket. This is often painful, and the tooth is sensitive to heat and cold; but sometimes it does not hurt, so x-rays are needed for diagnosis.

Root Canal Treatment

If the infected pulp is removed by root canal treatment and the germs are destroyed, fresh healthy pulp grows in to support and save the tooth in most cases. If the tooth has darkened, it can be bleached, and such teeth may last a lifetime—usually at less cost than replacing them with artificial teeth.

Broken Teeth

If the pulp is exposed in a fractured tooth, the nerve should be removed. The rest of the tooth can usually be repaired, sometimes with a porcelain jacket.

Teeth Knocked Out

Teeth knocked out of their sockets can sometimes be successfully re-emplanted. Wrap the tooth in a cool wet cloth and take the child and the tooth to the dentist at once. The sooner it is re-emplanted, the better the chance that the tooth will live. If a primary tooth is lost before the permanent tooth is ready to replace it, the teeth may shift, forcing the permanent teeth to come in crooked. Dentists often recommend space maintainers to preserve the space for the permanent tooth.

TEETH AND THUMBSUCKING

Will your child get buck teeth from sucking a thumb or pacifier? Perhaps your *child* will, but not your baby. Dentists say that thumb sucking is of no concern during the first several years; but thumbsucking beyond age five may affect the position of the permanent teeth and alter the shape of the jawbone. In order to understand and avoid damaging thumbsucking, you need to understand why babies suck their thumbs.

Dr. Richards points out the practicalities of thumbsucking in infants:

A baby who finds his thumb or finger during the first two or three months will usually enjoy it as a built-in pacifier and will continue sucking for several years, especially when bored, tired, unhappy, or hungry. Except for covering the hands twenty-four hours a day for three or four weeks, little can be done to stop the habit once it starts. Since covering the hands is both difficult and undesirable, one can only accept the situation and try to keep the baby well fed and entertained as much as possible.

Of course, some babies instinctively suck on something during most of their waking hours. After two or three months of age, it is a learned habit. When parents encourage extra sucking during the first year of life, the habit is almost certain to continue. Many babies don't need encouragement, and resist all efforts of their parents to discourage the habit. Others refuse to suck on anything after seven or eight months—and sometimes earlier.

All of this just re-emphasizes the theme of this book—that each child really is different. As the end of the first year approaches, most babies are too interested in the world around them to suck their thumbs, except when they are tired or unhappy. After two, sucking is usually seen most when the child is bored, especially in the winter time, when outdoor play is restricted. Sucking to go to sleep continues, but if the child is kept busy during the day, there is little reason to suck. At school age, the teasing of other children usually motivates the child to give it up completely during the day; and then it's not too much longer before the night habit is completely forgotten.

You *can* get your child to stop thumbsucking without harming him, says pediatrician McClellan: "The key is consistency. You should be for or against things and be so all the time. If you say 'no' today, make it 'no' tomorrow, and for all times. Don't confuse the issue by saying 'no' one day, 'yes' another, and 'maybe' a third. The child treated this way will learn to ignore his parent—and should."

However, Dr. Richards feels that scolding, bribing, punishing, teasing, and pulling the hand away from the mouth can only make a child more unhappy, and that it usually aggravates the problem. Dentists can at times convince older children to stop sucking the thumb—probably because they represent outside authority figures.

Emotional Thumbsucking

When do you decide that thumbsucking isn't just an infantile and physical problem but is a significant emotional problem? Pediatric psychiatrist Herman states:

> In my experience, some children suck thumbs; others are not at all interested in this natural pacifier. They become attached to thumbsucking while on the bottle and after weaning. There are no harmful effects from this practice; in fact, it has a tranquilizing effect. If it continues beyond age five, it would be wise for the parent to review how the child is spending time: does he have enough stimulation with other people? Many older thumbsuckers use it when they are tired, bored, or alone too much.
>
> When the habit continues into late childhood or adult life, sucking is invariably a sign of an emotional need. So get at the cause and don't look at the thumbsucking itself.

There is no question that continued thumbsucking after the age of five years will cause "buck" teeth and malocclusion. Maybe you can convince the child to stop if you follow Dr. McClellan's advice. Maybe not. Another out is to substitute a pacifier for the thumb.

The Pacifier

When babies cry between feedings or suck their thumbs, you can use a pacifier. Dr. Richards says:

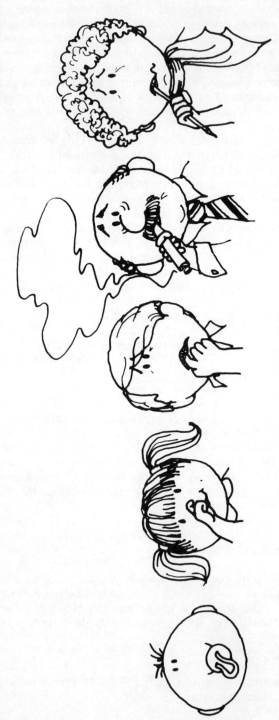

FIGURE 37

Used with discretion, a pacifier can be a real "mother's friend," but don't make it the first means of quieting the baby all of the time. During the first three months, a wakeful baby is usually a noisy crying baby who will continue crying until held or given something to suck. You can't hold him all of the time. When left alone to cry it out, he sometimes will have more endurance than you. When this happens, a pacifier may be all that is needed to help the baby relax and go back to sleep. So if you have nothing else demanding your attention, hold him. But, if your activities are piling up, or, at 2:00 a.m., when you just have to get some sleep, try the pacifier. It may work.

After three months of age, it's wise to begin taking the pacifier away, gradually. Use rattles, mobiles, and bright noisy toys to distract the baby. He will learn to play and entertain himself much more quickly if he is not sucking on a pacifier. One means of helping a baby learn to use his hands for play is to eliminate the pacifier completely by the fifth month.

When it is used too much of the time, many babies become "hooked," and after six months of age it is almost impossible to take the pacifier away. Save yourself and your baby a lot of unpleasantness by taking it away before problems develop. It's just not fair to a child to encourage the pacifier for a year or two and then suddenly tell him he can no longer have his best friend.

A word of caution to those who have older children. Often, it is a brother or sister who, upon learning that a pacifier works immediately to stop the crying, will be the one who is always putting it into the baby's mouth. So be on the alert to keep this from happening too much of the time.

Don't give a pacifier every time a baby cries. They cry for varied reasons. "In due time, a new parent will be able to recognize whether he is crying because he is hungry, wet, in pain, or is bored," writes pediatric professor Norman Kendall. "Each cry sounds different to the perceptive ear. Some babies may require a pacifier. They are not harmful." Pediatrician Hashim goes even further, and states: "The advantages do outweigh the disadvantages, so I am liberal in encouraging it at an early age. It may help prevent a potential thumbsucker. I think that stopping the pacifier at age five months may result in thumbsucking instead. I have had no trouble whatsoever in stopping the pacifier at age twelve months simply by throwing it in the garbage can and making it unavailable. Simply tell him the doctor said so and throw it away! This way of 'calling it quits' has worked well in my hands."

Perhaps, or perhaps not. Mother Nancy Cookson makes some very valid points against using pacifiers:

I have raised six children, and have found no need to use a pacifier. If babies are well fed, dry, stimulated through holding, cuddling, mobiles, musical toys, and so on, they are quite ready for the rest they need, and after a few minutes of fussing they usually fall fast asleep. Sometimes a buggy ride works wonders, and helps Mom get her figure back.

A baby will cry because he is hungry, wet, or dirty, or because he is getting sick. Giving him a pacifier can cover up the symptoms. I feel that a baby cries because he has a need, even if it's just to be held and cuddled. Holding and cuddling an infant, even several times a day, is not going to spoil him. Love him; he is young only once, and he is grown and gone before you know it.

Nail Biting

Nail biting is the next "best" thing to thumbsucking or pacifiers. It allows the thumb to be almost in the mouth in an almost acceptable manner. The traditional view is that nail biting is a sign of nervousness. "Try to find out what is causing the tension," counsels pediatrician Neil Henderson. "It usually is not a serious problem. If scary shows on television are causing it, they should be avoided. Constantly reminding the child not to bite on his nails is usually not successful, nor does putting foul-tasting materials on the nails work. Sometimes a mature two-year-old girl will do well by having a nail polishing set."

My view is that it is important for children to demonstrate to themselves that they can control their emotions and face up to the fact that nail biting is a substitute for thumbsucking, a form of oral gratification. There is nothing innately wrong with the habit, although it is hardly attractive. More to the point, it is a poor substitute for positive action toward fulfillment.

I have helped some older children stop biting their nails by explaining the genesis of nail biting. Ask the child why he bites his nails and don't accept "habit or nervousness." Point out that nervous means unhappy or fearful, and that the nail biting is a substitute for happiness. This started way back when all the little baby could do for himself for happiness was to suck his thumb. The habit continued until about school age when the other kids teased about the baby thumbsucker—so he stopped. And did what? The next nearest thing—biting the nails. The reason the child didn't know this is because he isn't running himself when he is biting the nails—his "baby part" is still controlling him.

Then ask whom he wants to have run himself: Does he want the baby part of him to be in control, or would he like to let his eight-year-old self run him? Most children say *I* want to run me, I don't want to have the baby part run me. Then print BABY with washable ink on the back of the four fingers, as a reminder to the child of "Who is running me now?" I have had remarkably good results with this technique. Most kids try to stop, and at least half or more succeed.

THE STRAIGHT FACTS ABOUT CROOKED TEETH

Thumbsucking, nail biting, and pacifiers all have an effect on the formation of the teeth. If all our fine advice is not read or taken seriously by your child, or if the child's jaws develop genetically in an unattractive or unphysiologic way, you may want the services of an orthodontist. We asked orthodontist Dr. Donald Hull, D.D.S., M.S., to give us the facts about the tooth straighteners.

Orthodontics deals with the correction of malocclusions—the irregular closing of the upper and lower jaws, and with the straightening of teeth.

1. Why is it necessary for a person to have "straight" teeth? Teeth that are crooked and crowded are difficult to keep clean and are more likely to decay. Crowded and crooked teeth can also be responsible for malocclusion, which can be very harmful to a child's general health. Teeth that don't meet properly interfere with chewing and put an abnormal burden on the jaw muscles. Improperly chewed food is often poorly digested. In addition, because they have difficulty chewing, many people refrain from eating the healthy foods their bodies need. Speech difficulties can result from malocclusion and its effect on the jaws. Dental deformities may also cause facial deformities, which may in turn cause emotional problems. An attractive smile is a great asset and helps a person present a pleasing appearance. Irregular or protruding teeth detract from appearance and can result in feelings of inferiority in some children and adults.

2. How can a parent know if his child will need orthodontics? Malocclusion is most obvious when the first teeth are being shed and permanent teeth are erupting. Specific signs include crowding, spaced or rotated teeth, protruding upper front teeth, a very prominent lower jaw, a weak lower jaw, or one swung to one side. Overly prominent lips due to protruding front teeth, front teeth which do not meet when the back teeth are closed, or a very deep bite are other causes for concern. If you are uncertain as to when you should consult an orthodontist, ask your dentist.

3. What is the difference between treating for cosmetic purposes and treating for health reasons? To the orthodontist, there is no such thing as treating for cosmetics alone. The patient sees the cosmetic improvement, but the orthodontist is striving to improve the function of the teeth and the supporting structures. Cosmetic improvement invariably follows improvements in tooth health.

4. Why are x-rays important? If the orthodontist is to diagnose the complete problem accurately, x-rays are an absolute necessity in the vast majority of cases. X-rays show many abnormalities otherwise unseen by the naked eye. A child may be congenitally missing a tooth or even several teeth—permanent teeth that never form. There are times when extra supernumerary teeth form and may block or divert the normal eruption of teeth. Sometimes, baby teeth do not resorb or dissolve properly, thus retarding the eruption of permanent teeth.

The orthodontist will usually need photographs, headfilms (a side view of the patient's head), study models, and x-rays in order to make a definite diagnosis. By using these aids, he can determine the treatment procedures to follow. Since no two conditions are identical, the treatment will be specific for each patient.

5. What determines the length of treatment? Many factors

influence the length of treatment. Inherited factors include the relative size of the teeth and the jaw, which determine the degree of crowding. A child who inherits a small jaw from one parent and large teeth from the other may have a more complicated and prolonged problem than other inherited combinations. Early loss of the baby teeth may cause drifting of the permanent teeth, which requires considerable time to restore them to the normal position. Tongue thrusting and finger and thumbsucking may prolong treatment.

The time estimates given for correction may be thrown off by lack of cooperation of the patient, who is responsible for proper wearing and use of elastics, neck straps, or headgear. If these are worn properly, the treatment time can be fairly accurately predicted by the orthodontist.

6. What determines the cost of orthodontic treatment? Some of the factors involved are: the complexity of the problem; the total time it will take to obtain satisfactory results; the number of visits the patient is to make; the cooperation of the patient; and the changes to be made in the appliance during treatment. Fees will, of course, vary from area to area, as they do for other commodities and services.

Most orthodontists require an initial fee to cover early visits, diagnosis, study models, x-rays, photographs, consultations, and banding. Payment for the remainder of the treatment can be arranged, usually as a monthly payment over a number of months or years. If a patient moves during treatment, transfers are made readily from one orthodontist to another, usually with very little cost to the patient.

7. Will "braces" cause cavities? Bands that are positioned and properly cemented can prevent decay on the portion of the tooth covered. An appliance in the mouth, however, can retain foods. The teeth should be kept scrupulously clean. The gums can become swollen during orthodontic treatment. This happens when the plaques on the teeth at the gum edge are not brushed off. If brushing instructions are followed, both the teeth and gums will be healthy during treatment.

8. Do orthodontic appliances cause pain and discomfort? Immediately following the cementing of bands and their adjustment, there is often soreness. A toothache type of pain is uncommon and should receive the immediate attention of the orthodontist. As the child becomes accustomed to the appliances, the discomfort and soreness will disappear.

9. Are retainers necessary? After orthodontic treatment, it is necessary in most cases to wear a retaining appliance. The teeth act almost as if they have memories. They try to return to their original position. The retainers hold them in their corrected position until the bone has "set-up" and the musculature has reformed to suit the teeth. The retaining portion of the treatment can be just as important as the active treatment phase.

10. Why is it more common now to see adults undergoing orthodontic treatment? The public is becoming aware that teeth will move at almost any age. Adults are turning to orthodontics as knowledge of the importance of good teeth to overall health becomes

more evident. The public is becoming accustomed to seeing adults in "braces," and this seems to give others courage to follow suit.

Orthodontics improves the esthetics, health, and hygiene of individuals, and adds a dimension of emotional stability to society. Your regular dentist is trained to detect approaching or present orthodontic problems; he will see that you are referred to a competent orthodontist for treatment.

A PERSPECTIVE ON THE MOUTH

As in other areas of *The Manual,* our emphasis is on the prevention of disease and the need for individual assessment of problems. The "teething time" illustrations are enclosed only to show the norms. Remember not to take it seriously if junior has nary a tooth in his head at the age of a year. If he is bright-eyed and alert, he may well beat you at chess before he is ten years old. But he may not have any intact teeth by then if you don't give him fluoride, or if you let him run around with a bottle of juice in his mouth. Those precious and expensive teeth can be kept intact if you use plaque discloser to help you learn proper brushing.

Dr. Hashim has blasted the reassuring nonsense that teething causes fever. We included the donnybrook about pacifiers and thumbsucking to point out that some of our expert advice often varies. It may contain a component of emotion as well as reason. At least we are honest about it. It may help parents to know that in spite of our differences in emotional attitude about sucking, we do agree on some things. The pacifier should not be used as a plug in lieu of love and attention. There is a time to quit thumbsucking, even if we don't agree on exactly when it should occur. And, if all else fails, Dr. Hull comes to the rescue with wire and bands and the sophisticated understanding that will produce a healthy million dollar smile.

9

THE CHEST,
ITS CONTENTS,
AND COUGHS

The ancient Chinese thought that the seat of the soul and emotions was the liver. Western culture favors the heart. Aside from congenital heart disease and very rare infections of the heart, most chest problems involve the lungs. The more common conditions are discussed here. Other infections that include the chest in their attack are discussed in Chapters 16 and 17.

INNOCENT, NORMAL, AND
FUNCTIONAL HEART MURMURS

Without reference to the soul, we include a short but clear description of heart murmurs in children by pediatric cardiologist Saul Robinson.

"Innocent," "normal," or "functional" heart murmur are words used to describe a sound heard by physicians with a stethoscope over or near a heart. It becomes louder with fever, excitement, or exercise. At one time or another, such a murmur is heard in at least sixty-five percent of all children as they grow up.

The exact cause of a functional murmur is not known. It is probably because we can hear the normal blood flow going through the heart with our excellent stethoscopes. The presence of this murmur in no way affects the normal life style of the child. Occasionally, a murmur will be somewhat different from the usual type, and the physician may wish to examine the child further before making a definite diagnosis. He can fortify his belief by doing an electro-cardiogram and an x-ray of the chest for heart size, as well as a blood count and urinalysis. If the murmur seems sufficiently atypical, further diagnostic studies may be recommended, such as cardiac catheterization, angiograms, or echocardiograms.

The diagnosis of an innocent murmur means that the child has no heart problem. No special restrictions of activity and no unusual nor more frequent examinations are indicated. The child does not need a special diet, added vitamin preparations, or special exercises. The presence of this murmur should not be used as a disciplinary weapon. Overemphasis on the aspects of the innocent murmur, or injudicious discussion regarding its presence, may give the child a tool to use against his parents or teachers when he or she wishes to avoid some unwelcome chore. A murmur is not synonomous with heart disease. Children may have a heart problem without murmurs, and, conversely, the presence of murmurs need not indicate a heart abnormality.

If the child is referred by his personal physician to a pediatric cardiologist for a confirmatory examination, the results of the normal examination should be given to the child and parents together, so that what is being told to the child is no different than what is being told to the parent.

The child with an innocent murmur is a well child who has no heart disease nor abnormality, and should be treated as any other well child.

ABNORMAL HEARTBEATS

The heartbeat is regulated by pacemaker cells in the heart that send electrical impulses to the heart muscle, causing the heart to beat—usually 60 to 90 beats a minute. Occasionally, hearts skip a beat; and this usually doesn't mean that anything is wrong, although you should let the doctor know. Rarely, the pacemaker gets confused, causing the heart to beat exceptionally rapidly, sometimes above 160 beats a minute. If this goes on too long, the heart may weaken; or the beat is so short that it becomes ineffective. Consult a physician who may want to get an electrocardiogram in order to determine what the problem is and to aid in treatment.

Do Chest Pains Mean Heart Trouble?

Children get chest pains, and mothers worry about whether this means heart trouble. The pain is usually localized discomfort over the breast bone or the left side of the chest. There are usually no other complaints, except maybe indigestion, and the child's activity, wind, and physical examination are all normal. Often, the pain and tenderness are due to a chest muscle strain. Often, they are due to soreness in the cartilage of the chest. Sometimes, these pains are due to a hyperacid stomach or to acid getting into the esophagus (the swallowing tube), and are relieved by milk or antiacid. They don't last long, and they don't mean heart trouble or anything serious. Rarely, chest pain occurs with an irregular heart beat or a heart rate, at rest, of over 180 beats per minute in older children. This can be determined by checking and counting the child's pulse.

To Check the Pulse

The pulse or heartbeat can be checked in several ways. The usual way is to feel it with the tips of the index and ring fingers touching gently on the thumb edge of the palm side of the wrist, about a half inch above the crease on the wrist. The pulse can also be felt high in the neck, in front of the ear, under the jaw, just at the edge of the muscle that runs from behind the ear to the breast bone. Usually you have to press the skin in about a half-inch at the edge of the muscle in order to feel the beat. A third way of checking the pulse is to put your ear flat to the bare chest over the heart. The pulse rate in children is normally a regular even beat, 60 to 90 times a minute, although when they are active it goes much higher. In infants, the average resting rate is 120, and in older children 80.

ENLARGEMENT OF THE BREASTS

One oft neglected part of sex education for young boys verging on adolescence is that their breasts may enlarge. As a normal stage of adolescence, the breast plate under the nipple becomes a hard, firm, dime-shaped lump. Occasionally, it gets sore; and often it frightens the boy who has wild fears about misdeveloping into a girl. Boys may be so ashamed of this abnormality that they say nothing about it. There are reported instances of breast enlargement and hormonal imbalance from heavy marihuana smoking and from a variety of prescription drugs in rare instances. Aside from that, you can reassure them that the breast plate development is normal, and that it will gradually vanish—and that if they quit smoking pot, their hormones will get back in balance also. It pays to tell them around the age of eleven to twelve that boys' breasts usually swell a little.

It is worth knowing that, when girls' breasts start developing, it is often on one side at first. This can cause a lot of unnecessary alarm. Later, as the breasts develop rapidly, the skin stretches—and linear marks develop, running along the breast. These stretch marks subside, and the skin will not show the marks once the rapid development slows down.

BRONCHITIS

Bronchitis is an inflammation of the lining of the bronchial tubes of the lung. When inflamed, they swell and excrete extra mucus, which reduces the airflow to and from the lungs. If the cause is allergy or viral infection, the cough produces a greyish mucus at first; but if the cause is bacterial infection, the mucus is usually yellow. Often, but not always, there is fever with bronchitis as well as the cough and spitting phlegm. Infants and children usually swallow the phlegm with no harm.

Although bronchitis may become chronic after a poorly tolerated infection, it is usually due to allergy in children, and to chronic cigarette smoking in adults. It is made worse by smog. Over a period of time, it may produce bronchiectasis.

Asthmatic Bronchitis

One type of bronchitis is asthmatic bronchitis. Dr. Hashim explains:

If your child huffs and has wheezy labored breathing, he may have asthmatic bronchitis. Even his stomach seems to work hard to help him breathe. The cough is usually tight, dry, hacky, and fairly frequent. His nose is runny, and his color is pale, occasionally with a bluish hue. His temperature may or may not be elevated, and his appetite is terrible. But the key sign of asthmatic bronchitis is the wheeze that occurs when the child is breathing out. Children who get it often have a family history of allergy. It is frequently triggered by a cold or an upper respiratory infection. Since a child is liable to pick up a cold easily, he may develop asthmatic bronchitis several times a winter.

Not every wheezer is asthmatic. A wheeze can be caused by conditions not related to allergy. Certain cases of pneumonitis look and behave like asthmatic bronchitis. Croupy children may seem similar to the wheezers if your ears are not trained well enough. Even a piece of a carrot stick or peanut aspirated into a bronchial tube can cause a wheeze.

Tracheobronchitis

When an infection primarily settles in the membranes lining the trachea, or windpipe, it causes a slightly different picture. While some of these infections may spread down into the bronchial tubes or further, most of the problem is just below the vocal cords. Dr. Hashim describes the clinical picture accurately.

His cough is barking, frequent, tight, and deep. He may or may not have fever. He usually looks and feels "lousy." These are the symptoms of tracheobronchitis. It occurs more frequently during the winter. If the cough is harsh, and if the child feels sick, don't wait too long before calling the doctor. Complications such as pneumonia may show up.

Coughs and Rattles

Some coughs or chest rattles are due to infections of the bronchial tree or lungs. Others which may sound as bad are due to allergy or mechanical causes, explains Dr. Charles Hoffman.

There is an allergic cough which is frequently a prelude to asthma, usually resulting from inhaled pollens or dust, but sometimes from food allergy. The membranes swell and the muscles constrict and a wheezy dry cough results. Sometimes, however, there is a wheezy loose cough, and a chest rattle, if mucus is excreted by the bronchial tubes. At other times there is a cough and rattle that have little to do with the chest. This is due to mucus from a postnasal drip puddling around the larynx. Some small infants who salivate a lot may have the same type of cough. When there is mucus around the larynx it often rattles with breathing and sounds as if it is in the chest. In a way it is like blowing on a horn, the sound is produced near the mouthpiece but is amplified in the horn itself. You can feel this by putting your hand on your chest when you say your name and feel the vibration in the chest wall.

Should You Stop Coughing?

Should you stop coughing? After all, that cough is dictated by bodily defenses that have helped mankind to survive. Usually, the cough is helpful. A cough is a reflex spasm of the diaphragm which expels air in short, intense bursts from the lungs. A successful cough will remove whatever is irritating the respiratory tract, whether it is peanuts, pollens, pus, or germs. Most soft or dissolvable foreign bodies will be coughed out. Some objects, however, like pieces of carrot, celery, apple, or nuts, do not dissolve and cannot get back through the narrow larynx. Children occasionally inhale irritating candy powder through straws; and, although the powder dissolves, it damages the mucosa and sets the lungs up for infection.

Infections of the mucous membranes of the throat, larynx, trachea, bronchi, and distal lungs cause cough. The cough is initiated by the mucosa, which has become so inflamed that it can no longer produce its healing and washing mucous. Then the cough is dry and nonproductive; in spite of all the effort, nothing is coughed up or out. A similar dry cough can occur from swollen lymph glands in the chest or dilated blood vessels.

When the mucous glands are irritated, or when the individual is dehydrated, the mucus produced may become thick and gummy. This is especially true for the asthmatic or fibrocystic. The body responds to the inflamed respiratory lining by sending white cells to combat the infection. These finally are able to help localize the infection and kill or neutralize the germs involved. The germs and white cells are coughed up with the mucus as pus. If the damage is deep, there may be serum oozing into the area, and on occasions small amounts of blood leak into the pus. It is essential that the mucus and pus which exudes into the tracheobronchial tree be coughed up, along with the germs and debris. If not, and if it sets in the lungs, the white cells die, and the high protein mixture is an excellent growth medium for many bacteria—thus perpetuating infection.

How Do You Stop a Cough?

From the foregoing descriptions it can be seen that coughing is an essential defense mechanism. Yet coughing is uncomfortable and at times unproductive and very fatiguing. There are several mechanisms which may help control or ease coughs:

Moisten the Dry Membranes and Moisten and Thin the Sputum

Water in one form or another is probably the best defense for inflamed, irritated respiratory membranes. When the membranes are inflamed, they dry out more quickly, and a thicker, less protective mucus is produced. The mucous cells are damaged by dryness, as they cannot function or survive without adequate moisture. The cilia, which sweep particles out of the lungs, cannot work without fluid. If dry, the membranes crack and open for deeper infection. Water can be furnished in three ways:

1. By mouth—it is absorbed and gets to the lungs via the blood stream. Dehydration reduces the amount of fluid available to the lungs, which use around thirty percent of our total daily water intake under normal conditions. Even if inhaled air is one hundred percent saturated with water, it is drying to the mucosa. Air is warmed by the mucosa prior to getting into the lungs; and the amount of water needed to saturate air is increased with increasing temperature. So a good intake of water is crucial, and if enough cannot be given by mouth, it will have to be given by vein.
2. Use expectorant cough syrups to increase the amount of water excreted by the mucosa, to thin the mucus, and to keep the membranes moist. The most common, and possibly the most effective, expectorant is potassium iodide. Other expectorants include small doses of syrup of ipecac, ammonium chloride, glyceryl guyacolate, and terpin hydrate.
3. Moisten the air:
   a. Steam is the old standby, but cool air has a higher relative humidity. Hot steam, however, has the added advantage, under some circumstances, of relaxing tense muscles in the throat and vocal cords.
   b. Fog is helpful, either through an open window if the outside air is foggy, or by the use of a cool mist vaporizer. The cool air has more moisture than the heated furnace air and dehydrates the lung less. At times, it may help by cooling and reducing the swelling of inflamed, congested respiratory membranes.

How to Use a Vaporizer or Humidifier

1. Use water only—never add medications to the humidifier. You can add medication to the hot steam vaporizer if you like the smell, but it will do no good.

2. Use it primarily at night or naptime.

3. Open the door to allow air to circulate. You don't usually need a sauna bath effect.

4. Set the vaporizer several feet away from the child and pointed at him.

5. If the vaporizer or humidifier seems to make the child's cough worse, which is rare, then don't use it.

6 A tent is needed only for some cases of croup (see page 151).

Soothe the Irritated Membranes

In the throat area where the membranes can be reached, there is nothing wrong with trying cough drops or a soothing solution of honey and lemon. Some physicians advocate candy or any thick sugar solution, which does temporarily bathe and relieve the irritated mucosa. A theory has been raised that the sugar encourages bacterial growth and "causes" infections. This is unproven, and seems unlikely, as there are always sugars in bodily secretions.

Medicated cough drops or vapors to put in steamers make an attempt to soothe the membranes by delivering smelly substances to the membranes deeper in the respiratory tract. These include menthol and tincture of benzoin, which can be classified as "counter-irritants." They are mildly irritating substances, although they don't seem to irritate enough to cause a cough. It seems unlikely that they achieve anything worthwhile. Yet many people swear by them, in spite of most physicians' skepticism. I don't know that they do any harm, unless one happens to be allergic to the chemical.

Suppress an "Ineffective" Cough

If there is nothing to cough up, the continued cough fatigues and unnecessarily congests the respiratory tract. Temporary relief is often obtainable by the use of sedative cough syrups. The most effective of these is codeine, and, like other narcotics, it is addicting. There is a nonaddicting, less effective, cough suppressant, dextromethorphan. Given routinely, codeine cough syrup becomes ineffective, because a tolerance to the codeine builds up. It is an excellent agent for the middle of the night, when a cough interferes with sleep and is fatiguing the patient. It is, however, irrational to use codeine to try to stop a cough all the time. Yet, for some severe nonproductive coughs, several days of suppressive cough syrup is logical to try.

How Can You Cure That Postnasal Drip Cough?

You may have postnasal drip when infected or allergic membranes in the back of the throat produce an irritating mucus that drips down the back of the throat. This initiates a cough which is frequently worse when you lie flat, since the mucus puddles rather than drains. It then has to be coughed away. Frequently, there are inflamed membranes around the larynx, which add to the problem. This type of cough at times responds to the following treatment:

1. Prop the head up at least six inches higher than the hips. (Use a wedge between the mattress and the box springs.)
2. Take an antihistamine decongestant that dries the nasopharynx and reduces the drip.

More About Treatments for Coughs

As you can see, coughs are not simple. Nor is treatment always clear-cut. Doctors can be more specific on an individual basis and can use antibiotics and other medicines, including prescription cough syrups. We find, however, that at times there are disagreements between doctors. Dr. Hashim, for example, offers a list of things you can do at home to reduce the cough of asthmatic bronchitis.

1. A central humidifier for the house or apartment will raise the humidity and give the respiratory tree a good break.
2. An electronic air filter is helpful.
3. Avoid sudden exposure to extremes of temperature.
4. Avoid irritants at home such as cigarettes, pipe, or cigar smoke; the smell of fresh paint; and kitchen fumes.
5. Avoid all dust collections, stuffed toys, rugs, drapes, and so forth.
6. Avoid animals—dogs, cats, birds, and so forth.

As is often the case, there are many ways of skinning a cat or of treating chest conditions. Dr. David Sparling notes:

Although asthma and asthmatic bronchitis overlap, there are differences that are important. If the wheeze is primarily triggered by infections, it is unlikely that an allergy work-up or an electrostatic air filter will be of as much help as in "pure asthma."

So you may still need your own doctor's advice. But what about grandmother's advice to use a chest rub? Here Dr. Hashim takes a firmer stand:

Although medicated chest rubs used to be very popular, and both your mother and mother-in-law still swear by them, they will do you no good. Scientifically speaking, there's little justification for their use. Room sprays are also of little value and may even be harmful. Don't waste your money, time, and effort on them. Stick to the good old vaporizer or humidifier.

I prefer the cool mist humidifier that produces a more effective mist to reach the deep areas of the bronchial tree where the moisture is needed. However, if you have an old-fashioned steam vaporizer, keep it until it breaks down. My enthusiasm for treating bronchitis by moistening the air is not shared by chest specialist Birt Harvey, who contends that there is no evidence that this affects the course of bronchitis and points out that cool mist units may become contaminated with bacteria and molds. Others believe that the increased comfort, reduced cough, and less loss of moisture from the lungs with cool mist units makes them valuable anyway. See page 275 for prevention of mold and bacterial contamination of the mist unit.

CHRONIC COUGHS

When coughs become really persistent and last over a few weeks, there are more conditions to consider. A chronic cough in a child may have no serious import, or it may be a portent of life-threatening illness. Pediatrician Birt Harvey, a pulmonary disease expert, discusses conditions causing chronic coughs.

It is not uncommon for the cough associated with the runny nose of a cold to persist after the runny nose stops. A cough such as this may last for several weeks. If there is no fever associated with the cough, the child acts well, and the cough gradually decreases in frequency and severity; a physician need not be consulted. In winter, young children often have one cold after another. The cough of one respiratory infection blends right into the cough of the next. Should the cough last more than several weeks, or should fever, lethargy, or increased severity of cough develop, it is wise to speak to the doctor.

Cough may also be associated with a runny nose due to allergies. This usually follows a seasonal pattern, primarily in the spring or the fall, but it can occur at all times of the year. The runny nose associated with an allergic cough generally remains watery and may be associated with sneezing, itching of the nose, eyes, and mouth, and tearing from the eyes. The allergy cough is more inclined to be a dry, nonproductive sounding cough, and may at times be associated with a wheeze on exhalation of air from the lungs. Such a cough and mild wheeze may be the forerunner of significant asthma.

When a cough occurs *without* an associated runny nose, consult a physician sooner in the course of the illness. If there is no fever, and if the child acts well, you may wait several days and treat the child with a cough medicine to loosen his cough. If there is fever (over 100°), and if the child acts ill, consult his doctor quite promptly, since such a cough may be due to a bacterial infection of the lungs.

Bacterial infection in the lungs can cause serious tissue damage. If severe enough it may destroy the inner lining of the bronchial tubes. The tubes then bulge out and mucus and debris accumulate in a condition called bronchiectasis. Special x-ray studies with a dye in the bronchial tubes is needed to diagnose and treat this condition. Chronic lung infection in a child with bulky, foul, and frequent stools may mean a child has cystic fibrosis, an inherited lung disease characterized by chronic cough and failure to grow well.

PNEUMONIA

We asked the prestigious and effective American Lung Association to give you the facts about pneumonia and how it is treated.

Pneumonia means an acute inflammation of the lung caused by an invasion of living organisms. As the result of the inflammation, the lung tissue and spaces become filled with liquid matter. Only a generation ago, pneumonia meant a terrible ordeal. It was a death sentence for one out of every four cases. Today, thanks to many varied and effective antibiotics, pneumonia no longer holds such terror. There are three main causes of pneumonia: bacteria, viruses, and mycoplasma.

Bacterial Pneumonia. Bacterial pneumonia can attack persons of any age. The pneumococcus is the most common cause of bacterial pneumonia. Today, mortality from pneumonia caused by the pneumococcus and streptococcus is low. That caused by the staphylococcus, which is usually contracted in the hospital, is quite high. Patients with pneumonia caused by the Klebsiella bacteria also have a high mortality rate.

Pneumonia bacteria may be present in healthy throats. Only when body defenses are weakened in some way do the bacteria multiply and do serious damage, working their way into the lungs and inflaming the air sacs. The tissue of part of a lobe of the lung, or even an entire lobe, becomes completely filled with liquid matter. (This is called consolidation.) The infection quickly spreads through the blood stream and the whole body is invaded. The symptoms of bacterial pneumonia are varied, and the onset can be gradual to sudden. The patient may experience chills, severe chest pain, and a cough that sometimes produces rust-colored sputum. The temperature often shoots up as high as 105.0 F. The patient sweats, and his breathing and pulse rate increase rapidly. He may have a bluish skin due to lack of oxygen if his pneumonia becomes severe.

Virus Pneumonia. Half of all pneumonias are believed to be of viral origin. More and more viruses are being identified as the cause of respiratory infection, and though most attack the upper respiratory tract, some produce pneumonia, especially in children. Most of these pneumonias are patchy and self-limiting.

The initial symptoms of virus pneumonia are those of influenza: fever, a dry cough, headaches, muscle pain, and prostration. Within 12–36 hours there is increasing breathlessness, the cough becomes worse, and sometimes produces a scant amount of bloody sputum. There is a high fever, and sometimes there is blueness of the skin. Often, virus pneumonias are complicated by an invasion of bacteria with all its typical symptoms of bacterial pneumonia.

Mycoplasma Pneumonia. Identified during World War II, mycoplasmas are the smallest free-living causes of disease in man, unclassified as to whether bacterial or viruses, but having characteristics of both. They generally cause a mild but widespread pneumonia. They affect all age groups but occur most frequently in older children and young adults. The death rate is low, even in untreated cases.

The most prominent symptom of mycoplasma pneumonia is a cough that tends to come in violent paroxysms but produces only sparse whitish sputum. Chilly sensations and fever are early symptoms. Some patients experience nausea and vomiting.

Prompt treatment with antibiotics almost always cures bacterial and mycoplasma pneumonia, and a certain percentage of rickettsia pneumonia. [There is some evidence that treating mycoplasma or "walking pneumonia" too early may interfere with the development of immunity, so doctors may elect to defer treatment for a time.] There is no effective treatment yet for viral pneumonia. The drugs used depend on the germ causing the pneumonia, and on the judgment of the physician. Drugs lower the temperature within a day or two and produce a dramatic recovery. After the temperature returns to normal, medication must be continued according to the physician's instructions; otherwise, the pneumonia may recur. Relapses can be far more serious than the first attack. Besides antibiotics, patients are given supportive treatment: proper diet, oxygen to relieve breathlessness, medication to ease chest pain, and, in the case of mycoplasma, some relief from the violent cough.

There is no way known to prevent pneumonia, and there are no specific measures for its control. There is little prospect that a vaccine can be developed that will be effective against all the different organisms that cause pneumonia. (An effective vaccine against pneumococcal pneumonia has been developed but will probably be used only for individuals who are especially susceptible.) Since pneumonia often follows ordinary respiratory infections, the most important preventive measure is for a person to be alert to any symptoms of respiratory trouble that linger for more than a few days. Good health habits—proper diet and hygiene, plentiful rest, regular exercise, increase resistance to all respiratory illnesses and help promote fast recovery.[1]

BRONCHIOLITIS

As bad as some pneumonias can be for infants, a condition called bronchiolitis can, at times, be worse. Under the age of a year the trachea and bronchial tubes are small; even smaller tubes called bronchioles branch off and lead to the alveoli (air sacks) where oxygen is absorbed. Some virus infections can cause the membranes in the bronchioles to swell. As there isn't much room to start with, this makes it very difficult for air to get to the alveoli.

Babies with this type of infection obviously will have trouble breathing. They sometimes grunt, become pale, and always have a very high respiratory rate—usually well over 60 breaths a minute. Sometimes they have fever with the infection and sometimes they don't. In either case they usually need the doctor's attention and may require special treatments to help reduce the swelling.

WHAT DOES SMOKING DO TO YOUR HEALTH?

- Doubles the heart attack rate.
- Increases blood pressure.
- Narrows the arteries to the hands and feet.
- May cause lung cancer.
- Causes emphysema.
- Creates indigestion.
- Slows healing of duodenal and gastric ulcers.
- Aggravates colds and bronchitis.
- May cause allergic symptoms.
- Annoys nonsmokers who therefore may not like you as much, which is depressing.

- Infants and children in families with smokers have more respiratory infections than those in nonsmoking families.
- May contribute to atherosclerosis (hardening of the arteries).

Remember that filters remove only some of the many harmful substances in cigarette smoke. Pipes and cigars are safer than cigarettes, but they too can lead to deteriorating health. The best approach to smoking is not to start—it's a lot harder to stop than it is to start.

SUMMARY: ELEVEN POINTS FOR CHEST HEALTH

The contents of the chest are wonderous indeed. The heart can murmur yet can work beautifully well. The lungs are far more than two complicated bags of air. Out of this chapter, there are some facts to be emphasized and some preventive steps to follow:

1. An innocent heart murmur should not be allowed to make an emotional cripple of a child because of misunderstanding fearful parents.
2. Pains over the heart in children and young adults are usually due to mild cartilage irritation or digestive upset.
3. A child with a long-term cough, recurrent infections, and foul frequent stools may have cystic fibrosis.
4. Bronchitis, or inflammation of the bronchial lining, can result from smog, allergy, or viral or bacterial infection.
5. Asthmatic bronchitis is discussed in Chapter 15 on allergy.
6. Tracheobronchitis is related to croup.
7. Chronic bronchitis or bronchiectasis seems to be partly due to personal smog —cigarettes.
8. Pneumonia is an infection of the tissue of the lung itself, and is due to viruses, mycoplasma, or bacteria, although special pneumonias can be due to the inhalation of foreign bodies, silica dust in coal mines, fungi, or rickettsia. Bacterial and mycoplasma pneumonias respond well to antibiotic treatment.
9. Smoking is stupid.
10. Chronic cough over a few weeks deserves a check by your doctor.
11. Don't just try to stop a cough: It is a friend. Help it with moist air and lots of liquids. Prop yourself up and take decongestants if it is caused by only a postnasal drip cough.

10

YOUR STOMACH AND BOWELS

This chapter concentrates on what happens to the gastrointestinal tract under a variety of common circumstances. Specific biological, physical, and chemical agents which incite "gut" reactions are discussed in the Enemies of Man section. Throughout *The Manual,* you will find diseases and conditions which can adversely affect the gut. Not only may it suffer insults of all sorts, but it reflects our own emotions. We hope that you will get a better view and understanding of this wonderful individualistic complex tube which sustains us in this world.

Figure 38 shows the anatomy and diseases of the intestinal tract. The numbers 1 through 13 refer to the anatomy as follows: (1) tongue, (2) esophagus, (3) diaphragm, (4) stomach, (5) liver, (6) gall bladder, (7) pyloris of stomach, (8) pancreas, (9) small bowel, (10) large bowel, (11) appendix, (12) rectum, (13) anus. The numbers 14 through 23 refer to diseases: (14) Choking sensations in the neck may be due to spasm of the esophagus. (15) Pain in the chest may be due to gastric juice from the stomach getting into the esophagus or the stomach being pinched from pushing into the hole in the diaphragm. (16) Yellow skin or dark brown or orange urine may indicate hepatitis-liver inflammation. (17) Pain after meals may indicate gall bladder disease or gall stones or gastritis. (18) Stomach pain before breakfast may indicate hyperacidity or ulcer in a child. (19) Loose stools and poor weight gain may indicate cystic fibrosis. (20) Poor weight gain, cramps, loose stools, blood in the stools may indicate disease of the small bowel. (21) Cramps after eating may indicate inflammation of the stomach or of the large bowel (colitis). (22) Cramps in the right lower side of the abdomen may indicate ap-

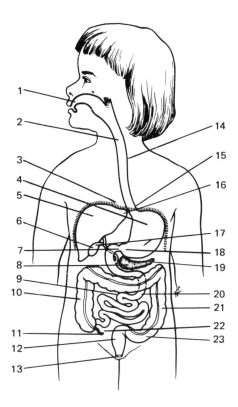

FIGURE 38 *Anatomy and diseases of the intestinal tract.*

pendicitis. (23) Blood in the bowel movement if black may indicate ulcers; if red and jelly-like, intussusception; if bright red, colitis or fissure. Pain on bowel movement may indicate fissures, constipation, or an inflamed bowel.

THE ANATOMY OF THE DIGESTIVE TRACT

The anatomy of the intestinal tract is complicated and wondrous indeed. However, it is made easy to understand by the deft pen of pediatrician A. S. Hashim.

The digestive tract is the tube that handles food from the time we eat until we expel the remnants in the form of a bowel movement. The system starts at the mouth and ends at the rectum.

This tube is indeed unique. It is straight in certain areas, such as the esophagus or gullet. It has many unusual and complex parts like the mouth and lips, teeth, tongue, palate, and the salivary glands. It bulges almost like a football to form the stomach. It curves on itself like a boa constrictor to form the small intestine. Then it curves like an upside-down U-shape to form the large intestine. Finally, it ends in the rectum and anus, where waste is disposed. There are places along the way where organs and glands, such as the liver and pancreas, secrete juices to help digest food.

In the mouth, food is lubricated, chewed, and treated with enzymes from the saliva. In the stomach, it is churned, mixed, and kneaded with acids and more enzymes. The food matter breaks down into fine particles and is prepared for further digestive steps.

In the small intestine, it is mixed with juices from the pancreas and liver. After so many hours of hard work by the intestine, the nourishing microscopic food particles are absorbed through the walls of the intestine. Other chemical changes then occur to help make these particles suitable as food for the organs. The roughage and remnants of the food, mixed with a fantastic number (zillions!) of bacteria, form the bulk of the bowel movement.

The special roles all these parts and processes play offer many opportunities for things to go wrong with the digestive tract. The teeth can decay; the tongue can be bitten; the throat can be inflamed; the parts down below can be attacked and infected by bacteria or viruses; the organs may not function in perfect unison, creating special problems; the digestive tube may become blocked in certain areas, posing a threat to life; the same digestive tube can come out through certain weak points in the walls of the abdomen, leading to hernia. The rectum can have its own special problems. In a baby, it can crack, resulting in a fissure and notoriously painful bowel movements. Or it may have some birth defect requiring corrective surgery.

After reading all these gloomy facts, parents should realize that although the places where malfunction can occur are many, the instances of serious abnormality are relatively rare.

Are Your Child's Stomach Aches Serious?

Parents often ask, "How do I know if my child's many complaints of stomach aches should be taken seriously?" We turned to Australian pediatrician Eric Sims for advice on this subject. He tells me that children have as many stomach aches in Australia as in the United States.

Very small children, of course, do not localize pain very well and are apt to say they have "a tummy ache" when in fact they have a sore throat. Children in this age group, therefore, need a careful examination to exclude the possibility of serious illness. A "tummy ache" is not likely to be anything very serious if there are no other associated discomforts, such as fever, cough, or a bowel upset.

The bigger problem for parents is the slightly older child, perhaps of school age, who always seems to be complaining of pains in the tummy. Probably the most common cause of this symptom is nervous stress; a clue is the timing of the pain, which is apt to occur in the mornings before school and diminish as the day goes on. It will rarely occur on weekends. As in the toddler, abdominal pain as a *solitary* complaint from an older child is not likely to be serious; it is rarely an ominous symptom if it is not associated with vomiting or some other objective evidence of real trouble. You can safely be guided by common sense: If the child does not look ill, has no urgent call for bladder relief, or bowel movement, and has no obvious tenderness or muscle tightness when you gently press the abdomen, you do not need to rush him to the doctor.

Nevertheless, the constant complaint of abdominal pain, even if it is a manifestation of stress, is still a "cry for help." While you are reassuring him about the symptom, it is necessary to consider both the school and home circumstances that might be causing unhappiness and stress. When he complains of tummy aches, stay calm, and see if you can "get under his skin," not only to exclude physical illness but also to unravel the real problem he has unconsciously revealed to you with his apparently physical complaint.

When Should You Suspect and How Do You Diagnose Appendicitis?

The appendix is a small hollow "thumb" hanging off the colon in the right lower side of your abdomen. Like the rest of the bowel, it can become infected and irritated. True appendicitis does not occur unless the membranes swell enough to block the opening to the bowel, or unless some object plugs the hole. When this happens, the muscles in the appendix cramp down, trying to push its contents out through the opening. This causes spasms of pain. Local pressure damages the mucosa and leads to infection, which spreads through the appendix, causing the organ to become red and swollen. White blood cells come to fight the infection and a membrane in the abdominal cavity called the omentum wraps around the area to seal it. The inflammation causes the general area to become sore. The muscles overlying the inflammation stiffen to protect it from outside pressure. If the inflammation continues, it may spread through the abdominal cavity and cause peritonitis. Actually, most cases of appendicitis do not cause peritonitis, and some will heal themselves without surgery. But do not take the risk, because a ruptured appendix and peritonitis can kill. Where there is reasonable suspicion of appendicitis, the conservative path is an appendectomy.

There are unnecessary appendectomies. Pain, guarding, and tenderness in the area, associated with low grade fever, lack of appetite, vomiting, and perhaps a bit of diarrhea are typical symptoms of appendicitis. But they can also occur from other causes. These include mesenteric adenitis or swollen tender lymph glands next to the bowel, a right ovarian cyst, an infected fallopian tube, or even intussusception in the right lower quadrant. Even the best doctors are not always certain.

Therefore, a percentage of appendectomies are justifiably done on normal appendixes. But it is better to err on that side than to chance a rupture. Another complicating factor is that an appendicitis can occur in the midst of another disease, such as intestinal flu, scarlet fever, or measles.

Ordinarily, an appendix requires around twelve hours to become fully inflamed. Sometimes, but not always, the diagnosis is apparent earlier. The signs and symptoms to look for are:

1. Low grade fever.
2. Lack of appetite and often vomiting.
3. Mild diarrhea or loose stools.
4. Colicky or cramping pain starting around the belly button and gradually settling out in the right lower abdomen.
5. Firm muscles which will not relax with gentle pressure to the right and below the belly button midway between it and the crest of the hip.
6. Pain in the area of inflammation on walking; frequently, the individual cannot straighten up without pain and walks like an old, bent-over person.

Here are two tests to perform on suspected victims:

1. Have the child lie straight on his left side. Pull his right knee backwards. If it causes pain in the right lower quadrant of the abdomen, be suspicious.
2. If gentle and steady pressure on the abdomen, followed by sudden release, causes a sharp pain, be suspicious.
3. Have the child stand high on his toes and then come down really hard (with the knees stiff) . If this causes pain in the abdomen, be *very* suspicious.

These tests are not foolproof. At times, appendicitis is very difficult to diagnose, even by experienced physicians. The appendix may be tucked away behind the bowel and cause back pain. In very rare instances, it is on the left side. Or it may be deep in the pelvis, covered well by omentum. Atypical cases do occur. If you suspect appendicitis, call your physician; do not give laxatives; do not use a heating pad on the abdomen; and do not offer the child anything to eat or drink until you have the doctor's permission. Dr. Hashim adds that, "During the intestinal "flu" season, many will think that the stomachache, nausea, and vomiting are from the intestinal bug going around. Sometimes, the cause is a ruptured appendix."

OTHER CAUSES OF RECURRENT ABDOMINAL PAIN

Stomach aches are not always easy to diagnose. Of the many different causes some are common; some aren't writes pediatric allergist Dr. William Crook.

For example, your youngster may be experiencing trouble with his reading at school. Or he may be afraid of his teacher, who has been

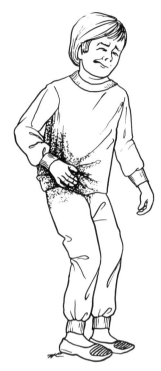

FIGURE 39 *The pain of severe appendicitis makes it hurt to straighten up and walk. Much of the time the pain is not that severe.*

criticizing him and making him stay in after school. Or he may feel insecure and tense because of something that has happened at home.

He could also have a heavy infestation of roundworms; or he could have a hidden kidney disorder. He might even have a chronic infection of his appendix (although most doctors feel this sort of appendicitis almost never occurs).

There is yet another cause for abdominal pain—allergy. You should especially consider the possibility of allergy if other physical causes of abdominal pain are ruled out by your physician. You should also suspect allergy if your child is irritable, looks pale, and has circles under his eyes, and if he complains of headache and aching in his legs or other muscles.

Physicians interested in systemic allergy advise: "Before blaming any child's recurrent stomachache on some ill-defined emotional cause, allergy should be ruled out. Often, such an allergy is caused by a food or foods the child eats every day."

Do Children Get Ulcers?

Children and adolescents get ulcers more frequently than most people realize. The most characteristic symptom is a stomachache on awakening. On occasions, there will be bleeding, with black tarry stools, and the child may be pale. Usually, the pain is relieved by eating or by antacids.

Why should children get ulcers? Because they lead very stressful lives. There are three peaks of ulcers in children and adolescents, around ages five, ten, and seventeen years. Each of these times is associated with peaks of emotional stress and concern over growing up and separating from parents and home. The five-year-old enters a new phase of life as he is pushed out into the jungle of kindergarten. The ten-year-old has usually made up his mind that he is not going to marry mother after all and is looking adolescence in the face. Those are causes enough for a stomachache. The seventeen-year-old has about finished blaming his folks for all his problems and is looking at the fact that he is responsible for his own life and must soon make gut-wrenching decisions about his future.

Naturally there are all sorts of stomach aches that are not from ulcers. Emotions may well cause colitis or spasms and weeping of the small and large bowel, as well as hyperacidity and stomach ulcers. One type of ulcer with pain and bleeding occurs in the small bowel if the small outpouching (a Meckels diverticula) which leads to the umbilicus during the fetal state has not vanished. This appendix-like thumb of bowel often has stomach tissue in it which excretes acid just like (and at the same time as) the stomach. As there is no food for the acid to work on, it can cause an ulcer in the bowel. This type of ulcer usually requires surgery, for it is difficult to diagnosis and treat.

CAUSES OF VOMITING

A whole host of things can cause vomiting in children. In toddlers you should first rule out ingestion of some household poison or plant. Check the material vomited to see if you can spot pills or plant parts, or smell chemicals. Beyond that Dr. Sims explains that the bowel has been described as the "sounding box" of the child.

Almost any illness that a child may get can cause vomiting. Vomiting instead of coughing, for instance, may be the presenting symptom of *pneumonia* (with or without abdominal pain). Usually parents are alerted because, in addition to vomiting, the child may have had "a cold" for a day or two, and may be breathing with some distress.

Vomiting may also be due to other things not directly related to the bowel, such as an *inflamed eardrum, tonsilitis, or meningitis.* There are several germs that can inflame the meninges (the membranes surrounding the brain), especially in young children. Recovery will be no problem if treatment with appropriate antibiotics is started early. The onset of *meningitis* can be quite indefinite: a "vaguely miserable" infant, with or without fever, who exhibits reluctance to feed, drowsiness, and vomiting. Usually, the neck is stiff or painful when an attempt is made to bend it, or to put the chin on the chest. The general condition usually worsens rapidly over the course of a day or so, with increasing drowsiness, perhaps convulsions, and irritability, suggesting severe headache. The diagnosis is established by a spinal tap (lumbar puncture), which your doctor will promptly do if he finds no other adequate explanation for the symptoms after his examination of the throat, ears, chest, urine, blood count, and so forth.

A urinary tract infection is a common cause of vomiting in children, especially girls. The doctor will probably want to look at a freshly passed specimen of urine under the microscope for any child brought to him with vomiting and "general misery," even if the common symptoms of infection (frequent urination and "burning") are absent.

Finally, vomiting may arise naturally from the various things that cause an "acute abdomen." The most common acute abdominal emergency in *early* childhood is *intussusception,* in which a segment of bowel gets forced into the segment ahead of it, like a sleeve being turned inside out. This usually happens in infants and toddlers, and starts with "colicky pain" (a gripping pain that comes and goes, and comes again) and vomiting. If the intussusception continues, blood may appear in the bowel movement. This is always an emergency, but if the condition is recognized promptly, it can often be cured by an enema under x-ray control.

The most common acute abdominal emergency after babyhood is *appendicitis,* which classically starts with abdominal pain around the navel, and, over the next twelve to twenty-four hours, moves to the lower right side, where the child is tender and rigid if touched. Vomiting is usually present, and there may be a disturbance of bowel function. The child may be feverish, and he looks genuinely ill. You are rarely in doubt that you need to call the doctor, although the severity of the symptoms can vary surprisingly, because the appendix can lie in different positions.

There are other possible causes: beta-hemolytic streptococcus infections, pneumonia, croup, appendicitis, nerves, head injuries, and several other conditions. Most vomiting occurs with many types of viral "flu" infections. At times, it is associated with diarrhea, which increases the possibility of *dehydration.*

Call the doctor if vomiting continues for several hours, or if there are other significant symptoms: heacache, stomachache between the spells of vomiting, or swollen tender lymph glands in the neck. Does it hurt to walk, or does the child walk bent over because it hurts to straighten up? Have the child curl up and touch his forehead to his knee to make certain that the neck isn't stiff. Read the earlier section on appendicitis.

How Should You Treat Vomiting?

Meanwhile, if the vomiting persists, the child may become dehydrated. Often, he will be able to sip and keep down a single teaspoon of Coca-Cola. A larger amount may be vomited. Give the child a teaspoon of Coke every ten minutes. If this is held down after one or two hours, offer an ounce every twenty to thirty minutes. Ginger ale or 7-Up will do, although Coke is best. Tea with sugar is another good fluid, but milk or plain water are poor. If vomiting persists for several hours, or if the child hasn't urinated in over eight hours, there is a danger of dehydration. Call his physician.

Furious Vomiting

Dr. Sims posed the question, "Should you be concerned about your child's tendency to vomit furiously for a day or two at various times?" This type of cyclic vomiting can be a real problem.

Some children, especially those whose parents have a history of migraine headaches, are very prone to sudden bouts of vomiting, often associated with fever. These continue for a day or two and then stop just as suddenly as they started. Some doctors call it "cyclical vomiting"; others "periodic acidosis"; still others "abdominal migraine." It seems to be the reaction of a particular sort of child to any sort of stress. Sometimes, it may be triggered by a typical childhood illness or infection such as tonsillitis; sometimes it may be by emotional excitement or other nervous stresses. This is the type of child who can never get to his own birthday party without throwing a fever and a bout of vomiting, in eager anticipation.

It is wise to call the doctor when your child first experiences "cyclical vomiting," if only to investigate the possibility of serious illness. But if the attacks recur and follow their typical pattern of sudden onset and offset with a quick return to bounding health, you'll gradually learn to live with it until he "grows out of it." Any child who reacts in this way to physical or emotional stress does slowly grow out of the cyclical vomiting pattern, but he is apt to grow slowly into the more adult type of migrainous sick headache with fuzzy vision.

The fact that a child is prone to react this way in his youth to even minor stress does not automatically make him immune to other coincidental illnesses. A child who usually has one of these bouts of vomiting with a sore throat or some minor ailment may one day have an attack of vomiting which is not following its usual pattern: It may be associated with more abdominal pain than usual, and with a tender tummy and tightness over the appendix. In this case, you would certainly *call the doctor;* this time it could be *appendicitis* rather than his usual "bilious attack." Similarly, children may have recurrent abdominal upsets from kidney troubles, so a doctor usually advises a few routine investigations early in a "bilious" child's life to make quite sure that nothing is being overlooked. After that, you can safely relax whenever your child "does his thing," unless any particular attack doesn't fit the pattern.

In some cases, dehydration (excessive loss of fluids) can be a problem. Some children with this type of vomiting almost routinely require intravenous feedings to rehydrate them and stop the spells. Watch for decreased or absent urination as one sign of dehydration.

DIARRHEA

Diarrhea, or loose watery stools, is an ailment common to small children. Normal stools of newborn infants (especially if the infant is breast or formula fed) are often watery, contain small yellow curds, and occur after almost every feeding. Homogenized cow's milk causes large formed stools. If, after the newborn's first week, the stools are green or contain mucus, it could be a symptom of diarrhea. One or two loose stools a day for a few days is usually not significant. A loose stool every hour or so in an older infant may be considered diarrhea—and *is* severe diarrhea in most children.

A mild diarrhea is five or less watery stools a day. When there are ten or more stools, and if the child looks greyish, vomits much, or has fever, call the doctor. Dehydration is a real danger.

There are many possible *causes* of diarrhea: poisons, nervousness, bacteria (salmonella, shigella), and viruses of many sorts. If there is tenderness to pressure on the lower right side of the abdomen, don't forget the possibility of appendicitis. Be certain to *call the doctor* if there is fever, if there is blood or much mucus in the stools, if the child's fluid intake is poor, or if the diarrhea lasts longer than a week.

Diarrhea Is *Good?*

An irritated bowel tends to become very active. It absorbs less fluid than usual from the stool and may actively excrete fluid and mucus into the bowel, prompting frequent and fluid bowel movements. Mother Nature's reaction to most poisonings and bowel infections is to "get rid of it." Research bears out the natural approach; according to one researcher, diarrhea in certain gastroenteric infections should be viewed as a protective medicine—like the cough in pneumonia. It keeps the patient from developing more severe illness.

Medicines which slow down the bowel and reduce diarrhea make patients more susceptible to some bacterial bowel infections. This research should do much to reduce the urge for the treatment of diarrhea with paregoric and other antispasmotics. Diarrhea may be good for you! Also stomach acid tends to reduce the chance of bowel infection by killing bacteria before they reach the bowel. Therefore, antiacids reduce this protective effect and increase susceptibility to infection—and perhaps should be avoided.

Checking the amount of urine output is one method of determining whether the child is dehydrated. Loss of body fluids is a dangerous aspect of diarrhea. It is not important that a child eat solid foods during diarrhea, but the *liquid intake* is important. Do *not* give milk, vegetables, laxative fruits (prunes, plums, apricots), greasy, spicy, or fried foods. If the child's diarrhea is mild and if he is hungry, offer Jello (avoid red or green Jello, as it may color the stool) , boiled or baked potato, rice, soda crackers, or lean meat.

There is more than water in the watery stools of diarrhea. Salts, especially sodium and potassium, are lost in quantity. This is made worse if only plain water is taken in to assuage the dehydration—it exaggerates the salt loss. So it is wise to give salt-containing fluids rather than plain water. Soft drinks are sometimes better than fruit juice in the early stages of treatment. Tea is high in potassium and is usually well tolerated. One cheap recipe for replacing fluids lost from diarrhea contains one cup of weak tea, four tablespoons of sugar, one-half level teaspoon of salt and one-fourth level teaspoon of baking soda in a quart container—with water added to fill the container. It is horrible stuff but many children like it! There are more sophisticated commercial mixes, and not all doctors approve of the home brew. Beyond that, every doctor seems to have his own favorite diarrhea diet. Pediatrician James Bramham suggests ice chips, tea with sugar, and soft drinks at first; then he offers soups and milk. Others of us believe milk should be the last thing offered. Probably the results depend on the digestive capacities of the individual patient.

What Causes Travelers' Diarrhea?

Many people develop diarrhea when traveling. This has been blamed on many things, mostly "the water." If it *is* the water, it is because the water contains human bowel bacteria. Infection with such bowel bacteria is more likely to be introduced by contaminated food rather than water, since most urban water supplies are adequately chlorinated. Yet the natives don't seem to have diarrhea; at least they don't advertise it. Probably most of them have had it in the past and are now immune to the disease-producing *E. coli,* shigella, or salmonella which reside in their intestines. Shigella and salmonella infections are often quite severe, while *E. coli* infections are usually mild in older children and adults.

We all live with the bacteria *E. coli* in our bowel. Aside from causing problems in infants, we do not seem to be bothered by such germs. The problem is that strains of *E. coli* may be as different from each other as are people; and local strains may have toxogenic properties to which outsiders have not become immune. Immunity comes rather quickly, but often not before runny bowels.

Viral infections probably account for many or most episodes of diarrhea; and if sanitation is poor, there are many forms of intestinal protozoa which can stir up the bowel. It pays to eat well-cooked hot foods and to make certain that the water is sterilized.

Causes of Recurrent Diarrhea

As one might expect, an allergist would think of allergy first as a cause of recurrent diarrhea. Dr. William Crook doesn't surprise us in this short section from his book, *Your Allergic Child.*

You may notice that a particular food, such as corn, seems to upset your child's stomach and cause diarrhea. Corn may provide a mechanical laxative by giving more bulk to the stool. Some children may have more stools than average, even on a bland diet. This may be from "celiac disease," a specific irritation caused by wheat gluten.

Your child may also show symptoms of diarrhea because of intestinal parasites or a dysentery infection. Finally, he may suffer from a specific intolerance to milk sugar. But, sometimes, a child or an adult who has none of the above conditions continues to have diarrhea. Such a diarrhea may be caused by a food or even by an inhalant allergy.

Dr. Joyce D. Gryboski of Connecticut has described a number of infants and young children with diarrhea caused by food allergy. Others have many patients, including both children and adults, with ulcerative colitis caused not only by food allergies, but by inhalant allergies as well.[1]

COLITIS

Another cause of recurrent diarrhea is colitis, here explained for us by Dr. Eric Sims.

Colitis is an inflammation of the colon, the large intestine in which fluid food residuals are reduced to a paste consistency for evacuation. The lining of the colon can become inflamed as part of a general bowel infection from a dysentery germ or similar microbe. The child may suffer fever, vomiting, and diarrhea. Bowel movements are fluid, slimy, and often blood-stained. Such dysentery or entero-colitis may result from a child's eating or drinking something contaminated with a disease-causing germ.

This germ is spread by the four F's: feces, fingers, food, and flies. Treatment includes a restricted diet, plenty of clear fluids, and appropriate medications from the doctor.

A more troublesome form of this illness is chronic ulcerative colitis. Bowel infections, milk allergy, and emotional stresses have been suspected as causes of this condition. The lining of the colon becomes extensively ulcerated, much normal mucous membrane is lost, and the bowel wall becomes scarred and contracted. There is a frequent and sometimes painful passage of small stools containing blood, pus, and mucus. Also common are bouts of severe diarrhea and accompanying anemia, a consequence of nourishment loss.

The physician diagnoses the condition by the use of a sigmoidoscope, an instrument inserted in the anal passage, confirmation of the diagnosis is provided by a barium enema x-ray. Treatment includes restricted diet or soft, non-bulky foods, vitamin supplements, sedatives, and antiseptics. In protracted cases, removal of the colon may be necessary. Most important in the successful treatment of colitis in children is the attempt by parents and physician to give understanding and support to the child during this difficult illness.

There are severe cases of colitis such as those described, but there are far more who have only a minor degree of this illness. Many people live a lifetime with an irritable bowel which responds to some foods, medications, or tension, with cramps and loose, mucusy, diarrheal stools. Even such mild cases may have ulcers, although it is more likely that the bowel wall is just tender with low grade inflammation. Often, there is a family history of colitis. At times, the symptoms overlap with those of sprue or celiac disease.

WHAT SHOULD YOU DO ABOUT CONSTIPATION?

Generally, not much. First, determine whether your child *really* is constipated. There is too much emphasis on "a stool a day is the only way." Constipation may exist if a bowel movement hurts, if there is blood in the stool, if the abdomen is too full, or if the child chronically has dirty pants. The child may be constipated even if he has loose bowel movements. A hard stool is held back, and soft stool from above will be forced around it. Some people will normally have a stool only once a week with no problem. Others will usually have two a day. If the child is uncomfortable, and if he can't get relief, call the doctor.

The most common cause of constipation probably is excessive milk intake. Over a quart a day is too much for most children. It is helpful to give extra water and juices as well as laxative fruits (prunes, plums, apricots). Routine times to go to the toilet should be encouraged, but should not be imposed on children.

The other common cause of constipation results from trying to force toilet training on reluctant two- and three-year-olds. These "midgets in a world of giants" have found that you can lead a horse to water but that you can't make him drink. This sets up circumstances where the "midget" can finally win a battle. He can, and often does, refuse to "produce." And the more pressure the parent applies, the more effort he'll expend to keep from having a bowel movement. He holds back; the result is a large, hard stool. This hurts when passed, even to the point of tearing the rectum and creating a painful fissure, with blood on the stool. Pain with a bowel movement naturally inhibits further bowel movements, leading to chronic constipation. Call your physician. For methods of toilet training see our companion volume, *The Parents' Guide to Child Raising.*

Temporary relief can be obtained by using a glycerine rectal suppository. They come in children's sizes that can also be used by infants. It would be unwise to use any laxative stronger than milk of magnesia unless you check with your doctor. For constipation with acute distress, you can give an enema. The easiest types to use are disposable enema containers available at the drug store. You can also use the regular enema can with hose and tube. In either case, the best physical position for an enema is as illustrated in Figure 41. Some small fry are a bit reluctant and have to be held down flat as shown. Administer as much enema fluid as possible before they sit back on the toilet. For the fluid, use one quart

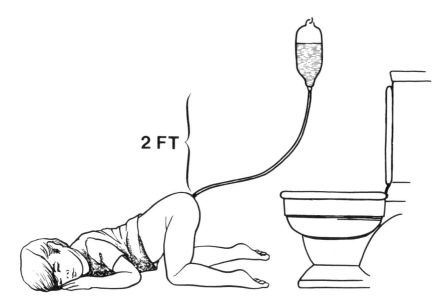

2 FT

FIGURE 40 *The "butt up" position is an efficient way of giving an enema. Use a heaping teaspoon of salt in a quart or liter of water for the enema solution.*

of warm water with one heaping teaspoon of salt. Do not hold the bag or can more than one to two feet above the tip of the tube. Grease the "business end" of the enema tube with vaseline or a similar lubricant.

About Giving Enemas

Giving enemas is no one's favorite occupation, but sometimes it is necessary. Pediatrician Marvin McClellan offers some other "tips."

An enema is the injection of a fluid into the rectum. The fluid may be injected by repeated applications of two to four ounce portions with a rubber bulb syringe, or it may be allowed to flow in by gravity from a can or rubber bag through a hose and an appropriate sized nozzle. Regardless of the method, the object is to get enough fluid inside the lower intestinal tract to cause the patient to evacuate that fluid and whatever else is in the lower portion of the intestinal tract.

If you use too small an amount of fluid, then the fluid may either be absorbed into the stool or picked up and absorbed by the body. Then the mother will say, "I gave an enema but it did no good." We cannot dictate an exact amount, but give enough fluid to make the child have a bowel movement.

An enema given to an infant may be done either on towels or diapers, on a table next to the sink, or on a pad in the bathtub. The older child must obviously be managed in another way, usually by having him lie down on the floor in the bath room, or by having him sit on the toilet.

There is usually a lot of disgruntled comment from the child about receiving an enema. The parent must overcome these comments by saying: "We are going to do it anyhow." To do a thorough job of cleansing out the lower intestinal tract, two or three enemas may be required.

Giving a Glycerine Suppository to Relieve Constipation

Lay the child on his stomach. Spread the cheeks of the buttocks so that you can see the anus. Push the suppository almost all the way in, but leave a little showing at the anal opening. The suppository melts and lubricates, and the part left in the anus causes the child to feel like having a bowel movement.

Giving a Rectal Suppository for Medication

A rather commonly used medicine to prevent or help control vomiting is given by rectal suppository. It is pushed through the anus into the bowel, where it dissolves and is absorbed, usually becoming effective after half an hour. If the suppository is pushed back out with a bowel movement before a half hour, it usually has not been absorbed. To use the suppository, lay the child over your lap. Remove the paper from the suppository (some people have forgotten to do this!), moisten the tip of the suppository with water or lubricating jelly, and spread the cheeks of the buttocks so you can see the anus. The key to getting a suppository to stay in is to push it all the way through the anus, which means you have to push your finger into the rectum about a half an inch. A rubber finger cot may be used to keep your finger clean if you wish. As you pull your finger out, squeeze the cheeks of the buttocks together and hold them firmly a few minutes in order to keep the suppository in.

THE LIVER AND GALL BLADDER

The liver lies under the heart and lungs at the bottom of the rib cage. It can be bruised or torn from severe trauma. Infection of the liver secondary to a ruptured appendix can occur. Worm larvae of various kinds can lodge in the liver, causing disease. The most common liver problems in childhood are from viral hepatitis A or B, or from mononucleosis, although smaller children develop yellow jaundice less often than teenagers and adults.

Gallbladder disease is rare in children, but it does occur. The gallbladder is a sack located under the liver that stores bile which, when released into the intestine, helps to digest fatty foods. The gallbladder can become infected with bacteria or can form gallstones. If one of these stones lodges in the tube that leads to the bowel, it can be very painful in the upper abdomen and the pain may spread to the back or shoulder.

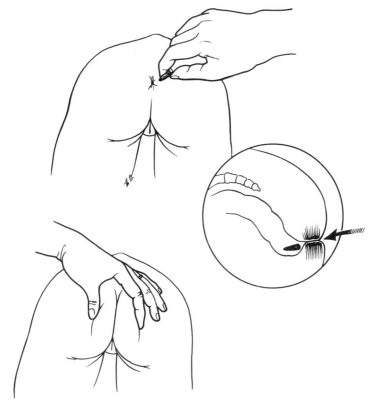

FIGURE 41   *Giving medicine by rectal suppository requires that the suppository be pushed completely through the anus, which is surrounded by a heavy band of muscle as shown above in the circular insert: a cross section of the buttocks, anus and rectum.*

Usually there are nausea, vomiting, fever, and maybe even yellow jaundice. Often the attacks are fewer if fatty foods are avoided.

YOUR STOMACH AND BOWELS: A SUMMARY

Gastrointestinal tracts, like people, are complex, senstive, and have great individual differences. We generally function on a "gut level" as far as decision making is concerned, harking to the feelings in our bowels rather than the logic of our intellect. Our "gut" is an end organ of our emotions—from ulcers to colitis we respond with spasms, vomiting, or diarrhea to gut-wrenching decisions, fear, and stress. Children are especially vulnerable to stomachache as a major symptom of a wide variety of ailments, from strep throat to stern teachers.

Vomiting and stomachache are usually caused by viral intestinal infections, or the "intestinal flu." However, keep in mind that such symptoms may be due to all sorts of diseases, from meningitis to appendicitis. Study the symptoms and signs of trouble so that you can seek early treatment and avoid the potentially serious complications of significant diseases. Read Chapters 17, 18 and 19 in order to make yourself aware of the phenomenal number of organisms that can cause stomach and bowel infection, and learn the rules on how to avoid such enemies. We spend a great deal of energy protecting ourselves from these germs and their waste products. Periodically, we are forced to entertain or fight new viruses, bacteria, protozoa, or worms with resultant nausea, gas, aches, pains, and diarrhea.

Whether from infection, allergy, or lack of enzymes, or from frank poisons and irritants, our intestinal tract does much of our suffering. That it, and we, survive and tolerate all this rather well is a tribute to our Designer.

11

KIDNEY, BLADDER, AND BOTTOM

This chapter is about urinary problems and how to avoid them. There is too little public education about the care of the urinary apparatus, and about its diseases. Considering the frequency of urinary tract infections in females, many of which are easily prevented, it is vital that women and girls study the simple subject of personal hygiene.

Figure 43 is a diagram of the urinary tract showing its anatomy and diseases. The numbers 1 through 4 refer to the anatomy as follows: (1) kidneys: behind and slightly below the liver in the abdominal cavity on each side of the spine against the lower ribs—they filter urine from the blood; (2) ureter: a muscular tube that pumps urine from the kidney into the bladder; (3) bladder: an elastic bag to collect and hold urine. Some people can hold over a quart. Two ureters feed the bladder urine through small holes surrounded by muscles which keep urine in the bladder from being squeezed back up the ureters when the bladder contracts to empty through the urethra. The bladder wall is resistant to bacteria and probably excretes antibodies that are somewhat effective if they are not diluted by too much urine. (4) urethra: the short tube from the bladder outlet to the end of the penis in the male, or to a spot in the vulva in the female just in front of the vagina about one inch from the anus.

The numbers 5 through 13 in Figure 42 refer to the diseases of the urinary tract, as follows: (5) Kidney disease may cause swelling (edema or retained fluid from nephrosis), high blood pressure (from kidney scarring), and anemia (from uremia or kidney failure, or bleeding in the urine from glomerulonephritis). Kidney disease is caused from: (6) Toxins, usually not identified, though occasionally from chemical

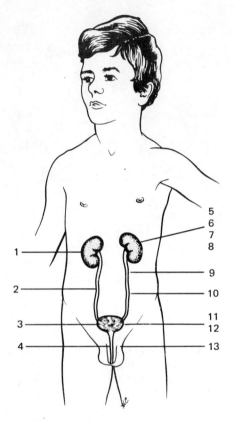

FIGURE 42   *The anatomy and diseases of the urinary tract.*

poisoning or allergic reactions to bee stings—causing nephrosis; (7) infections, usually from bowel bacteria causing abscesses in the kidney (pyelonephritis) and pus in the urine; or (8) mechanical obstruction may cause urine to back up in the kidney causing them to swell (hydronephrosis. (9) The ureters may swell if plugged or infected, or if the valve where they empty into the bladder won't close so the bladder urine is also pushed upward when the bladder empties. (10) Cystitis often starts from obstruction—bacteria may grow in urine remaining in the bladder after urinating. They can swim up the urethra. (11) Difficulty in passing urine, starting the stream or dribbling urine from too small an outlet from the bladder. (12) Infection of the urethra (urethritis) in the female is usually from feces being wiped frontwards from the anus, infecting the vagina and vulva and opening of the urethra. (13) In baby boys the opening at the end of the penis may rub on the diaper and become infected, scarring the opening and causing a very small urinary stream.

THE ANATOMY OF THE URINARY TRACT

The kidney's importance is emphasized by the fact that one fourth of all the blood in the body goes through the kidneys. Inside the kidneys, the blood courses through a network of small capillaries wound around the glomerulus and tubules. The glomerulus is a cup-shaped arrangement of cells that filter much of the fluid out of the blood. This fluid then passes through long thin tubules whose cells absorb back useful salts and water and excrete waste products. The remaining fluid passes into progressively larger tubes and into the renal pelvis, a sac in the center of the kidney.

A muscular tube, the ureter, moves the urine from each kidney to the bladder. Urine is periodically passed from the bladder through the urethra. In the female, the urethra is very short and empties just in front of the vagina. The opening is only around an inch, or two and one-half centimeters, from the anus in a young girl, and is thus exposed to the bacteria passed in bowel movements.

In the male, the urethra is longer and the opening in the penis is far away from the rectum. The testicles are formed in the developing fetus just below the kidneys in the abdominal cavity. They migrate to the bottom of the abdominal cavity and out through a hole in the muscle, carrying the lining of the abdominal cavity with them, coming out under the skin of the groin midway between the hip and the penis. They migrate under the skin into the scrotum on each side. Their blood supply is carried along with them from the abdominal cavity, as is the epididymis, a tube which carries sperm through the prostate into the penis. On rare occasions, a girl's ovaries will accidentally follow the same path and create a hernia into the inguinal area.

How Should You Use Toilet Paper?

It might seem silly to give advice on how to use toilet paper, but it isn't. Improper use of toilet paper probably contributes to millions of bladder infections each year. And who ever gives a course on "How to wipe yourself after a bowel movement or urinating"? So far, not even the *Ladies' Home Journal* or *Reader's Digest* has tackled that one. It is a subject not talked about in most families.

Unfortunately, most girls and many women use toilet paper incorrectly. They rather "naturally" reach between the legs from the front and wipe from the back to the front. This smears bowel movement over the vulva, vaginal opening, and urethra. The bowel movement is irritating as well as dirty. More important, half of it is made up of all sorts of bacteria and viruses. Many of the bacteria can actively swim, having little arm-like projections called cilia. They can swim up the short female urethra into the bladder and even up to the kidney. The infections they cause may provoke burning urination, abnormally frequent urination, and occasional fever and stomachache. At times, after the acute infection settles down, a girl will be left with a smoldering low-grade infection that may go unnoticed. If left untreated, this can lead to kidney damage. Others can get vaginal infections, marked by yellow pus and irritation from bowel germs.

The proper way to wipe is from the front to the back. Lean to the side and raise one leg. Reach under the leg and forward, then wipe backward. Throw the paper away after each wipe. This should become a habit.

Mothers, mark your calendar with a check once a week for the next three months. Show your daughter how to wipe, and when each check on the calendar comes up, have her demonstrate to see if she is doing it properly. Also look for staining from pus or bowel movement on the underpants.

Many girls who shower all the time never adequately wash the vulvo-vaginal area. Girls who haven't reached puberty have very tender vulvar (the area around the vagina) membranes and are naturally bashful and protective of their privacy. Mothers of infants and little girls who attempt to wash the area with a wash cloth usually give up. The child screams and holds the legs together. Naturally! A wash cloth on a little girl's vulvar membranes would be like a wire brush on a woman. The membranes toughen up markedly after menstruation starts. It is best to use cotton balls and a simple soap on the vulva membranes in girls. Then, be sure to rinse well.

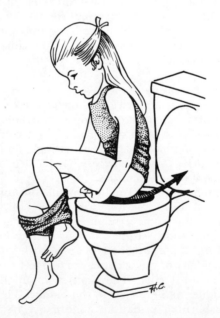

FIGURE 43   *Females should wipe from the front to the back and throw away the toilet paper after each wipe.*

Bubble Baths and Sore Bottoms

Some mothers settle for a bubble bath or a detergent to get their children clean or even to get them into the tub. One product has the advantage of dissolving the ring of dirt off the bath tub! However, none of these is advisable, for detergents are too strong for human skin, if not for enameled bathtubs! The skin can become excessively dry, rough, rashy, or irritated. And the detergent or bubble bath can get into the urethra and cause severe irritation and pain on urinating. Bathtub water frequently gets into the bladder itself in some girls; and if it carries an irritating detergent, it can cause considerable harm.

Other Causes for Irritation of the Vaginal Area

Colored or scented toilet paper may cause a rash in sensitive or allergic individuals. Moisture from failure to pat the vulva dry after urinating, or from chronic sweat and vaginal secretions, irritates the membranes and sets the stage for infections. Intestinal bacteria can swim around in this moisture. Another cause of irritation is tight garments: body shirts, tights, tight pants, panty hose or bathing suits. Synthetic material is worse than cotton in causing irritation. And don't forget pinworms. They may crawl up from the rectum and lay their eggs in the vagina or the urethra .

DIETHYLSTILBESTROL AND VAGINAL CANCER

If mother took diethylstilbestrol during pregnancy, will it cause vaginal cancer in the girl baby? Until late 1971, diethylstilbestrol (D.E.S.) was used in the treatment of threatened miscarriage. Without the use of this drug, it is probable that many children would not have survived until birth. After over twenty years of use, it has become apparent that there is a high correlation between in-uterus exposure to D.E.S. and vaginal or cervical cancer occurring fifteen to twenty years later. This was called to the attention of physicians in 1973. At this time, no one knows whether adolescent girls without symptoms who were exposed to D.E.S. during the fetus stage have a greater chance of developing cancer; however, the physician should be alerted, and the possibility considered in cases of irregular bleeding in adolescent girls, so they will be given routine physical and pelvic examinations and PAP smears when big enough.

BLADDER INFECTIONS

Is a "little bladder infection" important? Pediatrician William Misbach thinks it is. Increasing evidence over the years has made us more aware of the importance of urinary tract infections in children. We now know that these infections occur more commonly and are more easily missed than previously realized. They often result from an underlying abnormality of the urinary system.

Urinary infections occur more commonly in girls, due to the shortness of the urethra (the tube from the bladder to the outside) and the subsequent difficulty of keeping it clean. The infections are often characterized by symptoms of increased frequency of urination (urinating more often or more frequently than usual), painful voiding, abdominal pain, chills, and fever. These signs may be relatively silent. Consequently, a diagnosis can only be established by the analysis and culture of a carefully collected urine specimen.

Since low-grade infection may smoulder for many months without causing symptoms, periodic urine studies may be necessary. When infection is suspected, culture is mandatory. Culture is sometimes needed while the child is on medication.

Since urinary tract infections are so rare in boys, the presence of one may indicate an abnormality of the urinary system. Consequently, further studies may be necessary in order to diagnose the underlying cause. In girls, the same approach is indicated, depending on the number and severity of their infections.

In most instances, irreparable damage to the kidney can be avoided if an infection of the urinary tract is promptly diagnosed, correctly treated, and, most importantly, *carefully followed* to detect relapse or re-infection.

In order to diagnose a urinary infection properly, it is necessary to catch a good clean specimen. Ordinarily, if a girl or woman bears down to urinate, cells and bacteria may be pushed into the urine from the vulva and vagina. The urine than looks infected, for it is not always possible to tell outside contamination from bladder or kidney cells and bacteria. In order to avoid this, the following technique is used:

1. "Prime the pump" by drinking extra fluids.
2. Wash the labia gently, but thoroughly, with soap (Phisohex or Dial) and warm water. Rinse well.
3. Females should sit backwards on the toilet facing the wall or have the legs spread widely apart.
4. When the urine stream has started, let the first portion go, then catch a one-half to one ounce specimen by holding a small sterile jar under the stream. (The initial urine stream may be contaminated, so don't collect that portion.)
5. Cap the jar tightly, and place in the refrigerator until it is brought to the office (preferably within one hour).
6. Be sure to tell the nurse that it is a "clean catch" specimen so that it will receive proper attention.
7. You may prepare the sterile container by washing a baby food (or other small) jar and lid with soap and water and then boiling it for ten minutes.
8. A first morning specimen is desirable, but not necessary.

Treatment of urinary infections can be complicated. Although antibi-otics and cleanliness help, bladder infections frequently recur. The major reason for recurrence in some girls and women is a lack of antibodies in the cells at the opening of the urethra, which permits bacteria to grow and spread up to the bladder. Your doctor may be able to give medica-tion to take routinely to help prevent this local bacterial growth and subsequent spread.

PYELONEPHRITIS

We asked Dr. Eric Sims to explain the disease pyelonephritis—a bacterial infection of the kidneys which occurs mainly in girls.

Infection of the bladder lining, called cystitis, frequently ascends into the kidneys. Pyelonephritis may start quite suddenly—with fever, abdominal pains, backache, and frequent urination with a burning sensation. Microscopic examination of the urine reveals pus cells, and a culture of a cleanly collected specimen will grow a significant number of the causative bacteria (which are usually the same sort of germs as are found normally within the bowel). The infection always responds promptly to treatment with the appropriate antibacterial medication by mouth. However, special x-rays of both the kidneys and bladder may be recommended as soon as the child is well again, because pyelonephritis is the result of a minor abnormality in the urinary tract which causes stagnation of retained urine.

The bladder x-ray may reveal the defect of ureteric reflux, a squirting of urine back up the ureters from the bladder to the kidneys as the child urinates. It is most likely to happen if there is back pressure, which can result from a narrow opening that may have been present since birth, or which was caused by scarring resulting from infection. Such reflux results in stagnation of urine and in infection, because a child with this problem almost never has an empty bladder; as soon as she has urinated and has left the bathroom, the urine which squirted up to the kidneys drains into the bladder again. Urine which stays in the bladder too long tends to grow bacteria.

Minor degrees of reflux may respond to the long-term administration of antibacterial medications, combined with the technique of double urinating, emptying the bladder again a minute or so after the first voiding. A severe degree of reflux sometimes requires surgery to protect the kidneys from slowly accumulating damage over the years. If the x-rays reveal other anatomical abnormalities of the kidneys, ureters, bladder, or urethra, surgery may be essential.

Pyelonephritis is sneaky and may occur without the usual symptoms. It may be recognized only when a doctor examines fresh urine microscopically. There are times when the microscopic examination will be negative yet a urine culture will show the presence of large numbers of infecting bacteria. A child may be vaguely unwell, with no obvious "waterworks discomfort" at all, and yet have a chronic and damaging infection. This child requires a complete examination. If these special studies do not reveal any surgically correctable defect, medical treatment may have to be continued for years.

The kidneys have several vital functions to perform in maintaining the water, salt, and chemical balance of the body. If a child with chronic kidney damage ultimately develops kidney failure, uremia—a very complex disturbance of the body chemistry—will result. Recurrent or chronic pyelonephritis may cause such kidney damage. An attempt can be made to cope with this situation by dietary measures such as the restriction of protein foods, careful control of water intake, and the reliance on mainly carbohydrate foods for the body's energy requirements. If the damage is severe enough, dialysis will have to be undertaken. This involves the use of an "artificial kidney" that can remove various substances from the blood. The treatment is rather tedious and expensive, and has to be repeated at regular intervals indefinitely.

Eventually, one may have to consider a kidney transplant operation. This procedure is being done in increasing numbers in children, especially in adolescents. Two aspects of the problem pose special difficulties for young people. One is the failure of growth that may result from the powerful drugs that have to be given for the rest of a person's life after a renal transplant in order to prevent the body's rejection of the donor kidney. The other is the emotional disturbance, particularly in adolescent girls, caused by undesirable cosmetic side effects from these drugs. These problems can be helped and must be accepted as small prices to pay for the benefit of survival. Nevertheless, chronic kidney failure poses a difficult decision both for the parents and the doctor. Few parents would want their child to undergo heroic and protracted treatments unless they felt he was going to enjoy to the full the life that was to be gained by these measures.

ALLERGY AND URINARY PROBLEMS

Dr. William Crook writes that few think of allergy when a child wets the bed, shows albumin in the urine, or suffers from repeated urinary tract infections. Skeptical pediatrician Robert Burnett, in fact, suggests that, "If your child wets the bed, check with your doctor before you rush to an allergist." But Dr. Crook contends that allergy can be a factor in causing diseases and disorders in any part of the urinary tract.

Doctors James Breneman of Michigan and John Gerrard of Saskatchewan have clearly documented the relationship of allergy to bedwetting in many children. Apparently, when a child eats a food he's sensitive to, the bladder muscles have a spasm. This keeps the bladder from holding the normal amount of urine. When the bladder can't hold the normal amount, the child may have to urinate more often during the day and may wet the bed at night.

Allergy can also cause albumin in the urine and other types of genito-urinary symptoms, including vaginal discharge, urinary frequency, and, in little girls especially, contact sensitivity to bubble bath, soaps, and the like. Foods your child eats, including food coloring and additives, can also cause these symptoms.[1]

Why Is Urine Dark or Cloudy?

The urine color changes with the fluid intake. If it is a hot day, if water intake is low, or if there is vomiting and dehydration, the urine becomes dark yellow. If there is a large fluid intake, the urine becomes very light yellow or almost colorless. A cloudy urine usually means the presence of normal crystals and is not significant.

At times, however, a cloudy urine can be due to infection; then the cloudiness is from pus. This is often accompanied by other symptoms, such as discomfort on urinating, burning, stinging, or pain. Usually the child urinates more frequently than usual. A dark tea-colored urine can be a symptom of yellow jaundice, and may be associated with yellowness of the skin or eyes and stomachache. Reddish or coffee-colored urine can be due to blood from kidney disease or severe bladder infection. Any of these may be accompanied by stomachache. They all deserve a call to your physician.

GLOMERULONEPHRITIS

One of the diseases that can turn a urine dark is glomerulonephritis, explains Dr. Sims.

This is an acute inflammation of the kidneys, which sometimes follows a streptococcal infection of either the throat or the skin. Some particular strains of the *Streptococcus* germ are especially likely to produce toxins that may reach the kidneys and damage the glomeruli, clusters of intertwined blood vessels and tubules where fluids and substances are extracted from the blood as the first step in the formation of urine. The toxin damages the glomeruli slowly; so a child recovers from the initial sore throat or skin infection before the symptoms of glomerulonephritis appears. Days later, the child becomes unwell, with fatigue, headache, poor appetite, and a reduced output of urine. This reduced output causes a little water-logging, with puffy eyelids and edema elsewhere in the body. In the early stages, the urine may be dark brown and cloudy in appearance because it contains red blood cells that leak from the inflamed kidneys.

In the early stages of such acute kidney inflammation, the blood pressure is likely to be elevated, so occasionally a child may convulse. The fluid retention may cause some strain on the heart, and the kidneys may even fail to secrete any urine at all for a few days. In such an event, the child may have to be hospitalized for the continuous supervision necessary in order to minimize the possibility of these early complications.

The mainstays of early treatment are rest in bed, antibiotics to eliminate any persisting focus of streptococci, and some dietary and fluid restriction until good kidney function is assessed. Most children with this disease progress smoothly, without complications, and can convalesce at home with every prospect of complete recovery in a few months. [Pediatrician Ed Shaw cautions, "Rest in bed does not mean staying in bed all the time; in fact, absolute bed rest for a long period of time may have significant ill effects."]

UNDESCENDED TESTES

When the male fetus is forming in the uterus, the testes develop behind the abdominal cavity, and, in the seventh month of pregnancy, begin their descent into the scrotum. This process is normally complete by birth, but occasionally it does not become complete until six to nine months after birth. When this process is incomplete, the child has the condition known as cryptorchidism, or undescended testes. When this occurs the testicle cannot be felt in the scrotum. In older children sometimes the testicle will pull up into the groin when the child is chilly and will come down when he is warm.

If the testes do not go down into the scrotum, they may be damaged between the age of six to twelve years. This results in a reduction of male sex hormone and sperm, later may predispose to cancer, and often is associated with a hernia. Treatment may be hormone injections or surgery to fix the testes in the scrotum. Surgery is often recommended before the age of six years, but there are some differences of opinion about "proper" treatment.

What About Genital Pain and Swelling in Boys?

Injury to the penis or swelling of it should be checked by the doctor. If there is pain on urination, blood in the urine, very frequent urination, or coffee- or tea-colored urine, the child should be examined. If possible, collect fresh urine in a clean container and take it with you to the doctor. A discharge from the penis requires medical attention.

If there is a lump in the groin, it might be a hernia. Usually, such lumps are soft and will go away if the child lies down. At times, the lump may go down into the scrotum. Usually, you can feel the hernia slip silkily away if you push it toward the head. If possible, get the child to the doctor when the swelling is present but have him seen anyway. Firm lumps at the crease of the groin or below it may be swollen lymph glands. If they are sore or readily visible, the doctor should check them.

Pain in the scrotum, the sacks in which the testicles hang, should always be checked, whether there is an injury or not. On occasion, the testicle can twist around for no known cause, cut off its blood supply, and become gangrenous inside the scrotum. Usually, the spermatic cord muscles pull the very tender testicle up into the edge of the canal; the scrotum on that side is higher than the other. A small vestigial appendix

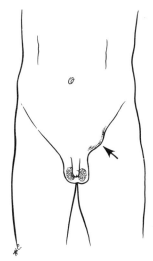

FIGURE 44   *Swelling of an inguinal hernia.*

testes can twist and cause severe pain. Mumps can infect the testicle, which becomes swollen, painful, and sore. All painful testicular swellings deserve prompt medical attention.

A diffuse "wormy" mass above the testicle in the scrotum, usually on the left side, is frequently from dilated veins or varicoceles. Although there is no urgency, inform the child's doctor if this is noted. A loop of bowel from a large hernia may get into the scrotum, but this can be felt in the groin area where hernias start.

Infant boys frequently have a sack of water above the testicle called a hydrocele. A flashlight will shine through the clear fluid. Most hydroceles will spontaneously vanish, but a few may persist and be associated with a hernia.

How Can You Help Your Child Stop Bed Wetting?
We all wet the bed until we finally outgrew it. Most children stop by two to four years, usually because they don't like a wet bed, or because they want to "be big" and out of night diapers. Some children, however, wet the bed far beyond that period. There are three basic causes for such prolonged bed wetting: physical disease, psychological problems, and sound sleeping. Most bed wetters are simply exceptionally sound sleepers, but before you accept such a diagnosis, it is vital that the other causes be ruled out.

Physical diseases that cause bed wetting include urinary tract infections, diabetes, and other conditions which produce excess urine, as well as debilitating diseases in which the child is too exhausted to get up or has developed excessive urine flow or mechanical bladder problems. Diabetics eat a lot, drink a lot, and wet a lot. They urinate more frequently and in larger amounts both day and night. The urine may smell sweet or fruity. Usually there is a family history of diabetes. Onset can be at any time from early infancy to old age. Another clue that a child may have diabetes is deep hard breathing with a fruity breath odor and often some fever from dehydration, in spite of excessive water intake.

Urinary tract infections are especially common in little girls. Often they do not complain of pain on urination, and the original infection, with fever and stomachache, may be passed over as "a virus." Around one percent of grammar school age girls have urinary tract infections which produce no complaints or noticeable symptoms.

Parents should follow a few brief steps in order to be aware of possible urinary problems: Note the number of times a child urinates, and whether or not the child has to rush to the bathroom. Listen to the child urinate to determine if it is hard to start a full stream or if there is dribbling afterwards. Check the pants for stains or wetness, indicating the child may wet himself. It should be realized that some children who do not wet the bed can have urinary frequency, urgency, and infection but simply get up several times a night to go to the toilet.

Before deciding that a bed wetter is in the sound sleep group, a child should have a complete history and physical with a urinalysis and a urine culture. In a few cases, the doctor may want x-rays of the kidneys, bladder, and urethra—or he may even have the child cystoscoped.

Psychological bed wetting does occur, although in my experience it is far less common than bed wetting from disease or from deep sleep. On the other hand, children who wet the bed often develop psychological problems from the embarrassment and lack of self-esteem the condition causes. Children who have been dry at night and then start wetting the bed again should be suspected of infection or psychological problems.

Two very common psychological causes of bed wetting are moving to a new neighborhood and having a new baby in the house. Fear of the dark is another cause. Perhaps the most unfortunate cause of bed wetting is when it is either used by the child to prove to himself that he can be accepted as a baby or when it is used to manipulate or punish the parent. Children who fear that they are being forced to grow up too fast and feel rejected will often regress to bed wetting. By wetting the bed they say, "I am a baby," implying that they are too young to be sent out into the world. Children who find that wetting the bed aggravates a parent may use it as a way of punishing or manipulating the parent by ensuring attention, even if it is negative.

Most children, and certainly most boys, have neither organic, physical, or psychological causes for bed wetting. They simply sleep so soundly that they lose control of their bladder and wet while in a deep sleep. Often there is an unsung family history of bed wetting by fathers, grandfathers, and uncles. The majority of children who bedwet after age four outgrow the tendency and establish night bladder control by age six. Of those who don't, some may still bedwet as teenagers. Overall, it does no good and much harm to shame or to punish a child for this condition. Limiting fluids at bedtime may reduce the volume of urine, but it rarely eliminates bed wetting. Waking children up in the middle of the night to urinate occasionally helps, but some can be up, go to the toilet, still never be really awake, and urinate shortly after going back to bed. But don't give up hope. There are other ways of helping the child stay dry at night, thereby regaining his self-esteem and reducing mother's laundry work. One is by the use of a mechanical conditioner. Another is medication that helps the individual to hold the urine all night. It is especially useful for temporary trips. Used long enough, it may help until the individual outgrows the need. It is, of course, a drug, and rare reactions have been reported. In many ways, it is inferior to mechanical conditioners. Proper use of mechanical conditioners results in about a ninety percent cure of the deep sleep bed wetter. Success, however, requires that the stage be set for real motivation. Pediatricians skilled in hypnosis often have good results with positive suggestion. I suspect that this is a factor in the success of conditioners.

Assuming that a four-year-old is bed wetting, has no indication of physical or psychological problems, and has been thoroughly checked by his doctor, operation "Dry Bed" can start. Around the child's birthday, it can be announced to him by his mother that he is now big enough to help in his own care by stripping the sheets from his bed each morning and putting them in the laundry room. By the fifth birthday, his responsibility can be increased to helping make his bed after school, and by the sixth birthday to making it himself and washing his own sheets. If he refuses to do these personal tasks, simply withdraw some of the privileges that he should have with his increased age—and do the tasks yourself without complaint. But until he does the required tasks, he should not be allowed the privileges of his age. It is most important that the privileges be withdrawn calmly, not in anger or disgust. It is the child's choice and business as to whether or not he wishes to act his age or act "grown up." He has to desire the respect of being treated appropriately for his age, and he has to really want to stop bed wetting for himself—not just to please his mother.

Around age six, take him to his doctor with the request that he be helped to stay dry all night. It is important that someone from outside the family be involved, but it is not necessary to spend a large sum of money for a commercial conditioner "package." If the doctor decides that it is the child's desire, not just the mother's, to stay dry, and that no physical and psychological causes are involved, he can offer the child the opportunity to condition himself to wake up and go to the toilet rather than to wet the bed.

The physician's role is as an advocate for the child. He not only determines the child's readiness, but he helps the child stay aware of this help by having him call the doctor or his nurse once a week with a report on his success or failure in staying dry. This outside motivation is undoubtedly significant in aiding the child to make the required effort to awaken prior to the alarm.

The conditioner itself can be purchased for a reasonable price through the catalog department of Sears, Roebuck and Company. It is simply a safe battery-operated bell which rings and wakes up the child as soon as he wets. The urine wets a mat between two foil pad receivers, completing a circuit which rings a bell. This wakes the child up. Usually, after a few times, he will begin to wake up, if he desires, just before he wets. A Pavlovian reflex pattern is established which finally enables the child to establish sleep control over his bladder. In my experience, ninety percent of all deep sleep bedwetters are cured within a month. Some of those not cured actually had hidden psychological problems and became angry at the machine and would disconnect it. Others slept so soundly that the alarm awoke the entire household but not the bed wetter. For the latter group, give them a few more years before trying again. For the angry children, psychological help may be indicated. But for any child who conquers bed wetting, regardless of help, it is a significant and productive psychological and practical victory well worth the time and expense invested.

VENEREAL DISEASE

Venereal diseases usually start in the area of the bladder and the bottom—in the penis or vagina. Of course, these diseases are rare in infants and children, but an infant can be born with gonorrhea, syphilis, or herpes infections, and good obstetrical care and early pediatric care are aimed at preventing these diseases. In women, gonorrhea may smolder along without symptoms, gradually causing sterility; or if an infected woman delivers, it infects her baby. If the infection is not diagnosed and treated early, the baby may become blind. Unfortunately, syphilis is also a very subtle disease. A person may go along for years feeling fine after the local sore on the penis has healed and the body rash has gone. Later, however, he can gradually develop blindness, insanity, or die of syphilis heart infection. Infants born of infected mothers are often retarded. (For further information see Chapter 16.)

As children get older there is more chance of contacting venereal disease sexually. Boys of grade school level, as well as high school, are occasionally targets for some homosexuals and have at times developed gonorrhea of the rectum after sodomy (anal intercourse). Young girls have occasionally been infected with gonorrhea or syphilis from sexual molestation.

Incurable Venereal Disease

Although the gonorrhea epidemic, which has left a trail of infertility and blind babies, has captured public attention, a potentially more serious epidemic of a different venereal disease has developed. The new V.D. is caused by the "genital" Herpes virus II and the common cold sore virus, Herpes I. Although the ordinary cold sore virus is not venereal, it, too, can cause venereal disease. Herpes II is currently more common than syphilis and is found more frequently in teenagers than in older age groups. More often than not it is silent, asymptomatic, and undiagnosed. In the male, it may cause a temporary "genital cold sore" on the penis. In the female, it may cause genital cold sores of the skin of the buttocks or thighs or the vulva. More often, it is unseen, in the cervix at the top of the vagina. What's so bad about a venereal "cold sore?" Plenty.

Women infected with Herpes II have a high incidence of abortions. Babies born of infected women may catch Herpes II and can be severely damaged or die from the infection. There is also a link between Herpes II infections and cancer of the cervix. Antibiotics do not cure viral diseases such as Herpes.

Women most likely to have Herpes II are those who start intercourse at an early age and who have intercourse with multiple partners. The chances of catching the disease increase with greater frequency of contact. Its relatively high incidence in teenagers may be partially due to a lack of immunity. There is some cross-immunity between Herpes I and Herpes II. Herpes I cold sore antibodies increase with age; the older you are, the more likely you are to have had many cold sores and a relatively high antibody level, which may partially protect against venereal Herpes II.

Another virus that is suspected to be genitally spread is the cytomegalovirus. This virus can infect the fetus and cause severe damage that may continue to progress after the baby is born.

Another new venereal disease is serum hepatitis or Hepatitis B. This viral disease of the liver, originally thought to be transmitted only by blood transfusions or serum on unsterile needles from shots, such as are used by heroin addicts, now turns out to be also transmitted through sexual intercourse. This is probably from minor genital friction, but there is recent probable evidence to indicate that the virus may be carried by the sperm.

Venereal warts, another viral caused disease, have become common in the sexually active group. This, at least, can be treated by the physician.

The solution to prevention of venereal Herpes, venereal spread of serum hepatitis, or venereal warts, may be a pragmatic return to the "custom" of intercourse only within marriage. Whether on a moral, historical, or medical basis, the value of marriage sanctity will undoubtedly reassert itself.

Will Rubbers Stop V.D.?

Rubbers, rubber sheaths, or condoms carefully used over the penis during intercourse will significantly reduce pregnancy and the transmission of venereal disease.

SUMMARY: KIDNEY, BLADDER, AND BOTTOM

Disease is better prevented than suffered and treated. Too little attention has been given to the prevention of urinary tract infections. It is worth repeating that simple processes, such as proper wiping habits and avoiding detergents in the bath, may well reduce the incidence of bladder infections. Early conscientious and consistent long-term treatment and follow-up of childhood bladder infections can prevent the asymptomatic smoldering kidney infections which lead to hypertension and renal failure in some young adults.

Glomerulonephritis may be avoided by early treatment of Streptococcal throats and especially of Streptococcal skin infections. These infections can start in a sore around the nose or from a bug bite or skin scratch.

Bed wetting is most often caused by very deep sleep, and can be successfully treated by a mechanical conditioner, without psychological harm if properly used. Care must be exercised to rule out bladder problems, diabetes, infections, and psychological problems prior to the use of a conditioner. Equally, care should be exercised not to damage a child's self-image, either by shaming him for bed wetting or by unnecessarily dragging him to a psychologist to find out "what's wrong" with the child.

Early awareness and treatment of hernias may help prevent the major surgery and damage which occurs if the hernia incarcerates or sticks in the inguinal canal and gangrene develops. (For more about hernias, see page 209.) And don't let passion overrule common sense; avoid venereal diseases! All told, this adds up to a simple principle: Take care of your plumbing, for it takes care of you.

12

THE GROWTH AND DEVELOPMENT
OF FEET, LEGS,
AND OTHER BONES

WHAT CAN YOU DO ABOUT LEGS,
FEET, AND OTHER BONES?

Quite a bit, actually. You should be aware of potential problems, especially in growing children and adolescents. Prevention of problems should start with a well-rounded diet, especially in the two most rapid periods of growth: infancy to age two years, and adolescence. During these times, there is an extra need for calcium and vitamin D in order to obtain maximum bone growth. The daily calcium requirements are one gram a day or above, and it need not just be from milk (see page 386). The vitamin D requirements are 400 to 800 I.U./day. Calcium and vitamins, along with phosphorous and a little fluoride, combine in the formation of bones which grow, usually at each end, by laying down soft cartilage, which is gradually replaced with bone. The more rapid the growth, the thicker the cartilage plates, and the more prone to damage are the bones. Luckily, in small children, the bones are relatively flexible, and although they may break, they often just bend. A description of various types of breaks and how to handle them is found in the section under first aid, Chapter 2. This chapter concentrates on the problems of growth and development of the feet, legs, and bones. A description of how to start your approach to the whole business is given by Stanford University orthopedist Dr. E. E. Bleck, who begins at the beginning.

Shoes For the Baby

First of all, shoes are not necessary for the normal growth and development of the foot. Shoes cover, warm, and protect the foot from pins in the carpet, stone on the ground, and snow in the winter. For fit and function, remember: Shoe is to foot as glove is to hand. In this light, you *can* buy a pair of shoes for your baby when he begins to walk. But there is nothing wrong with the baby walking barefoot; children in more primitive lands have been doing this for centuries. There is, by the way, no objective evidence that going barefoot (or wearing sneakers) causes fallen arches.

The best shoe is shaped like a baby's foot. Our studies on 2,000 feet show that the outline of the normal foot is almost straight. Therefore, the shoe should be almost straight, the leather soft, and the sole pliable. The only value of high-top shoes is that they keep the shoe on the foot; high-tops do not support the ankle or help develop a good arch.

The most appropriate first shoe is the sneaker (a canvas top and flexible rubber sole). It has a straight side, it is soft and pliable, and it does not cause flat feet. In a ten-year-study of children who wore sneakers 85% of the time, not a single case of flatfoot developed. As a matter of fact, feet appeared to develop even higher arches. The freedom of movement and the exercise obtained caused the muscle of the foot to pull the arch up and in.

You can leave baby barefooted, or a good compromise is to "not buy shoes when he begins to walk but only when his walking takes him places where his feet need protection," says pediatrician Tom Cock. If you do get leather shoes instead of canvas ones, Dr. Charles Hoffman cautions his patients: "The normal gait is heel, toe. If the sole is rigid, the foot is not strong enough to bend it and the baby learns to walk plopping his foot down in one solid piece. The sole should be soft and flexible enough for the *baby* to bend it."

Many so-called sturdy shoes are built like British army boots—it is almost like putting the feet in casts. We asked the opinion of the Chairman of The Board of The Juvenile Shoe Corporation of America, Gale Pate, Sr., about baby's shoes and he responded:

A shoe fit is good if the back part of the shoe, in the arch and heel area, fits fairly snugly, so that the shoe will not slip on the foot, allowing the toes to rub on the front of the shoes, and if there is plenty of room in the forepart for growth. Lace shoes rather than straps help keep the shoe on properly tight. It is extremely important to have a flexible sole at the ball of the foot. Leather is flexible and is best, but some newer sole materials are satisfactory if the material is buffed to a velvet finish. I personally do not like canvas shoes, aside from the fact that I am in the leather shoe business, because I think they hold moisture in the shoe because of the adhesive backing.

We are pleased and encouraged by Mr. Pate's candor. Take your choice; no shoes, tennis shoes, or soft flexible leather, or a substitute.

Toeing In

When babies begin to walk, they often toe in. We asked orthopedic surgeon Alan Merchant to tell us what causes "pigeon toeing" and how it may be prevented or corrected:

Some toeing in (pigeon toeing) is natural in infancy, since the lower leg is formed in an internally rotated position and then gradually "unwinds" during early development. During the first year of life, when the baby sleeps mostly on his stomach, there is not as much chance of the toeing in to correct itself. Later on, it most generally does.

If the child toes in noticeably by the time he walks, or at the latest by the age of eighteen months, night splinting may be recommended, and corrective treatment considered. It is important to start treatment by a year and a half, while the bones are still growing and pliable, and will "correct" more quickly, and before he reaches the "terrible two's," when a child will not accept the night splints easily.

There are three common causes for toeing in:

1. *Metatarsus adductus:* The foot—when viewed from the sole—has the curved appearance of a comma. It is "fixed" if it is always curved, even when lying down. It is "dynamic" if it occurs only when the child is walking—a strong muscle on the inside of the foot pulls the great toe and fore foot inward. If metatarsus is mild, simple stretching exercises done by the parents may correct it. If the foot is more resistant, prewalker corrective shoes may be necessary. For the very rigid foot, a series of plaster casts is used—they are not painful to the child.

2. Internal tibial torsion: An inward twist of the leg bones between the knee and ankle causes this condition. Although it is most noticeable after the child starts to walk, severe cases can be recognized earlier. Mostly, treatment involves splinting the feet in a turned-out position during the night and during napping hours. A simple method is to tie the heels of an old pair of high-top shoes together with a shoe lace. (Even "too small" baby shoes with the front end cut off will do.) You can also buy leather straps or have a bar attached between the shoes.

For the older child, twister cable braces are available, and can be worn during the day as well as at night. Some doctors also prescribe shoe wedges or special devices attached to the heel of the walking shoe to encourage a toeing-out walk.

3. *Internal femoral torsion* is a rare condition with an inward twist of the thigh bone between the hip and the knee. When viewed from the front, the entire limb turns in, not just the foot. The kneecaps seem to point inward as well.

In the older child, encourage such activities as ice or roller skating, ballet lessons, and exercise. The child should not be allowed to sit on the floor with his thighs and knees together and his legs and feet out to the sides. Instead, they should be encouraged to sit cross-legged in "the Indian squat."

It is possible for these, and other conditions, to occur in combination. Treatment must be determined by your physician.

Orthopedists don't all agree about treatment. Dr. Bleck says, "In general, pigeon toeing does not respond to so-called corrective orthopedic shoes, many of which have swung-in lasts. These frequently worsen the condition. The Thomas heels and wedges often do little to correct pigeon toeing. I believe plaster casts are the treatment of choice for metatarsus adductus." Part of this disagreement is because orthopedic specialists generally see only a very selective group—those screened out as having special problems. The majority of milder instances of pigeon toeing are never seen by orthopedists. For example, most cases of metatarsus adductus (turned in feet) seen by primary physicians do not require casting; they are corrected by early extension exercises, or by the use of open toed "corrective" shoes. Severe cases, or those which do not respond, are then sent to the orthopedist, who often does use a cast.

The use of Thomas heels, wedges, and other devices is still in vogue, and many pediatricians, family practitioners, and orthopedists still feel that such devices help. In any case, no single treatment works for all people.

Knock-knee and Bowlegs

Should you be concerned when the legs seem to bend in or out excessively? Orthopedic professor E. E. Bleck tells us:

> Knock-knees tend to correct themselves by the age of nine without any special treatment. However, when the knock-knee is severe after age ten, corrective surgery may be considered.
>
> Infants are normally born with bowlegs. When the bowing is severe in the toddler (three to four inches between the inner aspect of the knees when the ankles are put together), corrective measures are necessary.
>
> Often, an x-ray examination will be made in order to determine whether or not there is rickets due to lack of vitamin D, or hereditary vitamin D resistant rickets. These rare cases demand large doses of vitamin D and careful medical supervision—or even surgery—to correct the bowleg.

Orthopedist Alan C. Merchant calls attention to a different variety of bowleg: "A false 'bowleg' appearance can occur in children with severe tibial torsion (twisting) of the lower leg, who rotate the leg out at the hips to compensate. They look ready to ride a horse. Correcting the twist in the lower legs corrects the 'bowlegged' appearance."

WHAT ARE "GROWING PAINS"?

I don't know what growing pains are. Still I diagnose them occasionally. Probably Dr. Hashim's explanation is as good as any.

> Growing pains are not related to the *internal* bone and joint growth but to the whole process of growing up. From age three, children run, jump, and climb—and in a hundred other ways—exert their muscles. At the end of the day, the time most complaints come on, the weary bones, joints, and exhausted muscles are calling for help. These are the "growing pains"; and they are fairly common.
>
> The best help is aspirin, given according to the age. A good brisk massage of the aching part for about twenty to thirty minutes will do wonders, as will a hot water bottle, a hot, hard shower, or a hot bath.
>
> On rare occasions, these pains may be caused by some orthopedic problem. If the particular pain keeps coming back, it would be wise to have it checked out.

ACHES IN THE HEELS AND KNEES

Preadolescent and adolescent children often complain worse than grandpaw about various aches and pains. If it is not their knees it's their heels, and if not the heels it is the back. Usually this recurrent litany of complaints comes after vigorous physical activity that would make most adults have sore muscles. However, it usually isn't the muscles in youngsters, but the cartilage at the ends of their bones, that is the source of the pain. These are really true "growing pains," for it is their phenomenally rapid growth that leads to the problems which occur in the growth centers of their bones.

Bones grow by first forming a thick, relatively soft layer of cartilage which later gradually calcifies. When these cartilage plates become thick, they tend to bruise easily, and the bruised cartilage is painful. This bruise or cartilage degeneration is called osteochondritis. It occurs where the bone receives a lot of pressure or work. One area is the bottom of the heels, where the pounding of hiking or running produces a cartilage breakdown and soreness. Dr. John Richards calls attention to another sort of heel pain, "the week-end limp," which is caused by squeezing growing feet into Sunday-dress shoes that are too small to wear but seem to expensive to discard. Another area is just below the front of the knee, where the big muscle of the upper leg, the quadriceps, attaches to the bone at a growth center. This common condition, called Osgood-Schlatter's disease, is aggravated by running, by climbing stairs, or by hard pedaling of a bike. The same process can occur inside the knee joints, in the spine, and along the front of the hips. The pain usually slows the "growing one" down, and the cartilage heals and calcifies. Then, with more growth, more cartilage is produced. If the cartilage is too thick and the exercise too vigorous, it can all start over again.

Rest is the most important treatment—and, for this age, the most difficult to achieve. Extra vitamin D may help by encouraging slightly more rapid calcification. Some doctors disagree with me on this, feeling that a normal diet contains more vitamin D than needed. However, it is wise to let your doctor check it because there are occasionally other causes for the aches and pains. Anyway, the child is more likely to slow down for a doctor than for a parent.

CAUSES OF KNEE AND HIP PAINS AND AWKWARD CHILDREN

A large number of conditions can cause knee and hip pains. Some of these are as benign as constipation, and some are as serious as osteomyelitis or rheumatic fever. Some conditions are so gradual in onset and so subtle that they are frequently missed, even after examination and x-ray, until a considerable time has elapsed. One of the more difficult conditions, called Legg-Perthes' disease, is a softening of the bone in the upper leg where it turns to go into the hip joint. This creates awkwardness and falling, and, if it goes on too long, may shorten the leg.

Limps Without Injuries

Dr. Richard Mercer warns:

If an otherwise normal child develops a limp without an injury, he should see a physician right away. In the five-to-ten age group this is usually from Legg-Perthes' disease. This disease can lead to serious disability. It is often missed, for the limp seems to come on gradually and without pain.

The same type of limp in the ten-to-fifteen-year age group is usually a slipped growth center at the top of the femur. This, too, can have a subtle onset and may lead to permanent disability.

Another limp occurs when the child first starts to walk. Actually, it is more of a waddling gait than a limp. This might mean a congenital hip dislocation problem.

At any age, a limp with pain and fever may mean an infection in a joint and should be seen at once.

Another very subtle and often missed condition is "femoral torsion," a gradual slow twisting-in of the upper leg bone which causes the knees to point to each other, with resulting awkwardness, muscle strain, fatigue, and, occasionally, pain and limp. The onset of some of these diseases is so gradual and the symptoms so vague that they are usually not recognized or diagnosed early. To keep track of such potential problems, it helps to have repeated health supervision examinations during the rapidly growing years.

The most common limp in the preschool child is from an inflamed hip joint, presumed viral in origin. Often, there is little or no fever, and the complaint, if any, seems centered in the knee. These last a few days and heal themselves. However, the child should be checked by the physician, because the joint inflammation could be due to a bacterial infection which can cause severe and long lasting damage if not caught early.

The painless limp described by Dr. Mercer in the five to fifteen year old may be present a considerable time before it is caught. Early in the course of these problems, even x-rays may be negative. So even if nothing is found on the first examination, follow-up is necessary.

Limps From Injuries

A limp from an injury is frequently less of a problem, writes Dr. Mercer:

If a limp acquired from trauma is not painful or is only mildly painful, it can be watched up to a week. If it disappears, it is of no probable consequence. If it continues, it should be seen.

On the other hand, a painful limp from an injury should be seen if it lasts for over one to two days. Obviously, severe pain, inability to walk, much swelling of the joint or other areas of the leg or foot should be seen sooner.

The Dislocated Hip of Babies

In spite of our scientific approach to medical care we still don't have all of the answers. A case in point is brought up by Dr. Bleck:

We are not at all sure of the exact reason for a dislocated hip, but it has been theoretically linked with a relaxing hormone released in the mother before birth. In the baby, this hormone relaxes the ligaments, leaving the hip joint loose. It affects the hip more than other joints, and girls more than boys.

If it is present at birth, the pediatrician will most likely notice the condition and will recommend treatment.

Treatment involves spreading the legs apart by the use of splints. This forces the ball part of the hip joint into the socket, which in turn forces the socket to develop correctly—in a cup-shape instead of like a saucer. If the socket does not develop correctly by the time the child is eighteen months old, surgical treatment may be necessary.

Dislocation or dysplasia of the hip is not always present at birth; it can develop later. X-rays may reveal a normal thigh–hip relationship at four months of age and an abnormal one two to three months later. A slow tightening of the muscles on the inside of the thighs seems to pull the hip joint into an abnormal position in its socket.

Mild tightening usually causes no problems, but severe tightening may lead to dislocated or abnormal hip joints. This usually responds to a plastic diaper splint, which holds the legs in their normal growth angles during this critical period and prevents possible "congenital hip" problems.

POOR POSTURE

What can you do about poor posture? In general, stay off the kids' backs! Pediatrician Neil Henderson explains:

> Many children have poor posture because their muscles are not well enough developed to carry about their large frames. If a physical examination fails to reveal any disease process, exercises such as sit-ups, pull-ups, knee-bends, and weight lifting may be helpful. Often, the school provides special classes for this purpose. Regardless, it is best to avoid nagging these children about their posture.

More specific causes of poor posture are given by Dr. Bleck:

> A slumped posture with a humped back in teenage boys and girls can either be due to problems in the spinal column or to poor muscle tone and a lack of self-confidence.
>
> A child can have a true "round back deformity," due to so-called Scheuermann's disease, failure of growth of the vertebrae, or some abnormality which causes the vertebrae to become wedge shaped. No amount of exercise and nagging will correct the round back. These cases need treatment, which should be determined by the physician.
>
> Those children who merely slump, and who have no structural change in the vertebrae, may respond to postural exercise. I have found that these children also need a great deal of self-confidence. We call it the hang dog posture—it occurs when the child feels inferior for some reason, and at the low end of the totem pole.

Backaches in Children

Recurring chronic backache is not normal in children. Sometimes they have a temporary backache from such activities as tumbling or gymnastics, but persistent backache certainly ought to be investigated advises Dr. Bleck who describes here a variety of back conditions.

> In the teenage years, we do see backaches from herniated discs, as well as from a growth abnormality of the vertebrae, called Scheuermann's disease, which will usually heal uneventfully; frequently, doctors prescribe a brace for this condition. Another cause is a birth

defect of the vertebrae called spondylolisthesis. In this condition, the last lumbar vertebra slips forward on the sacrum or tail bone. If it is only mild, it can be managed with exercise and corsets. If it is more severe, a surgical spinal fusion will be necessary.

One frustrating condition in teenagers is psychogenic backache which seems to continue for no apparent reason. Emotional factors can often be found as the cause. Once recognized and treated with professional counseling, the backache, just like a headache, will disappear.

Sometimes I have noticed that parents who have had a history of chronic back trouble will transmit this sort of health anxiety to their children. It may be that these children select the back as the most acceptable way of expressing anxiety, hostility, or whatever emotional problem they may have. After ruling out physical causes for the backache, psychiatric counseling should be the treatment.

Swayback

Swayback (lordosis) is usually due to poor strength of the abdominal wall and buttocks muscles which control posture. This lack of muscle strength could be from physical causes or from poor habits. One physical cause is short muscles and ligaments on the front of the hip, which hold the body in a bent over position, causing the pelvis to rotate, and bending the spine forward, causing "swayback." Other causes include a weak abdominal wall and congenital deformities of the vertebrae.

If the swayback is simply postural, due to poor muscle control, exercise is needed under the direction of a physical therapist.

To Prevent Low Back Strain

Low back strain, fatigue, or pain results from many causes. They can be as simple as swayback, too much exercise or strain, or as complicated as a ruptured disk in the spine. Your doctor will help to diagnose the cause, but much of the treatment will be in your hands. In fact, you can prevent much of your trouble by following a few simple rules to PREVENT BACK PROBLEMS:

1. Sleep on your side with your hips and knees flexed, or on your back with bolster (pillow?) under your knees. A pillow under your head is fine.
2. Don't use a sagging or an excessively firm mattress.
3. Sit with your knees raised a bit off the floor, on a stool.
4. When driving a car, sit fairly close to the accelerator and brake pedals.
5. Bend your knees, not your back, when you pick things up.
6. Don't lift things above your hips.
7. Stand with one foot a bit higher than another.
8. Don't sit or stand with your head and neck bent forward.

Exercises for Low Back Problems

Exercises of any sort should build up slowly. Do not try to do the more tiring or stressing exercises until you can handle the easier ones. Check with your doctor to see if these exercises are indicated or not for your particular problem. To be of real value, such exercising must become a "way of life" and continued indefinitely depending on your status.

Lie with your back and hips flat on the floor:

a. Draw your knees up to your chest and "curl into a ball."
b. With one knee bent and that foot on the floor, raise the other leg straight and point your toe to the ceiling.
c. Draw both knees to the chest, and then straighten the legs, pointing toward the ceiling.
d. With both knees bent and the feet on the floor, lift the hips off the floor a few inches and hold them there for a short count.
e. With both knees bent and the feet on the floor, grasp the knees with your hands and pull yourself to a sitting position.

Scoliosis (Crooked Back)

Scoliosis is a condition of the spine that causes it to curve sideways and twist on itself. The twist carries the ribs with it so that they push out and cause a hump on one side of the back. The cause is generally unknown, although there is strong evidence that it can be inherited. We see more girls than boys with scoliosis.

Other causes of spinal curvature include paralysis from poliomyelitis, cerebral palsy, and muscular dystrophy. A few children are born with abnormally formed vertebrae, or congenital scoliosis.

Treatment starts with a thorough exercise program, but for many cases, a Milwaukee brace must also be used. It corrects and prevents the curvature from progressing until final bone growth stops.

The object is not to get a straight spine, which is impossible, but to compensate the curves so that the curve to the right equals the curve to the left. If the curves are equal, then the shoulders will be level and the appearance is often such that you cannot tell that a girl has scoliosis, even when she is in a bathing suit. Invariably, the x-ray looks worse than the patient.

The brace is not always successful, and some curves will progress despite the brace, requiring surgical treatment.

A new experimental treatment looks good for some cases of scoliosis and may replace some braces. The muscles on the weak side of the back are stimulated with a low voltage electrical current, which strengthens them and tends to pull the back bone straight.

Parents Can Check for Scoliosis

Scoliosis sneaks up on growing children, usually from the age of eight to twelve years, and this disabling and unsightly condition should be found and treated early. It is one of many reasons for routine health supervision examinations by the child's pediatrician or family practitioner. However, between examinations, parents can check this at home every few months. Be especially on the lookout if anyone on either side of the family had scoliosis.

Have the child stand with both legs straight and facing straight ahead. Station yourself directly behind him. If you cannot clearly see the back bone, feel it and mark it with a felt pen. Look for a curve. Then have him bend over, with the knees straight, and touch his fingers to the floor. Look for a hump on one side of the back. Sometimes the curve is low in the back and may cause an unequal waistline rather than unequal ribs. If you suspect scoliosis, take your child to the doctor promptly.

OSTEOMYELITIS

Osteomyelitis is a very serious bone disease of children. Pediatrician Eric Sims sees more of this relatively rare disease than most of us in his consulting role at the Adelaide, South Australia, Children's Hospital. Dr. Sims writes:

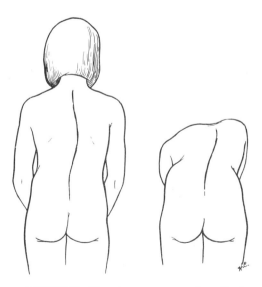

FIGURE 45 *A severe case of scoliosis.*

Osteomyelitis is an infection of a bone, usually occurring near the growing end of a limb bone. Most often it is due to the pimple and boil germ (*Staphylococcus aureus*). A squeezed pimple may cause staph germs to get into the blood stream, and they are likely to lodge in a growing end of bone, where they produce an acute inflammation with pus. The onset is usually sudden, with fever, acute pain in the affected limb, marked tenderness on touching the area, and reluctance to use the joint. X-rays do not help in the all-important early diagnosis, as changes in bone structure do not become visible for a week or more. By that time, damage may be severe. When not diagnosed promptly, swelling and redness of the skin and other soft tissues may appear over the affected bone, especially if it is a bone close to the surface, such as the shin bone.

Strangely enough, children with inflammation in or near the hip joint often complain first of pain in their knee—so-called "referred pain." The same sensory nerve that serves the hip goes down to the knee, making it difficult for the child to pin down the exact area of pain. Osteomyelitis in the hip region, therefore, can be misleading. It can be a tricky diagnosis to make.

Whichever bone is involved, the disease is always an emergency which usually requires surgical drainage, especially if there is pus in a joint. Splints or casts will be required, and antibiotic therapy may be continued for several weeks. Although it is a serious condition, you can usually expect complete recovery, provided that there is early diagnosis and adequate treatment.

HOW NOT TO CUT TOENAILS

If you like sore toes, you will cut the toenails back at an angle. This is especially true for the big toe, because the tissue on either side of the nail tends to push over the nail. If the nail is cut back, or is torn back, the tissue springs in front of the nail. Then, when the nail grows out, it pushes into the tissue in front of it and acts like a foreign body cutting the tissue. The usual result is infection, which causes the tissue to redden, swell, and become very painful. This infection, called a paronychia, is difficult to treat, and a cure may take months or years. At home, treating it early with hot water soaks and local antibiotic ointment may help. The doctor may culture pus if present, cauterize away proud flesh, give an antibiotic, slice the nail back, or even remove the entire nail in order to encourage healing.

Most of the time this is preventable if you cut the toenails straight across. Of course infections in this tissue can come from other causes too, from hangnails to blisters, or from shoes that fit too tight.

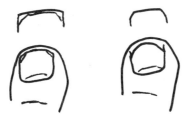

FIGURE 46   *Cut toenails as shown on the left instead of back at the corners because the tissue may bulge up over the nail as shown on the right.*

SPRAINS AND FRACTURES

Sprains and fractures can occur with almost any sort of activity. You can learn some specifics in the Chapter on First Aid, Second Aid, and Emergency Medical Care. Here, we concentrate on the sports aspects of sprains and fractures in growing children. Odd as it may seem, the California Medical Association Committee on Sports and Health, believes:

> The young athlete who incurs a bone fracture is better off than the one who is aware of only vague and persistent pains, particularly around the joints. Almost any youngster, whether engaged in organized or unorganized play, runs the risk of a fracture. There is very little danger of the injury being neglected, and it usually heals uneventfully. The young player is, it is true, removed from the game for the season, but that's a disappointment from which he or she recovers.
>
> The more threatening injuries are those which are too often ignored. They usually involve the portion of the bone adjacent to the joint, which does not complete its growth until the child is past the mid-teens. The child often engages in great muscular exertion in the course of competitive activities, and the undeveloped bone is not equal to the pull of the muscles. As a result, the ends of the still unfused bone may be pulled out of line, causing great discomfort, including swelling, tenderness, and pain upon movement.
>
> Often, the young athlete is being coached by a volunteer—perhaps someone who is engaged in sports at college and who is not making allowances for the fact that boys and girls are still in the developmental phase and cannot take the same rough-and-tumble that adult athletes tolerate very well. The youngster, encouraged by adults to behave like a Spartan and to smother his complaints, does not report the joint discomfort which, unless promptly and properly treated, may result in permanent damage.

THE SPRAINED ANKLE

A sprained ankle is probably the most common injury facing athletes. There are some good "rules of thumb" to decide whether or not the sprain should be seen by the doctor.

When Should a Sprained Ankle Be Seen by a Doctor?
1. If the ankle hurts enough that it cannot be walked on.
2. If it is so painful that it wakes you up during sleep.
3. If the swelling extends across the front of the ankle joint.
4. If the swelling is excessive.
5. If the pain and swelling do not start to subside within three to four days or if they last beyond six days.
6. If the area of the sprain is markedly black and blue.

Can You Prevent Sprains by Taping or Wrapping Ankles?
Many sports physicians believe that taping helps, but physical conditioning will do more to prevent sprains than either of these methods. The best protection for a joint is strong muscles. However, properly done, wrapping can help prevent some sprains. Once the young athlete has had a bad sprain, I would tape them for practice or competition, and would continue physical conditioning. Extend the tape above and below the joint for greater support. Try to make the tape do the job the ligaments, muscles, and tendons were going to do for the joint being taped.

However, as with many things in medicine, there is no "one way." Orthopedic surgeon Bleck writes: "Many question the real value of the standard ritual of ankle taping. We have no evidence that taping reduces ankle injuries. It takes emphasis away from the important exercise of muscles to prevent ankle sprains." Other orthopedists disagree. Some even suggest that high-top tennis shoes have been shown to reduce sprains.

When Physicians Disagree about Sprains

A not uncommon problem facing child athletes and their parents is what to do about a sprained ankle. Some of our contributors objected to putting this disagreement into *The Parents' Medical Manual,* saying that it is always the child's physician who makes the choice. However, the situation arises where the team physician and the family physician disagree. There are not only 1,001 ways of raising children but of practicing medicine. When physicians disagree, each obviously thinks he is right. Dr. Marvin McClellan, who functions as both a team physician and personal physician, explains:

> In a way, both physicians are right. Athletic youths want to return to competition as soon as they can. With proper healing, proper taping, and a strong desire to participate, one may return to active athletics safely after four or five days when the initial swelling and initial insult of the sprain have subsided. This does not mean that the sprain has completely healed, but that it is healed sufficiently so that active competition may be resumed under proper supervision and with proper continued medical assistance. If you wish to heal the sprained ankle 100%, then you must listen to the family doctor and wait for two or three weeks until the wound is entirely and completely healed. However, with

the short athletic seasons in most high schools and colleges, two or three weeks out may be the end of a particular season; and, in any case, the training would have been lost; and before training and conditioning can be resumed, the season would be over. Therefore, it is not expedient to wait two or three weeks for injuries to heal under these circumstances.

Orthopedist Mercer comments that this is a tough one. "I believe parents should listen to the physician who has the eventual final responsibility for the child's care."

KNEE INJURIES

Knee injuries are the most common injuries in sports such as football, skiing, gymnastics, and basketball. "Most of those I see from football," says team physician Marvin McClellan, "are caused by clipping, which causes some damage to the cartilage and often tears the ligaments of the knee. Players should realize the seriousness of such an injury and make every effort to avoid clipping. Some football shoes contribute to knee injuries. Long-cleated shoes planted firmly in the ground won't give when the player twists to move or when he is hit. Pop Warner football teams emphasize short and wide cleats. A cleat shaped like a wedge pointing sideways toward the edge of the shoe is said to help." However, Dr. McClellan points out that a player wearing no shoes at all could get a football knee injury. Proper physical conditioning and strength, as well as care to avoid clipping, are better assurances against knee injuries than the kind of shoes worn.

In general, the same principles mentioned concerning ankle sprains apply to injuries to the knee. When in doubt, consult with your physician.

13

BLOOD

WHAT IS BLOOD?

Pediatric hematologist David Rosenthal explains four major components of blood:

1. *Red Blood Cells.* These small disc-shaped cells, without a nucleus, are the predominant cells in the blood. The red material in the cell which gives blood its color is known as hemoglobin; it supplies oxygen to the body cells and removes the waste gas and carbon dioxide. In normal health, the total number of red cells in the body remains relatively constant.

2. *White Blood Cells.* These cells, also known as leukocytes, are one of the body's primary defense mechanisms. All leukocytes are not the same, and each cell type has a special purpose. The total number of white cells will vary, depending on the type of body stress. The polymorphonuclear leukocyte (P.M.N.) is the major component of pus, and serves the body in defense of bacterial infections. The lymphocyte carries some of the body's antibody defenses, the main protection in viral illnesses. Monocytes are cells which remain relatively constant in number. Their main function is to help the body get rid of dead and damaged cells and cellular debris. Eosinophiles increase during an allergy attack or parasite infection.

3. *Platelets.* The main function of these very small cells is to prevent bleeding. By actually plugging small holes and by producing certain substances known as phospholipids, they help to form blood clots. The lack of these cells leads to various degrees of bleeding including *petechiae,* small red pin-points of bleeding in the skin;

purpura, larger reddish purple or blue areas in the skin; or frank
hemorrhage, the loss of great amounts of blood.

4. *Plasma.* This is the fluid material of blood. It acts as a carrier of
the cellular elements, nutrients, and chemicals to the body cells, and
takes waste to the appropriate body organs.

As a readily accessible body fluid, the blood reflects what is
happening in the body. Appropriate analysis of the condition of the
blood is a great help to the physician in his determining the body's state
of illness or health.

ANEMIA

The most common "blood" problem is anemia or a low hemoglobin
or too few red blood cells. This usually occurs because a child has too
little iron in his diet, although it can be due to bleeding in the bowel,
chronic infection, heavy menstrual bleeding, and many other causes. The
most common basic dietary cause is too much milk. The child then has
little appetite for other foods and because milk is iron poor, he develops
iron deficiency anemia. Dr. Hashim describes the anemic child:

> He is fretful, pale, and not happy at all. He may look chubby and
> be of good size, yet you suspect there is something wrong. Take a good
> look at him and you will see that his lips look pale and his ears look
> waxy. You take him to your doctor, who checks his blood and says, "The
> baby has low blood." You shake a little bit, and ask him, "What is it?"

Sometimes the cause of anemia from cow's milk isn't that there is too
little iron but is that the child is sensitive to milk. Such a child may
actually lose small amounts of blood into the bowel and thus develop
anemia. Such anemias will usually respond to iron drops your doctor can
prescribe and to stopping milk.

Iron-rich foods include baby cereals (that have iron added), meat,
eggs, and some fruits and vegetables. A list of the iron content of foods
will be found on page 388. For premature infants, twins, or infants born
of anemic mothers, a formula with extra iron in it may be advised.
Untreated anemia may affect the child's entire system, even to the point
of heart failure. Prevent this by proper diet and periodic health supervision checks by your child's doctor. Some children have a naturally pale
skin and look anemic but aren't. Others may look pale because they are
allergic.

Sickle Cell Anemia

Many black people inherit a condition called sickle cell anemia. The
cells are crescent-shaped rather than round, and they do not move easily
through the blood vessels. This can result in episodes of severe body

pains, anemia from broken-down red cells, and other symptoms such as swollen hands and feet, slow growth, jaundice, and fever.

Every person has two hemoglobin genes—one from each parent. If both parents are carriers, there is a 25% chance that the child will have sickle cell anemia. Potential parents can have their blood easily tested to determine the risk.

A similar condition called thalassemia, with abnormal red blood cells, occurs in persons of Mediterranean extraction. In this disease the symptoms are primarily anemia.

HEMOPHILIA

Hemophilia is an inherited condition in which the blood doesn't clot well and the person has problems from excessive bleeding. Women carry the defective gene and pass it to their children but don't bleed themselves. This condition usually is found when a baby is circumcised or a child has his tonsils removed and won't stop bleeding. If there is a history of blood relatives who have bled excessively from these causes, tell your doctor.

WHAT IS LEUKEMIA?

Leukemia (acute and chronic, Hodgkin's disease, lymphoma, and multiple myeloma) is a cancer-like disease of the blood-forming organs which produce an overabundance of abnormal white blood cells. These unhealthy cells interfere with red cells and with blood clotting. Acute leukemia in children used to be rapidly fatal. Newer treatments, however, offer survival for as long as ten years and, recently, some apparent cures. Ninety percent of leukemias can be put into remission.

Chronic leukemia is the more common form in adults, and often lasts well over ten years. Lymphomas, Hodgkin's disease (of the lymph nodes), and multiple myeloma are somewhat similar. Early treatment of Hodgkin's disease by x-ray is proving successful. There is no known prevention. These diseases are not considered contagious.

Early signs are unfortunately vague, but they include undue weakness, fatigue, bruising, and bleeding. Other signs are swollen lymph nodes in the neck or above the collar bone, bone and joint pains, blood in the urine, pallor, jaundice, and skin lesions. Many symptoms of ordinary illnesses mimic those of leukemia.

When the disease strikes, families need more than technical and leukemic specialist help. A physician must assume the role of protagonist for the child and involve himself in family feelings. The parents as well as the rest of the family must form a cooperative team. Without such support, the child will suffer more. Unfortunately, the stress and sorrow, with their resulting feelings of guilt and anger, increase the chance of a broken home. Parents go through highly individualistic and personal expressions of grief and mourning which may be expressed by:

- An unwillingness to face facts.
- Hostility toward those who confirm the diagnosis.
- Guilt for some unknown failure.
- Sadness in anticipation of an acute and total loss.

Facing these feelings forces emotional growth in parents. Often, counseling is required, and can be of great value. There is help available *through your doctor,* through teams of leukemia specialists, or through your local chapter of the Leukemia Society of America, which may even be able to offer some financial aid. Don't forget friends, relatives, and your church. Have the courage to ask.

JAUNDICE

Jaundice is a condition in which the skin turns yellow and the urine dark because of bile pigment in the blood. This is not rare in newborn infants. Usually no harm results, and the jaundice just disappears in a few days. Other times it can be a serious problem. Dr. Eric Sims explains.

When the red cells become worn out and useless, they are removed from circulation. In the process, they split up into two parts: the *iron molecules,* which are used again in the formation of new blood, and the *pigment residue,* which is carried to the liver, where it combines with a chemical substance and is excreted as part of the bile. The bile leaves the liver through a duct and enters the adjacent bowel. Some of the bile pigment can then be absorbed back into the blood stream, but most of it passes out from the body in the bowel movements. Jaundice occurs when there is either an excessive breakdown of red blood cells, causing a "jam up" in the system, or a block to the excretion of bile from the liver to the bowel. Either of these can cause an accumulation of bile pigments in the tissues of the body, which gives the characteristic yellow color to the skin and whites of the eyes.

Normal newborn babies are often yellow for a few days because their systems are destroying the surplus red blood cells they are born with. The excess bile pigment, bilirubin, brought to the liver as a result of this normal mild blood destruction, tends to accumulate because the liver is still a little immature and inefficient in excreting it. This so-called "physiological jaundice" cures itself in a few days. However, if the baby is born prematurely, then the greater immaturity of the liver is likely to make this sort of jaundice even more prolonged, and sometimes it is sufficiently severe to require treatment. This jaundice of immature liver function is the sort that nowadays may be treated by exposure to visible light rays (phototherapy) under carefully controlled conditions.

Another condition that is partly due to the obstruction of the fine bile ducts within the liver is the jaundice of hepatitis. As a result of inflammation and swelling of the ducts, the bile cannot get out of the ducts into the bowel. This obstructive jaundice is characterized by very pale, even white, bowel movements and dark urine, due to the retention of bile, which overflows into the urine. Such an obstructive jaundice in the newborn also may be due to actual failure of development of the bile ducts, a rare congenital anomaly.

It may be difficult to determine whether a baby has neonatal hepatitis or atresia of the bile ducts, as both conditions can cause an obstructive jaundice that persists through the early months of life. Consequently, an operation is often advised after the first three or four months so that the adequacy of the bile ducts can be properly assessed by studying a piece of the baby's liver under the microscope.

A more serious form of blood destruction (hemolysis) can occur when the mother has a different blood group from her baby and has been stimulated to produce antibodies against the baby's blood. These antibodies filter back into the baby before birth and can damage his blood. Indeed, this is the most likely cause if a baby becomes significantly jaundiced on the first day of life. Appropriate blood testing will be done, and, if necessary, replacement transfusion scheduled immediately. Fortunately, this form of blood incompatibility is becoming less common now, because if the mother is known to be Rh negative, then an appropriate injection of protecting antibody can be given to her shortly after delivery in order to prevent future Rh disease.

Sometimes persisting jaundice in the newborn may be due to a bacterial infection in the blood stream, the kidneys, or elsewhere in the body. Jaundice is not a disease in itself—it is merely a pointer to possible causes in the blood stream, in the liver, in the body chemistry, or in the immaturity of the organs. Only expert investigation can sort out the cause in your baby. Fortunately, the vast majority turn out to need a simple treatment and do well.

14

KEEP YOUR SKIN HEALTHY

Skin feels good; I don't blame the Eskimos for rubbing noses. But although skin sensations may transport us to ecstasy, they can also be the bane of our existence. Such an important part of us deserves more consideration, and fewer medications, than it usually gets. The human urge to pet, pick, stroke, scratch, apply, and cover skin is phenomenal.

Most books on health advice for parents are relatively "skinless." There are good reasons for caution in offering printed advice for the layman reader. First is the danger that we will be taken literally. As an example, in one spot in *The Manual,* you are advised to use U.S.P. plain calamine lotion rather than fancier calamine products that include, in addition, many other medications. The reasoning is that each additional medication increases the risk of sensitizing and irritating your skin. But that doesn't mean that U.S.P. plain calamine lotion alone can't sensitize someone's skin, or that you should continue to use it if the results are not good. The other major reason for professional reluctance to offer general or specific advice on skin in a book is that everyone's skin is a little different—and some skins are a lot different. So as you read this chapter, keep in mind the bell curve variability discussed in the introduction, and remember that your skin is unique.

Our basic goal is to help you to prevent skin disease, or to help you control or cure any skin disease you may have. In any case, if you read this chapter, you will come to know your hide better—and you will probably take care of it better in the future.

All of us wish we could offer you more specific advice for your problems—but that will take personal examination and thought from your physician. We do, however, offer some good preventive advice that may reduce your need to take you or your child to a doctor for skin problems.

SKIN CARE

How clean should you be? Can you really wash *too much?* Cleanliness is nice. It reduces smell, scabies, and impetigo. However, the great American custom of a daily bath is excessive for most skins. This is especially true if soaps are used, for they remove protective elements from the skin along with dirt. Al Jacobs, M.D., professor of pediatric dermatology, explains:

> Skin, especially the outer horny layer, is a barrier between you and your horrible environment. This horny outermost layer consists of flakes of hardened dead cells that contain some water. If they contain too much water, from constant exposure to moisture, they become water logged and ineffective. If they dry out excessively, they flake off, the skin cracks, and the skin barrier is broken. Normal skin oils protect the horny layer cells from losing or gaining too much water. The oils also keep the skin flexible and form a barrier which protects against infection. Soaps, solvents, and bathing remove their vital skin oils. The average person doesn't need a thorough bath every day, especially a hot bath or the prolonged soaking kids get playing in the tub. A quick warm shower is better for the skin.
>
> If you wish to *produce* a rash, just add detergent or bubble bath to the bathwater. Bubble bath is especially sensitizing, and causes not only a skin rash but irritation in the urethra or even in the bladder of girls. Pure detergents are bad enough, but the more chemicals are added to them, the more business the dermatologist gets. The same applies to various additives in facial "soaps." Each additive—such as enzymes, and "cold power," "biodegradable," and "antibacterial" materials—contributes an additional sensitizing agent. Certainly not everyone becomes sensitized, but those who do often have a rash.

I am appalled at the practice of putting things like detergent for dishes in the bathwater with the child because "it keeps the ring off the tub." Why not take the poor kid to the car wash where he *really* can get cleaned?

How Much Sun?

> Sun is fun
> But son of a gun
> While sun is nice
> It can shorten your life.

How much sun should you get? Actually, sunshine on the skin helps manufacture vitamin D and is good treatment for acne and psoriasis. The sun is warm, it feels good, and a tan looks nice, yet the same sun is damaging as well as tanning. Dr. Jacobs explains:

You wouldn't think of lying under an x-ray machine for hours at a time, yet sun irradiation causes the same kind of damage to the skin as x-ray irradiation. Sun also ages the skin prematurely. The tanned and proud bathing beauty of today will be the first to suffer early aging and wrinkling that comes from skin atrophy and loss of elasticity. The next unhappy result is skin cancer, which is directly related to the amount of exposure and the complexion. Redheads and blond Scandinavian types suffer more skin cancers than the average person, while the disease is rare among blacks. If you have the fair skin of a redhead, you should protect yourself from sun as much as possible.

Skin can be more sensitive to sunburn when exposed to photosensitizing agents. The most common is sulfacilanalid, a common agent in antibacterial soaps. Some antibiotics of the tetracycline type cause increased sunburn. Photosensitivity in some people has been caused by oral contraceptives, barbiturates, aspirin, some diuretics, cyclamate, benadryl, selenium, hexachloraphene, sulfonamides, quinine, and many other substances.

Tanning lotions have little protective value against the sun. Effective sun screens are available, starting with the inexpensive but messy red petroleum jelly. The best sun screen contains paraminobenzoic acid in 50 percent alcohol. This combines with the horny layer of skin and gradually builds up a residual concentration that increases sun resistance. Paraminobenzoic acid in smaller concentrations of alcohol or in ointments is far less effective, but is certainly better than nothing, because "today's tan is tomorrow's wrinkle."

The photosensitive rash is hard to recognize. The skin's resistance to the sun is reduced and eczema-like reactions occur when it is exposed to the sun later. Such rashes can occur from minor sun exposure; and it takes less than ordinary exposure to get a sunburn. A considerable number of photosensitive rashes are caused by various plants being rubbed on the skin or eaten (see page 382).

From sunny Nebraska we are cautioned by Dr. Hobart Wallace that:

During the first eighteen months of age, most infants do not develop much protection from tanning. When outdoors, the use of protective lotions may be needed; remember that a baby can be sunburned by reflected sun rays even in the shade.

And from sunny California, another pediatrician Dr. Richard O'Neill advises that:

An ounce of prevention is worth a pound of grease: Insist that your small fry put on that old gray sun bonnet, and the older kids a baseball cap. Tee shirts are stylish and will reduce the exposed skin surface.

Light cotton long pants are great to prevent the legs from being fried, but you have to be the kids' watch dog from too much sun. Everyone loses sleep with sunburn, so don't be afraid to yell. Remember that you can get a bad burn even on a foggy, overcast day at the beach. If it's a mild sunburn, I advise a cool shower as soon as possible and for as long, and as often, as possible. Then, follow with one of the soothing sunburn sprays. (The rubbing on of cream is too painful and sticky.) A loose Hawaiian-type shirt will cover the burn, and not make it too hot when you have to dress. If you are going to apply an antibiotic ointment and need a dressing, a clean white cotton tee shirt is usually available and is easy to launder.

SKIN RASHES

When Should the Doctor See a Skin Rash?

Call at once and arrange to be seen if:

1. Blue, purple, or blood-red spots occur. These could represent serious infection, even if no fever is present.
2. A rash becomes progressively worse day by day, even if you think you know what it is.
3. There are signs of infection: yellow pus or red streaks going from the rash.
4. The itch is severe.

How well you describe the rash on the telephone may be of help in deciding whether it needs to be seen. However, even trained observers have difficulty describing a rash. The same agent may cause different types of rash or no rash on different types of people. Before you call:

1. Take all the clothes off and check all parts of the body for the presence and distribution of the rash. Is it on the scalp, the palms, or soles? Is it mostly on the trunk, or is it on the arms and legs? Is it mostly on the upper part of the body or the lower?
2. What color is the rash: whiter than the skin, grey, light pink, dark pink, bright blood-red, purplish, blue, yellow, or brownish?
3. Can you feel the rash or just see it? Is the border or the center raised?
4. Are the spots clustered or separate?
5. Are there blisters, oozing, scabs, or scaling?

I have trouble telling what a rash is by looking at it. Over the phone, it is harder. I know of a professor of dermatology who called in another dermatologist to help him decide if his own child had flea bites or chicken pox. And we all keep learning year after year. Some viral rashes are new, or at least are never described in the literature, or have never been seen before by a particular doctor. When in doubt, have the rash seen.

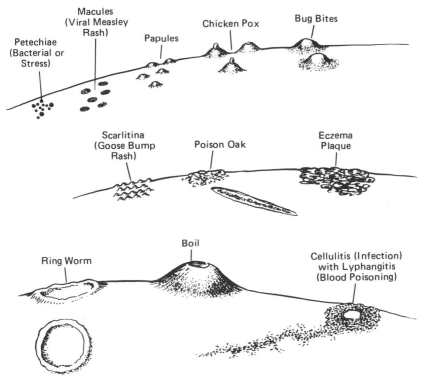

FIGURE 48 *Types of skin rashes.*

WHAT IS SKIN ALLERGY?

Skin allergy usually results from something your skin touches. It may not be a true allergy, sometimes it is a reaction to a chemical substance in a plant, or to an industrial product. But whether the skin is allergic or just sensitive, certain substances will cause rash in some people and not in others. It requires a lot of detective work to track down such allergies. You may get clues from Figures 48 and 49 illustrating various things that can cause rashes in various areas of the body—called contact dermatitis. You can also get help in the book, *Your Allergic Child,* where Dr. Crook tells us what can be done at home to reduce contact allergies on the skin.

1. Don't bathe as often, and don't use soap. Your doctor may suggest a soap substitute.
2. In the winter, the air in heated homes is very dry. Moisten it with some sort of humidifier or vaporizer, using plain water.
3. Coat your skin with inexpensive protective ointments like petroleum jelly or zinc oxide. They soothe the skin, reduce water loss, and

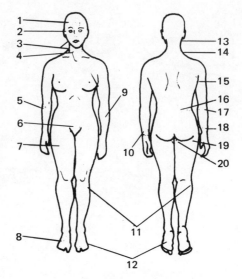

FIGURE 48   *Location of skin rashes caused by contact. (1) Hair oils, etc., (2) Eye make up, (3) Sun-sensitive dermatitis, (4) Bibs on babies, (5) Mother's cosmetics on children, (6) Ammonia urine or detergent burn on babies, (7) Permanent press pants, (8) Tongue of shoe, (9) Carrying a dog or cat, (10) Coat sleeve or bracelet, (11) Carpet or house dust on children, (12) Shoes, (13) Soap left behind ears, (14) Necklaces, collars, (15) Deodorants, or sweat dissolving detergents in clothes, (16) Weeds in garden where shirt creeps up, (17) Leaning on laundry tub or plastic surface, (18) Wrist watch, rubber gloves, (19) Rubber from panties, (20) Colored or scented toilet paper, Kotex or mini pads.*

protect it from contact with chemicals. Some skins, however, will react even to petroleum jelly with a rash, so be cautious.

4. Wear smooth cloth next to the skin, and long sleeves and pants to protect against contacts.

5. Be suspicious of detergents, fabric softeners, permanent press clothes, and various dyes in cloth which may chemically irritate or sensitize your skin.

There are other types of skin rashes due to allergy, including hives and eczemas. These are discussed in Chapter 15.

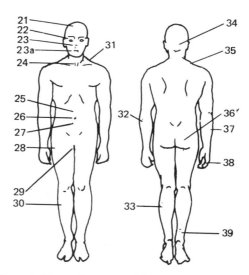

FIGURE 49   *Location of skin rashes caused by contact. (21) Hair oil, shampoo, or cradle cap from not washing the soft spot in babies' heads, (22) Eyedrops, (23) Eczema from mother's cosmetics on child, (23a) Impetigo under nose, (24) Dog tags or necklace pendants, (25) Rugs or grass where shirt and pants work apart, (26) Soap left in belly button, (27) Belt buckle, (28) Articles in pockets, (29) Poison oak from holding penis while urinating, (30) Weeds, bug bites, (31) Violin, (32) Armchair, table varnish, oil cloth, (33) Chairs, (34) Hair oils, shampoos, etc., (35) Suspenders, (36) From cleansing or sterilizing solutions on toilet seats, (37) Poison oak, (38) Rings, (39) Socks.*

ACNE

Teenagers suffer more than most parents realize. Acne can affect their personality and disposition. Even relatively mild acne can be a major problem to the self-critical adolescent, warns dermatologist Jacobs:

Parents should recognize that *acne is a very bad disease.* For some, it can be an irreversible physical and psychological disaster. In the words of an intelligent professional man, "Acne changed my whole life, because I was embarrassed and ashamed. I became an absolute loner and was afraid to try to date. It persisted through college and ruined my enjoyment of life during that period."

Yet, parents often despair and wonder if their acned teenagers will ever take care of themselves, eat the right foods, and follow the doctor's instructions. Parental heckling and storming usually just causes the kids to rebel. Mothers must accept the fact that it is the teenager's acne, not theirs. Let the child go to his or her doctor alone. Start this early enough so that physical or psychological scarring will be prevented. Then remember that good results cannot be accomplished in just a few visits. Each skin is uniquely individual, and its reaction to various medications and treatments must be evaluated over a considerable period of time. Acne is complicated and many myths are spread about along with the facts.

Dr. Jacobs continues:

Facts and Fallacies About Acne

1. Blackheads are not dirt. They are the result of air oxidizing the thick greasy oily material at the opening of the skin glands and turning it black. If the glands are not open to the air, the oil remains white, hence causing whiteheads.

2. Excess skin oil is produced in acne, as can be seen during the day when the face gets oilier and oilier. But this isn't the whole story—in fact, the whole story isn't known. Why do the skin glands get plugged? Perhaps there is a genetic factor.

3. Most acne pustules or cysts are not infected abscesses but are reactions to an irritating chemical, called a fatty acid, formed from the material in the oil glands by a normal skin bacterium.

4. The skin normally produces oil that serves as a protective mechanism to keep the skin from drying out, keeps it flexible, and protects it from chemicals and germs. There is an excess of oil in acne, but the oil itself is not all bad.

5. Acne is not caused by foods, and in most cases foods do not make acne worse. "Bugging" a kid about foods is usually counter-productive.

6. There is no relation between acne and sexual activity. It is not caused by masturbation or lack of masturbation. It occurs equally in boys and girls.

7. It is all right to wash the face to remove dirt and *excess* oil. Usually, a good face-wash twice a day is all that is needed. Washing four times a day may remove so much of the protective coating of oil that the skin will become damaged and inflamed. It is reasonable to remove excess oil once or twice a day, using one of the across-the-counter foil-wrapped cleansing and treatment pads which can be carried in the pocket. It is unreasonable and impractical to expect a high school student to wash the face twice a day in school.

8. Teenagers (or their parents) frequently try too much self-medication. For really mild acne, mild across-the-counter preparations are sufficient.

9. Sunshine or an ultraviolet lamp, if properly used, helps by mildly peeling the skin. The peeling opens the pores of the oil glands and allows cysts, pustules, and whiteheads to drain.

10. The skin in acne should be repeatedly rechecked by the physician in order to evaluate the results of past treatment and to plan future treatment. Everyone's skin is individual and requires individual assessment.

Dr. Jacob's advice about acne is "right on." We must emphasize that each individual's skin *is* individual. So what works for one doesn't always work for another. For example, teenagers often tout their favorite lotion or cream just like some neighbors who want you to take a pill that works "for them." In another instance, a few people have skin that won't tolerate soap. Your doctor can recommend a soap substitute. But our prescriptions do not always work. Your skin may be supersensitive to a treatment that works for "everybody." The proof of the pudding is in the eating; either it works or it doesn't work.

Foods by themselves don't cause acne, but some foods in some people will make acne worse. Watch for an outbreak after you have eaten certain foods. *If* a food aggravated your acne, quit eating it! For some individuals, the following foods are a problem: chocolate, cola drinks, peanut butter, nuts, spices, seafood, iodized salt, and greasy foods. There may be other foods that can affect you. Watch for them.

Dr. Blackburn Joslin suggests that we add eggs and milk to the list. Some people claim that no foods are truly implicated in acne. This may be so for many, but some seem to have flare-ups of acne after eating certain foods. However, Dr. Jacobs objects, saying: "Cutting out foods merely makes kids rebel! I especially object to including eggs and milk." He sees the severe cases where kids have rebelled and refused to even wash their faces. Dr. Joslin and I have seen diets occasionally help. That really has to be up to the individual adolescent.

SKIN INFECTIONS

Skin Diseases from the Staphylococcus Germ

Pediatrician A. S. Hashim explains:

The "Staph" bacteria on the skin can lead to impetigo, abscesses, and styes. Impetigo lesions are dull red, small, variable in size, and may have a yellow crust on top. They spread slowly and are ugly looking. They rarely itch. If the infection is deeper, it can cause a slight swelling of the skin which may last a long time; this is called *echthyma*. Boils are familiar to most people. They tend to come out sometimes two or three at a time. They have cores. An abscess is bigger than a boil, and a carbuncle is like a big abscess with many openings or "eyes" (cores full of pus on top of a "tunnel"). Styes are boil-like sores of the eye lids.

There are effective treatments for these horrible-sounding skin infections. For a spot of impetigo, use an antibiotic ointment (no prescription needed) twice a day for seven to ten days. It should improve within two to three days. If there are many spots of impetigo or if it doesn't respond promptly, see the doctor. In some cases, internal antibiotics will be needed, since about half the cases of impetigo are caused by strep germ. Boils often have to be opened and drained.

How Do You Get Skin Infections?

The majority of skin infections are from the bacteria staphylococcus and streptococcus. We are born into a sea of bacteria, and the staph germ becomes a normal inhabitant of our skin and nostrils. It lives on us in an almost friendly way, and we respond only by forcing the germ to stay on the outer layers of the skin by reacting with antibodies and germ-fighting white blood cells if it penetrates deeper. This balance can be upset in several ways.

Physical damage to the skin may introduce germs into areas where they are poorly tolerated. From a scratch to a bug bite or sunburn, the deeper layers are opened up for invasion. Skin resistance is also decreased from a variety of other causes. The diabetic has extra sugar in the skin, which encourages germ growth. Immunity may be decreased from drugs and disease. Or a child may be born with a genetically defective skin having less resistance than most. Chronically wet skin may be more easily infected, and a large variety of skin rashes lower local resistance to infection.

A different strain of nonfriendly staphylococcus may get on the skin and create trouble. You may not be immune to this staph, which is new to your system—and this is especially so for infants and children, who lack much immune experience. Some bacteria are bad actors and excrete damaging enzymes that allow them to penetrate the skin and get into juicier and more damaging areas. Where do these bad actors come from, and how does your infant or child get them?

Nebraska pediatrician Hobart Wallace points to a common source: "I am amazed at parents allowing a child who has a skin infection to play with children in the neighborhood. The skin infection of impetigo is transmitted from the infected child to another child's skin or throat."

Asking where they come from originally is like asking what came first, the chicken or the egg. We do know that if a staphylococcus germ gets into a good nourishing growth area like muscle or bone, it multiplies like fury. Every twenty minutes, each germ divides and there are twice as many as before. The body responds by sending bacteria-engulfing white blood cells, which form yellow pus. The reaction causes local swelling and a boil may appear. Each bit of that pus may contain hundreds of thousands of bacteria. They spread and are ready to infect again. If pus with staphylococci in it get onto your overstuffed furniture and dries, two years later the staph will still be alive and can be cultured from that spot. But take heart; soap and water will wash them away.

Perhaps the most common source of bad-acting germs is the hospital.

People who become sick because of staph often have to go to the hospital for care. Those who care for them become infected also—but usually, because of very high immunity, they do not become ill. So, hospital personnel can become staph carriers. A newborn in the hospital, for instance, may acquire not the usual friendly staph but instead a bad-acting staph. These are brought home with the baby and can spread to the family. On occasions, they may make a baby seriously ill. It was because of this experience that hexachloraphene-containing soaps were and are still used in many newborn nurseries in a successful attempt to reduce serious staphylococcal infections of the newborn.

Another source of staphylococcus is from animals. Even as adults, we may have little experience and poor immunity to animal strains of this germ. Butchers sometimes become infected from handling meat, and animal handlers may be infected directly. Pets may, of course, be infected by us—so it isn't a one way street.

Another source of bacterial skin infection is from insect bites, especially those of yellow jackets, which feed on garbage and then may bite you. Early use of a good antiseptic on insect bites and stings is helpful.

The most common source of skin infection in children is the nose and throat. Both streptococcus and staphylococcus skin infections may spread from colds or sore throats. Often the runny nose cold irritates the skin around the nose and the bacteria grow in the area, causing impetigo. A child who picks his nose and then scratches a bug bite may infect the bite area with bacteria. Streptococcal skin infections are especially bad, spreading rapidly and occasionally causing the kidney problem of glomerulonephritis.

Rules That Will Help You Avoid Skin Infections

1. Pus contains infective germs and should be washed off of anything it touches —you, your clothes, bedding, furniture, towels, and other items.
2. Picking the nose should be avoided.
3. Watch for signs of infected skin if your child has a cold, and treat it early by washing with an antibacterial soap, and treating with an antiseptic (containing iodine or mercury) or an antibiotic ointment.
4. Take special care if:
    You are around someone with boils or impetigo.
    You are around an infected animal.
    You are bitten or stung by insects, especially yellow jackets.
    If you have a cold or sore throat.

ATHLETE'S FOOT

Wash your teeth twice a day
Change your shoes before you play
Don't forget, your stockings smell
So go ahead, change them as well.

How Can You Prevent or Treat Athlete's Foot?

Sweating and chronic wet feet lead to soggy skin. This encourages the growth of fungi and bacteria. Excessive sweating may also cause vesicles or blisters on the skin of the feet, just as some deep fungus infections do.

Keep the feet clean and dry. A good rule is to have two pair of shoes; change shoes and socks immediately after school or work. If you are in an office, slip your shoes off under the desk while you work. Wiggle your toes and cool your feet. Sandals are great, and allow a lot of airing. Pure leather sandals are far less likely to contain sensitizing chemicals than shoes are.

It is reasonable to try an over-the-counter preparation for a few weeks before seeing a doctor for athlete's foot, as long as the feet don't get worse or sore. I prefer a liquid or powder preparation that will dry on the skin after the bath. Athlete's foot medication in ointment base tends to keep the skin too moist. In any case, the toes must be washed and dried thoroughly. The fungus spores will remain in the feet a long time, so continue routine use of the foot powder for months.

Not all rashes between the toes or on the feet are athlete's foot. A common cause is allergy to some material in shoes. Changing to a cheap all-plastic shoe or wearing leather sandals may allow this condition to heal. Psoriasis can appear on the feet, and bacterial infections can occur in any open skin lesion. If your feet are uncomfortable or sore, walk them to your doctor.

Pediatrician Lendon Smith offers a simple and rather accurate approach to the diagnosis of foot rashes:

> In general, if the rash is between the toes, it is a fungus. If it is on the top or bottom of the feet, it is a contact to shoes or stockings. Clean, white cotton stockings must be used.

ITCHING

The skin may itch from many causes. Contact with irritating plants, such as poison oak or ivy (and 184 others), is covered under poisonous plants (see page 382). Other common causes of itching are contact dermatitis from chemicals in clothes, soaps, cosmetics and so forth. Scabies from mites causes severe and chronic itching and is often not easy to diagnose (see page 336). At times, and in some people, the skin can itch from viral infections in the respiratory tract or from allergy to foods. In rare instances, itching can be caused by liver or kidney disorders or even by malignancies.

General rules about itching include, keep cool: Don't overdress, don't keep the house too warm, don't exercise and get overheated. Keep the fingernails cut down and smoothed with a file so that they don't damage the skin as much when you scratch. In severe cases, it may be warranted to pin a child's long sleeves to his pants so he can't scratch the

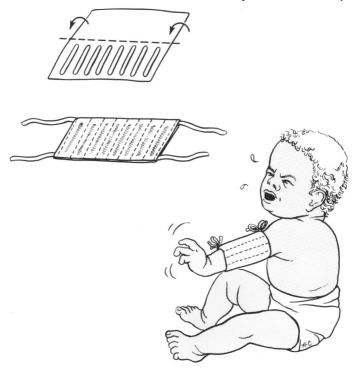

FIGURE 50   *Sew your own elbow splint from an old dish towel and popsickle sticks or tongue depressors. It keeps the arms straight and therefore the fingernails away from the head. Babies get used to it quickly (usually!).*

face. For infants, a splint can be made with tongue depressors and a dishtowel to tie around the arms. A cool shower or a bath in a tub with baking soda often helps. Many dermatologists recommend against calamine type lotions because they can sensitize the skin. An alcohol gel (topic) is sometimes useful. There are prescription cortisone lotions and creams for the skin, and fairly effective anti-itching medicines that can be taken by mouth.

PLANTS CAUSING SKIN RASHES

Skin rashes may be caused in several ways by plants:

1. Direct irritation or contact dermatitis of the skin from a chemical in the plant. This may vary with the age or portion of the plant, but usually doesn't bother the thick skin of the palms or soles, and usually starts within a short time after exposure.

2. Allergic dermatitis varies with the individual, and requires previous exposure

which has made the particular person sensitive. The rash usually doesn't occur for up to five days. Plants in this group include those as diverse as poison ivy and celery.

3. Some pollens have a chemical which causes a rash even if it lands on the skin. This is from a different chemical than the one which causes hayfever in allergic individuals. These rashes are on portions of the skin exposed to the air. Examples are pollens from elm or maple trees.

4. "Light" rashes may follow exposure to certain plants. Some sort of chemical reaction occurs when the skin is exposed to light; even artificial light results in "sunburn." Plants known to cause this variety of rash include parsnip, celery, and figs.

5. Mechanical injury which hurts and may introduce various infections. Various cactus thorns and nettles are examples.

6. Systemic or internal poisoning from some plants which cause rashes may be caused if a plant is eaten, or, in the case of pollens, inhaled. Even internal shock can occur from very severe rashes, that is, rolling in nettles. (See page 382 for lists of potential rash-producing plants.)

15

ALLERGY

A recent estimate indicates that about twelve percent of the population suffers from some form of allergy. However, I suspect that under the right conditions most of us are susceptible. As an example, during the exceptionally high pollen season in California in 1973, huge numbers of people who had had no prior problems became acutely aware that they were allergic.

Like many other conditions in medicine, allergy is a matter of degree; that is, many people have or develop severe allergy, most people may have a touch of allergy, and some may have absolutely none at all. We are aware, too, that allergy is a "great masquerader," often mimicking symptoms of other illnesses.

We are fortunate in this chapter to have a mixture of excellent contributors representing several views and fields of allergy, general pediatrics, and family practice. They offer a rounded look at a complex field, and a wealth of information, helpful to any who may:

Suffer and sneeze
itch and wheeze
with every breeze.

We have put allergy at the end of the part concerning the location of disease because most people think of locations when they think of allergy: the nose, the chest, the skin. It could just as easily go into the part on causes, because the disease or discomfort is caused by allergens such as pollens and dust. However, allergy can also be caused by emotional upsets, cold air, and even sunshine. So really, allergy is the body's reaction to an outside cause, whether it is an overbearing husband or a sophisticated cat with fur and dander.

WHAT ALLERGY IS ALL ABOUT

As you will see, the chemical and cellular details about allergy are slowly being discovered. What we know now, simply put, is that, for reasons we do not understand, some people seem to inherit a tendency to be allergic. Those people react to some substances they breathe, eat, or touch almost as if the substance is a poison or an infective virus. They produce antibodies to the allergen and release a bunch of chemicals which cause all sorts of complicated reactions which mimic the body's reaction to infection. So, some of us who are allergic sneeze with a cold or when we inhale pollens; we have diarrhea from a salmonella infection or from cow's milk; we wheeze from viral bronchitis or from inhaling dust; or our skin becomes red and swollen from a boil or from a chemical. These allergic disease reactions and the causes vary with the individual. There are thousands and thousands of things that can cause allergic reactions in various people. We start with a series of discussions about "what allergy is all about" by a group of knowledgeable practitioners leading off with some basics from Dr. Blackburn Joslin:

An allergic reaction consists of three basic mechanisms:

1. A dilation (swelling) of blood vessels which leak out serum.
2. Contraction of the smooth or circular muscles.
3. Stimulation of your mucus glands.

Allergies can affect many different systems. In the upper respiratory tract, the result of allergy is usually runny eyes, itchy nose, and hay fever. Reactions in the lower respiratory tract produce bronchitis, cough, and asthma. The skin response is eczema, hives, swelling, and itch. Intestinal tract allergies cause abdominal pain, diarrhea, vomiting, or intestinal upsets.

Allergies may be present at birth or may develop at any time during a person's life. They may change, but the old adage that "a person will outgrow his allergy" is not entirely correct. Usually, a person learns to live with his allergy or to avoid his allergens. He does not, however, outgrow the *allergic state:* The tendency is inherited, but specific allergies usually are not.

Here we have some expert disagreement from Canadian pediatric allergist Dr. John Gerrard who writes:

Even specific allergies may be inherited—the more you look for them, the more frequently you find them.

Dr. Joslin continues:

The number of allergic patients we see is increasing. In part, this is due to changing life styles and to environmental conditions. A man used to live in one location and adapt himself to the allergens in that area. Today, he is exposed to "foreign" allergens daily: He uses oranges from Florida, pineapples from Hawaii, and lobsters from Maine. He flies to other areas where he is challenged by other new allergens. In addition, he is surrounded by air pollution, aerosol bombs, and insect sprays.

The intensity of the allergic reaction is quite variable. To a degree, it depends upon the amount of the allergic substance around. When the level of allergens is low, even a very allergic person may have no significant discomfort; but as the level increases, the allergic individual shows increasing symptoms. Allergic reactions may increase during fatigue or illness. Conversely, when a person is feeling well, and is well nourished and without worry, he is more likely to handle allergens without symptoms. Nonspecific irritants, such as paints, odors, peppers, and mustard, also lower the threshold of resistance to allergens.

Allergies are noted for their chronicity and periodicity; that is, they will reoccur year after year and be highly evident in their own season. Treatment, however, can change this and make the allergic person more comfortable.

Our look at allergy continues with Mayo Clinic allergist (retired), Dr. George Logan explaining the overall course of allergy.

The course of allergy over a lifetime may not be plotted exactly, but we can recognize some sequences. Eczema, hayfever, and asthma may begin at any age. However, most eczemas begin during the first year, mostly the first two months, and most hayfever and asthma begin before age five.

About half of those who begin to wheeze in childhood no longer wheeze after adolescence. They may, however, begin again at a later date. Studies show a higher incidence of allergic nose problems in older adolescents than in grade school children.

As you can see, we had a good number of experts from all over working on this chapter. Pennsylvania allergist Stephen Lockey, Sr. adds a comment here:

Atopic dermatitis or eczema frequently starts before three months of age and continue through the first three years of life. This condition often transforms into childhood asthma.

If this looks like disagreement perhaps the following explanations contributed by Dr. Crook will help.

Allergy is often controversial and confusing. Different doctors have different ideas about allergy: how to define it, how to diagnose it, and how to treat it. One observer commented: "The different viewpoints in the field of allergy remind me of religion and politics. In fact, at times it's like the Tower of Babel."

Many conscientious physicians working to solve the riddle of allergy feel that the term "allergy" should be limited to those conditions in which an immunological mechanism can be demonstrated.

But other conscientious allergists feel that allergic diseases are much broader in scope. Such allergists feel that while immunological mechanisms are undoubtedly important in explaining allergic disease, they don't tell the whole story.

Food allergy is especially controversial. Some allergists feel it is of great importance, while others feel otherwise. One reason for the controversy about food allergy is the inconsistent results shown by foods on allergy skin testing. For example, you may show a positive skin test to egg, yet you may eat eggs without experiencing any allergic reaction. On the other hand, your skin test to milk may be negative, yet milk may be the major cause of your headache and nasal allergy.

In commenting on this situation, Dr. William C. Deamer said, in effect: "It would certainly clear up some of the confusion among both doctors and patients if we had a laboratory test to identify food allergy. But we don't. Yet I do not believe we need to sit back and wait for such a laboratory test. Instead, we can identify and successfully treat the patient with systemic food allergy by using a simple elimination diet."

Allergies can change. For example, egg or milk may cause your baby to break out when he is a few months old. But by the time he's two, he seemingly may be able to drink milk or eat an egg without trouble.

Then, when he reaches school age, milk may cause him to suffer from headache and nasal congestion, and to complain, "Mama, I'm tired." Your youngster may get rid of these symptoms by avoiding milk. But when he goes on a picnic in September, he may develop violent sneezing because of ragweed hay fever. He may also wheeze when he goes to the attic (house dust), or sneeze, wheeze, and itch when he's around a cat. In fact, most allergic individuals have multiple allergies which may affect various parts of their bodies at different times in their lives.

By learning what you can about allergy, you may be able to avoid things you're now allergic to and lessen your chances of developing new allergies in the future.[1]

What this all adds up to is that a lot of people are allergic, as documented by the Allergy Foundation of America:

Allergy is a major health problem. One out of seven people in the United States suffers from some sort of allergy. About thirteen million suffer from hay fever; nine million from other allergic conditions.

Allergy victims pay over $135 million for medications. One million victims pay $100 million to receive injection therapy for ragweed pollen hay fever. Twenty-five million man-days a year are lost at a cost of more than $400 million. Approximately 600,000 workers in the U.S. are victims of occupational dermatitis.

Surveys have shown that one in every five children has a major allergy, yet only one in three receives medical attention. Children with known allergic disorders lose over 36 million days from school and play and spend about 13 million days in bed. Further, allergies are the leading chronic disease in children.

Allergic patients require three times as many medical visits as patients with other illnesses. Allergies rank sixth as a cause of doctor's visits for children under one year of age and fifth up to the age of fourteen.[2]

WHAT CAUSES ALLERGY?

The following is a technical discussion and explanation of a significant area of allergy. Allergy antibodies, as you will see, can be measured and identified, and scientific and medical understanding has grown until the field of allergy no longer should suffer from the derisive skeptical term "witchcraft" once widely used to describe allergy and its treatment. Dr. George Logan gives us the scientific background.

When exposed to a pollen such as ragweed or grass, the pollen protein is absorbed through the lining membrane of the nose and goes by way of the blood stream to nearby lymph nodes. There, small lymphocytes—a kind of white blood cell—make the antibody "immunoglobulin E" (IgE) to work against the pollen. IgE flows into the blood stream, where some of it circulates. Most of the IgE is pulled out of circulation and stored on special white blood cells called basophils and mast cells.

When pollen enters the system again, after a delay of ten days or more, the basophils and the mast cells, loaded with the antibody, confront the pollen protein. The pollen–antibody confrontation causes the cells to release several chemicals: *histamine,* which causes the skin to flush and form hives; *bradykinin,* a slow reacting allergy substance; and *acetylcholine,* which affects nerves and causes sweating, bowel cramps, and salivation. They also release a substance collectively called *prostaglandins.* One of the prostaglandins causes narrowing of the bronchial tubes, which causes wheezing, while another evidently can cause relaxation of the bronchial tubes. Perhaps the constriction is an effort by the body to keep the lungs from breathing in more of the pollen? In any case, it seems to do more harm than good for some.

Research scientists now have developed antihistamine drugs, some of which also act against acetyl choline. Further research has led to the discovery of disodium chromoglycate, which, when taken by inhalation, blocks the release of histamine from mast cells in the lungs. It remains for science to find medicines which will neutralize the effects of bradykinin and the protaglandins. Epinephrine (adrenalin) is an excellent drug for the emergency treatment of asthma. It can, however, cause a rapid heart beat, a pallor, or a feeling of faintness. Such adverse reactions, though unpleasant, are not dangerous. Researchers have found drugs that are effective but which do not have such frequent adverse reactions; but these discoveries are not yet available for use.

[Sodium chromoglycate promises to be helpful for more than asthma. Recent research indicates that it may be useful in treating hayfever by nasal spray and in treating food allergy when it is taken by mouth.]

Hyposensitization treatment (allergy shots) helps the patient to develop an antibody called blocking antibody, because it seems to block the reaction of IgE and the pollen antigens in the sensitized basophils or mast cells. But the best of all treatments for allergy is to avoid contact with the substances to which one is allergic.

WHAT SORT OF THINGS CAN YOU BE ALLERGIC TO?

"Such a list would fill a book," writes Dr. Crook in his very full book, *Your Allergic Child*. His outline of the various causes is presented here:

1. Things you breathe: Weed and grass pollens, molds, animal danders, house dust, and chemical fumes.
2. Things you touch: Chemicals, fabrics, soaps, poison ivy.
3. Non-specific factors:
   a. Physical environment.
   b. Emotional state.
   c. Immune state.
   d. General health.
4. Things you eat: Chocolate, milk, egg, corn, citrus, sea food products, and other foods.[3]

Things You Breathe

The most easily recognized allergens are those that cause an immediate reaction when we breathe them. If you are allergic to dust, you may start to sneeze the minute you climb into a dusty attic; if you are allergic to roses, you may sneeze when you smell a rose. Other respiratory allergens are less easily recognized, for they are widely spread in the air and almost impossible to avoid. The most common offenders are pollens from plants. These can be divided into two types:

1. Heavy pollens from flowering plants, such as lilies or magnolia blossoms, which require insects to carry the pollens from plant to plant. Rarely are these windblown any distance, and they can be avoided by avoiding the blossoms.
2. Light pollens from nonflowering grass, weeds, and trees which are produced in enormous quantities and are spread for miles in the air.

Light pollens are especially hard to avoid and are a major cause of hayfever, asthma, and accompanying symptoms of fatigue and irritability. They are the major reason that people take allergy shots and antihistamines. These allergies are, of course, seasonal, and knowing in which season the symptoms occur is a help in identifying which pollens the individual is allergic to.

Non-pollen inhalant allergies include a wide variety of substances:

- Mold spores in damp places, grass, and dust.
- Animal dander (flaked-off skin) from all sorts of animals, including pets, and hair in rug pads.
- House dust, which may be due to an allergy to a microscopic mite that grows and dies in lint or in dead and shed scales of human skin.
- Insect dust from dead insects or discarded insect wings and so forth.
- Cloth fibers of many sorts—from wool to nylon, from rugs to stuffed toys.
- Feathers from pillows, down jackets, and sleeping bags to pet birds.
- Powders and cosmetics.
- Newsprint and paper.
- Various sprays, such as hair spray, insect sprays, paints, and so forth.
- Chemical odors, whether irritants or true allergens, cause similar reactions, from smog from a tire factory to house paint to perfume.
- Grain dust on farms and silos and bakeries.
- Cigarette and tobacco smoke.
- Smuts, rusts, and other types of molds.

To determine just what an individual is allergic to requires considerable detective work from someone experienced in allergy. At times, skin tests are required in order to determine what allergens cause the problem and thus to direct the treatment to avoiding the allergens or desensitizing the patient with vaccines (allergy shots) .

NONSPECIFIC ALLERGY

1. Your physical environmeat: Heat, cold, weather change, humidity, and atmospheric pressure may influence the type and severity of allergic reactions. For example, you may develop an attack of asthma if you become chilled and on the same day exposed to a heavy amount of house dust; whereas house dust alone might not have precipitated the asthma. Or, in the warm weather, your allergic child may tolerate a food which in cold weather causes allergic symptoms. Also, a change in the barometric pressure may produce and accentuate such allergic symptoms as headache, fatigue, and muscle and joint pains.

2. Emotional factors: Most physicians feel that emotional upsets trigger allergic attacks only in individuals who are already specifically allergic. A mother will report, "When Johnny gets angry or upset, he'll break out with hives. When he's really disturbed, he'll even develop an attack of asthma." Fortunately, when the allergy has been treated properly, it will not be affected by emotional disturbances. Most physicians feel that emotional upsets trigger attacks only in individuals who have already been specifically sensitized to dust, pollens, food, or other allergens.

3. Infections: Infection may make your allergy worse, and vice versa. Many children who "keep a cold" all winter suffer from combined allergy and infection. Allergy makes the lining membrane of the respiratory tract swell. Such swollen membranes are less able to resist germs. For this reason, respiratory infections occur frequently in allergic children and tend to "stay a while."[4]

Allergies from Things You Eat

Among the things that can cause allergy symptoms are things you eat. Knowledge of food allergy goes back to ancient times. "One man's meat is another man's poison." Yet food allergy is very controversial. People who eat a common food without harm often have trouble really believing that "their meat" really is someone else's "poison." "It's all in his head," some say. I know mine was; celery caused a sudden allergic swelling high in my throat and almost killed me by cutting off my air supply. And I had eaten celery all my life without any prior symptoms. Some people claim all sorts of problems from food allergy, and discussions of these problems in relation to food are included throughout *The Manual*. Others are very conservative and believe there is little or no relation to food. Here we present two viewpoints, one from Mayo Clinic pediatric allergist Dr. George Logan and another from Canadian professor of pediatrics Dr. John Gerrard. Dr. Logan says:

Yes, there is food allergy. However, some physicians feel that food allergy is a common occurrence; others, including myself, do not. Still, food allergy is very real. It produces nasal discharge, wheezing, hives, eczema, vomiting, diarrhea, and abdominal cramps. These symptoms may come on minutes to hours after the food has been put in the mouth or swallowed. Our testing mechanisms in this area are inadequate.

Skin testing with food extracts has been a commonly used practice for years. Unfortunately, the results are no more than fifty percent accurate. A positive skin test may mean that the patient is allergic to the material being used for testing. It may also indicate that the patient has been allergic to that food in the past, will become allergic to it, or is simply allergic to a related food. (George Logan, M.D., F.A.A.P.)

And Dr. Gerrard adds:

Dr. Logan is absolutely right when he says that food allergies are difficult to sort out—they are. They differ in this respect from inhalant allergy, where the patient can often give his physician valuable clues, and the physician can usually confirm his suspicians by skin tests. With food allergy, skin tests are usually not helpful, so the clues become more important:

1. Children who first develop colds and bronchitis, with or without wheezing or eczema, while still on the bottle, are often sensitive to cow's milk. Foods tend most often to cause symptoms in infancy and early childhood, while inhalants assume greater importance as the child grows older.

2. Children whose symptoms are most troublesome in winter are often sensitive to both foods and inhalants, and the inhalant is often house dust. The food in the summer does not cause runny nose or

bronchitis, but it does if taken in winter while the child is also being exposed to house dust. A few people find the reverse: Chocolate, for example, may cause headaches, but only if taken during the ragweed season.

3. Children with food allergies usually have very finicky appetites, refusing many foods, and insisting that others be prepared in special ways. They may like raw vegetables or fruit, even raw potato and turnip, and refuse them if they are cooked or canned—and vice versa.

4. Strange to say, the reverse of the above is also true, for some children, and adults for that matter, are sensitive to the foods they crave. The adult with a chronic wheezy bronchitis who smokes and consumes a litre of milk a day is more likely to be sensitive to the milk than to the tobacco.

5. Food allergies, and probably inhalant allergies, often run in families. This observation is sometimes helpful in unravelling food allergies. A parent may know, for example, that he has to avoid milk because it causes nasal stuffiness and bronchitis. If his child has a similar problem, it is probable that he, too, is sensitive to milk.

6. It is not true that foods to which a person is sensitive usually cause gastrointestinal symptoms, bloating, discomfort, diarrhoea, and vomiting, in addition to causing nonintestinal symptoms, such as wheezing and headaches. The food may cause no gastrointestinal disturbance whatsoever and still cause respiratory problems.

The proof of the pudding lies in the eating. Only when it has been shown that symptoms are relieved by removing the food or foods from the diet and that they return when the foods are once more included in the diet, can a person be said to be allergic to this food. Dietary elimination and challenge are, unfortunately, the only way of clinching the diagnosis.

Allergies from Food and Drug Additives

Due in considerable part to the pioneering efforts of Dr. Stephen Lockey, our appreciation, knowledge, and understanding of allergies due to food and drug additives is increasing. Many of these exist in hidden forms, both naturally occurring and man made.

Types of Allergic Reactions

Allergy to drugs usually involves an immediate reaction from antibodies to the drug, or a delayed hypersensitivity from immune cells. Anaphylaxis is an immediate reaction with swelling, frequently around the face; shock, with pallor, great uneasiness, anxiety, restlessness, sweating, and faintness; and, occasionally, wheezing and difficult breathing. Other reactions include:

Bleeding under the skin	Inability to urinate
Blisters	Itching
Convulsions	Peeling skin
Diarrhea	Runny nose
Eczema	Sea sickness-like reaction
Hives	

Toxic reactions may be due to an overdose of the drug or to hypersensitivity. Examples of overdose are ringing in the ears from aspirin, or blurred vision and dry mouth from belladonna. Patients who have reactions to a drug must know what the drug is and where it is found.

Cross-reactions often occur; an individual who is sensitive to one drug becomes sensitive to a similar chemical compound. Low molecular chemicals of coal tar or petroleum origin frequently produce reactions. They have the facility to combine with body protein to form a protein–chemical antigen which induces antibody formation. Possible sensitizing groups of drugs include: Acetylsalicylic acid (aspirin) derivatives, analgesics and antipyretics, antihistamines, artificial coloring and flavoring agents, barbiturates, iodine, mercurials, penicillin, phenolphthalein, sulfonamides, sulfones, tetracycline, tranquilizers (phenothiazine group), and zinc.

Why Are Additives Used?
Physicians who study allergic reactions find that the problems of food and drug additives are complex. Chemicals and drugs are added to food and medicines for many reasons, and frequently the same chemicals occur spontaneously in nature. Foods are adulterated with coloring, flavoring, and preservative agents made from coal tar, petroleum, and their derivatives, which cross-react with each other. If you are allergic to one, you may react to the other. Most additives are unknown to the consumer; their harmful effects are seldom mentioned. Yet the use of additives in foods processed in the United States has almost doubled in the last seventeen years, approaching one billion pounds of additives a year! The average American eats five pounds of food additives per year unknowingly. These chemicals are added to foods for a variety of reasons:

1. To enhance the appearance and consumer acceptance with coloring agents.
2. To prevent food spoilage.
3. As flavoring agents.
4. To thicken, firm, foam, emulsify, and gel foods or to prevent fermentation and oxidation.
5. To change the moisture content of a particular food: for example, adding calcium silicate to table salt to prevent caking ("When it rains, it pours.")
6. To control the amount of acid and alkali in foods and soft drinks.

7. To control physiologic activity: that is, as ripeners for fruit or antimetabolic agents to prevent potatoes from sprouting.
8. As supplemental nutrition: that is, vitamins, minerals, and amino acids.

Examples of Allergic Reactions and Their Causes

To better appreciate the scope of the problem and the problems that can occur from unsuspected additives in foods and hidden additives in drugs, Dr. Lockey presents an actual case.

> A twenty-year-old woman ate a spoonful of crisp cornflakes. After she had placed the cornflakes in her mouth, her throat swelled and she was short of breath. She felt very tired and could hardly move.
>
> An allergist tested her for sensitivity to corn, cow's milk casein, and cow's milk lactalbumin, but she failed to react. The source of the severe attack remained in doubt until one day she sat down to dinner and had a couple of bites of reconstituted dehydrated potatoes. She suffered the same type of attack. She was tested for sensitivity to potato extract. The results were negative.
>
> Puzzled, her physician examined the labels of the box of corn flakes and that of the dehydrated potatoes. The corn flakes had been treated with butylated hydroxyanisole food additive (BHA) and the dehydrated potatoes contained butylated hydroxyluene food additive (BHT), a relative to BHA; both are preservatives and antimold agents.
>
> All symptoms disappeared when she stopped eating foods that contained BHA and BHT.

Foods Containing BHA or BHT

- Beverages and desserts prepared from dry mixes
- Active dry yeast
- Lard and shortening
- Unsmoked dry sausage
- Chewing gum base
- Dry breakfast cereals
- Emulsion stabilizers for shortenings
- Mixed-diced-glazed fruits
- Potato granules or flakes (regular and sweet)
- Defoaming agent component (used in processing beet sugar and yeast)
- Enriched rice

Dr. Lockey describes another case:

> M.A., a very active seven-year-old school boy, developed hives and swelling around his eyes and tongue whenever he chewed certain

brands of bubble gum. To date, I have been unable to determine exactly what ingredients in various bubble gums he reacts to. He now avoids chewing all types of bubble gum, and experiences no difficulty when he chews standard brands of chewing gum.

Chewing Gum Additives

- BHA (butylated hydroxyanisole)
- BHT (butylated hydroxyluene) as antioxidant
- Butadiene styrene rubber
- Butyl rubber
- Chewing gum base includes at least 17 natural gums as constituents
- Chilte
- Glycerin ester of partially hydrogenated wood resin
- Glycerin ester of polymerized resin
- Isobutylene-isoprene capolymer
- Isobutylene resin
- Lanolin
- Latex (butadiene styrene rubber)
- Paraffin wax
- Polyvinyl acetate (mol. wt. 2,000 minimum)
- Rosin (polymerized, partially hydrogenated, and/or partially dimerized, glycerol esters)
- Rubber (natural) smoked sheet and latex solids
- Sodium sulfate
- Sodium sulfide
- Terpene resin (synthetic polymers of b-pinene and natural polymers of a-pinene)

HIDDEN DRUGS

A person allergic to a common chemical such as aspirin has a difficult time determining which particular preparation he can safely consume, because many prescription items and over-the-counter preparations contain aspirin or substances which will cross-react with aspirin. The number of compounds in medicines or in foods is so great that it takes painstaking work to identify a causative agent. If a reaction appears after the use of a specific drug, disappears on discontinuation, and returns when you retake the same medication, the problem may or may not be the drug; the cause may be a substance used as a flavoring agent. Drugs may also be part of foods or beverages and cause life-threatening reactions when taken inadvertently.

R.T., male, age five, is known to be clinically sensitive to aspirin (a salicylate), phenacetine, and members of the Sulfonamide series of drugs, which cause generalized hives and localized swelling. He also develops bouts of generalized itching and hives after he ingests artificially flavored jellies or beverages.

Episode 1: Became extremely ill with nausea, vomiting, generalized hives, and swelling around and in the mouth after he drank homogenized milk, a known brand which he drank daily, plus toasted bread covered with butter. Treated by family physician. *Episode 2:* Came home from nursery school hungry. Mother gave him a half of a sweet bun covered with butter. The child again became extremely ill with shock, generalized hives, swollen lips, and swelling in the throat. He required emergency treatment with adrenalin, cortisone, antihistamine, and oxygen.

The cause of his reactions was eventually traced to *Diacetyl,* a carrier of the aroma of butter.

What Can You Do About Hidden Additives?

One substance, tartrazine (FD and C yellow No. 5) is a widely used dye that can cause allergic reactions, such as hives, in some people. It may also sensitize them to salicylates that are mother nature's additives and have been eaten by man since things like apples and cucumbers existed (see lists on page 401). Most people are not harmed by these substances. On the other hand if you have recurrent hives you should consider salicylates and tartrazine. Or if your child is hyperactive, even though it probably isn't from man's or nature's food additives, they are worth considering as a cause. For more information see Chapter 8 in our companion volume, *The Parents' Guide to Child Raising.* If you are bothered by tartrazine you have a job cut out for you (page 401). It is in over 37,000 processed foods. It would be of tremendous value if the Food and Drug Administration could require full disclosure of all additives present in drugs, foods and cosmetics. Meanwhile Dr. Lockey has had magnificent cooperation from the private pharmaceutical firms in the United States. He has gathered from them a list of over 1,200 drugs and vitamins, douches, mouthwashes and suppositories, plus allergy medications designed to treat hives, and medications designed to treat hyperactivity, all of which contain the allergen tartrazine. This is available from the Allergy Foundation of Lancaster County, Box 1424, Lancaster, PA 17604.

If you are sensitive to a particular drug you should carry a pocket card (Life Card) or a standard dog tag (Medialert), plus a list of drugs and proprietary preparations which contain that particular drug or drugs.

DISEASES CAUSED BY ALLERGIES

Asthma

Asthma causes a wheeze in the chest on exhaling or breathing out. Usually, it is started by an allergic reaction that causes the muscles encircling the bronchi to constrict and the lining of the bronchi to excrete a thick viscous mucus. The constriction and mucus interfere with the air being expelled from the lungs, for air is forced from the lungs by the rather weak elasticity of the lungs and the rib cage. Inspiration, on the other hand, is accomplished by the strong muscular diaphram at the bottom of the lungs and the sturdy muscles between the ribs. As the air goes in with more force than it goes out, there is a tendency for the lungs to overfill and not empty completely, "ballooning out" the chest.

In children, the most common wheeze mistaken by parents for asthma is the wheeze or "crow" of croup, which occurs on breathing in, rather than the asthmatic wheeze on breathing out. A rare but important cause of wheezing is from inhaling a foreign body into the lungs whether it is a peanut or a piece of carrot stick. So don't jump to the conclusion that because your child wheezes he has asthma.

Hayfever

Tennessee allergist Dr. William Crook takes a broad view of hayfever, both in time and geography. He notes that:

Almost 2,000 years ago, doctors observed that certain people sneezed when they smelled a rose or picked up a cat. It wasn't until 1819 that Dr. John Bostock of London presented a medical paper describing accurately what we now know as "pollen hayfever." Dr. Bostock said, in effect: "Every spring and summer I develop a peculiar sort of illness. My nose and eyes run and itch and I sneeze repeatedly." Dr. Bostock mistakenly blamed his symptoms on the sun, although he didn't know how or why the sun caused his symptoms. But he had made a beginning.

Actually, hayfever is an allergy in the lining of the nose. You know it is present when:

1. You are bothered with an almost continuous cold and a runny or stuffy nose. If there is a nasal discharge, it is usually clear, white or gray, rather than yellow or green. However, many people with allergy of the nose have little or no discharge, but instead have a stuffy or stopped-up nose or a postnasal drainage to mucus (phlegm).
2. Your nose itches so that you rub it, wiggle it, twitch it, or push it up.
3. You tend to sneeze, sniff, snort, and clear your throat. The parents of an allergic child will often complain: "My child doesn't know how to blow his nose," or: "If he would only blow his nose, he wouldn't have to make those noises."

Hives

Hives are bumpy swellings on the skin that vary in size from as small as a pencil eraser and almost flat to large egg size bumps which can merge together into big patches of swollen, itchy, skin with irregular borders.

They are caused by a typical histamine release from mast cells, causing dilation and leaking of the blood vessels. Usually, they can be relieved with an antihistamine medication. The cause is frequently due to allergy to food, although hives can occur from pollens, and, at times, even from viral infections.

Eczema

Eczema is a reddened itchy thickened skin that becomes dry and flaky. It is often attributed to allergy, and I have seen numerous cases of eczema which resulted from allergy shots which were too concentrated. Often, such rashes quiet down if less soap and water are used on the skin, if a simple protective ointment such as vaseline is used on the skin, and if rough clothing is avoided. Early treatment with cortisone prevents eczema from becoming too severe; check with your doctor. If your doctor is dermatology professor Alvin Jacobs he will tell you that atopic dermatitis (a form of eczema) is not an allergy but does occur in some people who are allergic. It is, he believes, due to an abnormal skin caused by an abnormal gene which seems closely linked to the gene or genes which make a person susceptible to allergy. This may be, but it acts like an allergy to me. I have often seen it flare from foods, whether it is allergy or not.

THE ALLERGIC TENSION FATIGUE SYNDROME

This unlikely sounding name represents a very real disease. I became partially convinced that it existed after hearing it described by Dr. Crook, and I was completely convinced after trying elimination diets on a lot of problem children, some who responded beautifully. Examples of this disease are described for us by Dr. John Gerrard of the Saskatchewan University Hospital in Canada.

Dr. Crook, who is very adept at identifying the tension fatigue syndrome, has pointed out that children with this syndrome often have stuffy noses, pale cheeks, circles under their eyes, headaches, and tummy aches. These are all vague, rather indefinite symptoms, but when they are associated with lassitude and tiredness or irritability, restlessness, or hyperactivity, they indicate that the mental disturbance is probably a manifestation of allergy.

Allergic individuals are so often emotionally unstable that many assume that their emotions are responsible for their allergic reactions. I don't think that this is so; rather, the emotional disturbance is part of the allergic reaction, as the following case histories illustrate.

I first met Sarah when I was giving her well-behaved brother a preschool examination. Sarah climbed over the furniture, opened drawers, and spilled bottles with the destructive drive of a tornado. I was about to complain when her mother said, "Don't worry about Sarah.

She is only behaving like a maniac because I let her have a little butter for breakfast." Apparently, Sarah could be gentle, quiet, and docile if she avoided milk, dairy products, chocolate, and cokes, but with these foods she became disobedient, cried if reprimanded, drove her teacher to distraction, and made silly mistakes in school. She would be restless at night and even have nightmares. Her reaction to dairy products was as predictable as that of an asthmatic who wheezes whenever he comes in contact with a cat.

She was lucky that her mother, who had allergic problems of her own, discovered the allergy when she noticed abrupt changes in Sarah's behavior. By a process of trial and elimination, she found which foods made her bad-tempered.

We do not know why allergens are capable of altering human behavior, but they do.

C.P. was noted to have an allergic nose. I had his mother stop milk and dairy products. Two weeks later, his school teacher asked his mother if her son had been put on any new medicine, "because his behavior in class has been transformed. He used to be restless and inattentive. He was a distraction to the whole class, but for the last ten days he has been as good as gold. He has become the perfect pupil." Milk made this child's nose run and, in ways that we do not yet understand, also made him restless, fidgety, and inattentive.

Adults can also be made miserable by foods. One of my colleagues has to avoid wheat, egg, and milk and dairy products, for all these foods make him behave "like a bull in a china shop." In other people, foods can also have the opposite effect, making them almost uncontrollably sleepy. One baby under my care would sleep for twenty-four hours if rice was added to his formula. A student whom I saw recently with an allergic rhinitis also had difficulty in keeping awake during lectures. He was a great milk drinker, and the milk was one of several factors that not only made his nose run but also made him feel drugged. However, inhalants can also make patients tense or drowsy, as witnessed by a patient seen recently who, during the grass pollen season, develops not only hay fever but also profound mental depression.

It was Dr. Speer who first drew attention to the changes in mood induced by foods. He called this disorder the "tension fatigue syndrome." Many doctors find it difficult to acknowledge that mood changes can be due to allergy, but such changes are, in fact, quite genuine. Some allergic children can be made hyperactive or somnolent as easily by giving them foods, just as normal children can by giving them stimulants or sedatives.

Other Allergy Problems

As you can see, there is a broad spectrum of diseases caused by allergies. Dr. Gerrard noted examples of emotional reactions and hyperactivity from foods. Dr. Crook believes a commonly missed cause of hyperactivity is cane sugar allergy.[5] I have seen children whom the parents firmly believed had infectious mononucleosis or low thyroid turn out simply to be allergic to milk. San Francisco allergist Ben F. Feingold claims learning problems and hyperactivity in children are due to food additives.[6] In my experience this seems to be true for at least a few children. For more information on hyperactivity and learning problems see our companion volume, *The Parents' Guide to Child Raising*. For elimination diet lists for food additives, milk and milk products and so forth, see pages 396 to 401 of *The Manual*.

What other sort of illnesses do allergies cause? In most of us, they cause no illness at all, but in some individuals they can cause a wide variety of illness. Scattered throughout *The Manual* you will find reminders from Dr. Crook that allergy is the great masquerader and evidently can affect almost any part of the body in particular individuals. Some don't believe that allergy can cause such diverse conditions as school failure, bedwetting, constipation, behavior problems, and many more. The odds are that they won't in you or your child, but the odds don't count if you are on their wrong side. A friend of mine recently found that she has been suffering from diarrhea for over ten years because she is allergic to coffee which she guzzled in great quantities routinely. So be aware that an allergic cause is possible, and do some detective work to try and figure out if it is a cause in you.

TREATING ALLERGY

The most logical way to avoid problems caused by allergy is to avoid the allergen. Pediatric allergist Joseph E. Ghory counsels that the offending allergens must be removed:

A concerted attempt must be made to eliminate or avoid all known allergens. If it is impossible to remove an antigen completely, such as omnipresent house dust, then efforts must be made to reduce its access to the patient. For dust, this means clean furnace filters, a humidifier, or an electronic filter. For Kapok, a nonallergenic cover for the mattress will provide an adequate barrier. For pollen, air conditioning may be interposed as a filter. Such items are considered tax deductible as a medical expense. Your proof is a prescription or statement from your physician to this effect.

Sometimes it is necessary to remove the patient from undue exposure to the antigens. The grass-pollen sensitive boy should not be permitted to mow the lawn; the dust-sensitive girl must be excused from doing the housecleaning.

Many physicians not only provide meticulous directions for environmental control measures, but also insist on a home visit to make absolutely certain that the family has complied with these directions. The patient's bedroom is most important; he spends at least eight hours a day there. Check the effectiveness of your own efforts with the following list on how to avoid house dust.

To Avoid House Dust

In the bedroom:

1. No stuffed chairs, no rugs, no drapes. May have linoleum or wood floor, wood or metal furniture, washable cotton curtains or curtains made of plastic or plexiglass.
2. No blankets, woolen goods, felt hats, or other dust catchers should be stored in the bedroom.
3. Furnace vents must be covered with three layers of cloth; nylon stretch fabric works well.
4. Doors to the room must be shut and tight-fitting.
5. Windows must fit well.
6. Every week, the floor, ceiling, and walls must be washed completely; every day the furniture must be damp-dusted.
7. Pillows must be foam or dacron, or encased in a plastic cover.
8. Blankets must be double-washed, fuzz-free cotton or dacron, and sheets must be used next to the patient's body.
9. Mattresses must be completely encased in plastic with a zipper closing.
10. Springs must be vacuumed, washed, and covered with plastic.
11. No fuzzy toys.

In the rest of the house:

1. The patient must not sit or lie on overstuffed furniture or on rugs. Rugs are better if they are cotton or nylon and backed only with rubber.
2. No pets other than fish or turtles.
3. No house plants.
4. No room deodorizers, mothballs, or bug sprays.
5. Regular furnace cleaning and covers for furnace vents.
6. The allergic patient should not be in the house while the house is being cleaned.

Avoiding allergens isn't always easy nor are the experts always in agreement as to how you do this. Dr. Ghory suggested that the grass pollen sensitive boy not mow the lawn. Dr. Logan comments:

Patients who are grass-sensitive seldom seem to be sensitive to freshly cut grass. Those who react to mowing the lawn, which often contains many mold spores, are usually mold-sensitive rather than grass pollen-sensitive.

That, of course, depends on the length of the grass. If you have as much trouble as I did getting my boy to mow the lawn, it pollinates.

Then, whether you are either pollen or mold sensitive, it will bother you. Dr. Logan brings up another source of molds—humidifiers:

> Many parents feel that if a small amount of extra moisture is good, more is better. Under these circumstances, cool mist vaporizers are run to the point of allowing mold growth to flourish in various parts of the room or the home. In order to avoid this, use a humidity indicator and follow the directions to balance the inside humidity with the temperature outside. This is especially important where winter temperatures range from +15 degrees to −40 degrees F.

Cool mist vaporizers should be cleaned and sterilized weekly. Put in one inch of water in the container with three tablespoons of liquid bleach. Plug the opening with a towel and run the machine for fifteen minutes so that the entire inside of the unit is saturated with the bleach solution. Empty it and put in fresh water and run it until the clorox smell has gone. This kills the bacteria and mold which might grow in stagnant water. With all of this, you may decide not to use a cold air vaporizer, but actually it does work well if proper precautions are taken.

Family practitioner Raymond Kahn, who is aware of some of the practical aspects of our advice, added that if you don't have a humidifier or vaporizor, there are substitutes.

> A pan of water put over the floor register of a furnace is an inexpensive way of helping to humidify the air. Even having a child breath through a hot wet washcloth for a few minutes every hour is helpful.

Then, when I suggested that if your child is allergic to dogs that you get a pet turtle instead, Dr. Kahn reminded me that even turtles are not safe; they can carry Salmonella infections, a cause of fever and diarrhea! But what do you do when you are driving back after giving away your dog and your turtle and you still have sneezing and wheezing?

Sneezing and Wheezing When Driving

If you or your child have allergic symptoms when in the car, consider the following steps to make your rides pleasanter:

1. Use plastic seat covers to reduce dust and mold. (But if your skin itches it could be caused by the plastic.)
2. Avoid pillows with feathers, kapok, or foam rubber (which grow mold when damp).
3. Vacuum floor mats frequently and air the padding often, especially if it is damp. Spray with anti-mold substances such as Lysol.
4. Vacuum car heater outlets and operate heater occasionally when windows are open in order to expel dust.

5. If possible, use only air conditioned cars, and keep windows up and air in-lets closed.

6. Don't transport fur-bearing animals in the car.

7. Avoid driving from 11 A.M. to 6 P.M. or during windy days when pollen is high.

8. Avoid fumes from factories, freshly tarred roads, rush hours with heavy traffic; keep windows closed when refueling with gasoline, and stay well back from busses, trucks, and smog-producing cars.

9. Keep fumes from your car at a minimum by steam cleaning the engine yearly, checking all parts to prevent leakage, changing PCV valve frequently, and adjusting the automatic choke properly, and so forth.

10. Use a horse instead—if you aren't allergic to horses!

What About a Change of Climate?

In the long run, points out Dr. Ghory, it is more important to treat the patient's allergy than to move the patient to a different climate.

It is true that the ragweed sensitive person will obtain relief by taking a vacation to Florida or California; but if he is, in fact, an allergic individual, he can become sensitized to new pollens within three years' time. Each area has its allergy-causing pollens. As one west-coast allergist facetiously remarked: "No, we do not have ragweed in California, but thank God for the sagebrush!" It is wiser, therefore, to help the child to "outgrow" his allergy by improving his immunological tolerance.

There is one change in "climate" that can be achieved in the home without moving. The wheezing of asthmatic children is aggravated by cigarette smoke: They may even become allergic to it. Don't allow smoking in your house!

Allergy Shots

If you can't avoid it, and if there isn't enough help from antihista-mines and other medications your doctor may try, you may have to be skin-tested and start on a long course of allergy shots. Are they worth it? Dr. Logan discusses this objectively, but it is a decision that you and your doctor will have to reach, as every case is somewhat unique.

How Does Hyposensitization Cure Allergy?

Hyposensitization, or "allergy shots," is a technique of injecting gradually increasing doses of an offending pollen under the skin of the allergy victim. Presently, we think that the goal is to create a sufficient supply of blocking antibody. This form of treatment, over sixty years old, works best for those with hayfever or asthma due to pollen, mold, or house dust. Such treatment should not be used for hives, eczema, or food allergy.

If an allergic attack is mild, this treatment may not be necessary. Parents should not automatically plan for hyposensitization. There is very little evidence to suggest that severe disease will develop from untreated mild hayfever. If an allergy sufferer becomes progressively worse, or if his attacks were severe from the start, then one should consider hyposensitization.

Treatment proceeds in the following manner: The patient receives injections of hyposensitizing pollen once or twice a week, beginning with very small doses. Dosage depends upon individual tolerance, not upon the age or size of the patient. The dose is gradually increased, to the highest dose tolerated. After the top dose is reached, the interval between injections may be increased to every two, three, or even four weeks. The reason doses are increased gradually is to avoid both local (skin redness, itching, or swelling) or systemic (sneezing, generalized itching, or wheezing) reactions. Treatment extracts made with a watery solution are preferable to those made with glycerin or other materials. In my opinion, hyposensitization by mouth or under the tongue has no value.

THE TREATMENT OF ASTHMA

The early home treatment of asthma is outlined in the book *Your Allergic Child* by Dr. William Crook:

If you are an asthmatic, you will know the symptoms of a threatened attack. When you do:

1. Stay at home.
2. Drink plenty of water and other liquids.
3. In the winter-time, start your vaporizer or humidifier (containing only water), if you aren't sensitive to molds. (Ask your doctor.)
4. Stay in a room which is free of dust, feathers, pets, and odors of all sorts.
5. Avoid foods you are allergic to (especially milk, egg, chocolate, peanuts, popcorn, or citrus fruits).
6. At the first sign of a "head cold," take an antihistamine or antihistamine decongestant combination or other medication, but only if prescribed and recommended by your doctor.
7. If you develop symptoms of a cough or tightness in your chest, stop the antihistamine decongestant and take medicine by mouth, as prescribed, to open up your bronchial tubes and loosen the mucus and phlegm.
8. Take asthma medications prescribed by your doctor.

Some doctors recommend an asthma spray or nebulizer; others don't. Dr. John McGovern says: "I do not recommend that an asthmatic child be allowed to take an asthma spray around with him. He may develop a psychological dependence on it. He also may so overuse it that he may develop an attack of asthma which won't respond to adrenalin or other medicines."

If, in spite of all you have done, you begin to wheeze and become short of breath, you should check with your doctor. He may give you medications by mouth or rectum or an injection of epinephrine (adrenaline). The sooner treatment is given, the more effective it is and the less you have to suffer.[7]

Most cases of asthma are mild, and can be well handled by avoiding allergens and by following many of the preventive techniques already discussed. However, asthma can be a debilitating and prolonged disease.

Care of the severe asthmatic is a drain on a family, and at times it can cause resentment in parents who really love their afflicted child. This can lead to guilt feelings and overconcern, or it can lead to "blocking out the disease" and refusing to admit that it is bad. It is critical that you have your child under the overall care of a personal physician, that you keep him well appraised of the child's status and your feelings, and that you follow his advice. Make certain that he sees the child at least twice a year for check-ups when he is relatively well, rather than only when the child is severely ill. The chronic severe asthmatic is a real problem. This section, written by asthma specialist Dr. Joseph Ghory, covers some of the general things which can be done for the asthmatic.

What Can Be Done For a Child With Chronic Asthma?

First, we must dispense with two notions: (1) "Don't worry about it, your child will outgrow his asthma," and (2) "A chronic asthmatic child will become a chronic asthmatic adult and will develop emphysema."

Both of these notions are false. Waiting for a child to outgrow his asthma is like holding a lighted firecracker, waiting for the wick to go out: Sooner or later you will get burned! As soon as the diagnosis of bronchial asthma is clearly made, this patient deserves an allergy work-up.

Since bronchial asthma is the number one chronic disease of childhood, it is important that both the patient and his parents realize the implications of this chronic illness. It is imperative that they recognize all the causative factors, the long-term value of prevention, and the necessity of treating attacks as soon as they start. Parents are a vital part of the team needed to treat the child.

Unfortunately, some ten percent of children with chronic asthma reach the unmanageable stage. The one fear often cited by parents is that emphysema may develop. True emphysema is rarely, if ever, seen in childhood. Rather a reversible condition of hyperinflation will be encountered. This should be treated, so that the patient can be rehabilitated. Rehabilitation is just as important to the person with severe bronchial asthma who is a respiratory cripple as it is to the patient with broken bones who is an orthopedic cripple.

The key people in the total rehabilitation program are the individual patient and the immediate family. The education of the patient and the family are paramount. The more you know about your own problems, the better equipped you are to cope with them. It is not uncommon for children with this condition to be hospitalized four to five times a year, thereby creating family and school problems. Our approach to this unpredictable absenteeism is long term institutional rehabilitation.

Three groups of children should be considered for admission to an institutional program for asthma:

1. The child experiencing increasingly frequent and severe asthmatic attacks, necessitating multiple hospitalizations and school absence;
2. The child on maintenance cortisone therapy who should be weaned from this potent drug;
3. The child who has an intolerable home situation and is unable to cope with his repeated severe episodes. Frequently it is not a case of uncontrollable asthma, but rather an uncontrollable domestic situation.

What are the Advantages and Disadvantages of Institutional Programs for Asthma?

First, they provide a controlled environment, as free as possible from the house dust and emotional dust which provoke his asthma. Second, they provide school facilities so that the child does not lose out on his educational progress. Third, they provide a team approach to therapy with emphasis on the whole child, not just the disease.

The obvious disadvantage is the length of hospitalization—usually a minimum of two months to a year. Finances are a major issue, but some institutions accept free patients. If the program is located in an accredited hospital, rather than in a convalescent home, it is usually covered by health insurance. Whatever the institution, there must be round-the-clock medical coverage and ready access to an acute hospital for emergency care.

Another program that is gaining importance is camping for children with asthma. It is of great value, both for recreation and rehabilitation for the child. Camps which take asthmatic children are acquainted with their potential problems and are equipped to handle them early. The counselors help each child in adapting to separation from his family, and in camp problems such as sharing and cooperating.

Should an Asthmatic Child Compete in Sports?

All sports that permit a rest period between peaks of high activity are well tolerated by asthmatic children, but sporting events demanding endurance, such as distance running, should be discouraged. Swimming is an ideal sport for asthmatic children. It is important to have an understanding coach or physical education teacher so that the asthmatic child may take part in all that he is able but not be pushed beyond that point.

PART THREE

ILLNESS: THE CAUSE

We have discussed many causes of disease in the preceding chapters. It may well be that half of all disease is caused by emotional stress and insecurity. Then there is built-in disease that is inherited, such as diabetes or low immunity, and congenital disease, which some unlucky children are born with, such as congenital heart disease. This part of *The Manual* concentrates on infections and physical agents that are more susceptible to our efforts in prevention and cure. Included in these are the diseases that most children suffer in growing up. And much of this suffering from the various enemies of man can be avoided in our day—possibly more so in the future. This was not so in the past.

Man's dominance on this planet was threatened severely many times in the past. During the Middle Ages, the black death—bubonic plague, caused by a bacteria—stalked Europe, wiping out nearly a quarter of the population on several occasions. When the plague was quiet, viral diseases like smallpox, and bacterial diseases like cholera and typhoid took their heavy tolls, ravaging Europe, Asia, and America, unchecked by efficient ways of treatment or prevention. During World War I, more American soldiers were killed by disease than by the opposing armies. Diphtheria, meningitis, pneumonia, influenza, and streptococcus infections killed men in training camps by the battalions. Yet we have survived.

This survival is an important point to remember when looking up the various causes of disease. Mankind is so variable in resistance that a deadly killing bacteria like plague can be tolerated or rejected without harm by some of us. And there are some viral infections that can be tolerated or dismissed by most of us yet can kill a few of us. So when you read about all of the various biological and physical enemies of man, remember that you and your children will not likely suffer as much as the descriptions imply, if you suffer at all. In other words, don't panic when reading about all these hazards. You are probably tougher than you think. Further, by knowing about the spread, prevention, and treatment of diseases, you will be able to better protect yourself and your family.

16

BACTERIAL DISEASES:
THE CURABLE CAUSES

Scientists have not succeeded in producing many antibiotics that will kill viruses without killing us. They have, however, been very successful in producing agents which will kill or suppress bacteria. Thus, bacteria cause curable diseases.

MEET YOUR BACTERIA!

You may not be interested in unseen organisms with strange names, but you personally have hundreds of billions of bacteria living in and on you. If you are going to get really seriously ill from an infection, it will most often be from a bacteria, or rather a few bacteria growing to billions in numbers. When your resistance is down, whether from a cold or from a cut in the skin, bacteria can move in and set up housekeeping. These microscopic dots, rods, or spirals, only 1/25,000th of an inch big, are indispensible to, and occasionally damaging to, humans. One pinch of dirt has billions of bacteria. They survive in environments as different as ice, hot sulfur water, or our blood stream. Some develop seed-like spores even more resistant to destruction. They have remarkable reproductive ability, doubling in number every twenty minutes. They make rabbits look like nuns!

How Do You Get Bacteria?

Bacterial diseases can be caught in all sorts of ways, including by skin contact with germs, by food and drink, and by airborn droplets assisted by contaminated hands.

Spread by Skin Contact

The bacteria that usually live on the skin are harmful only if accidentally introduced deeper into the tissue. The harmfulness of the bacteria must be measured against the immunity and resistance of the individual. Most bacteria on the skin do not cause infection, but some strains are potent and can cause severe IMPETIGO, BOILS, OR ABSCESSES.

Almost all bacteria can be transmitted from person to person by direct skin contact. For this reason, it is necessary to use careful hand-washing when you have an infection or are in contact with infected individuals. Staphylococcus is the most notorious germ which spreads by this route. Staph is also able to exist on clothing or furniture for over a year and still be infective. There are many strains of "staph," most of which never cause disease in man, and, in fact, are useful in suppressing the growth of other more virulent bacteria. Some staph can only produce infection when the resistance of the individual has been suppressed by other disease conditions, or, as in the newborn, when there is not enough immunity to stop the growth of the germs. A few very virulent strains of "staph" cause serious disease in most people, and can quickly develop resistance to many antibiotics. These are the strains of staphylococcus which give it its well deserved reputation as a germ to be feared and respected.

Penicillin treatment of staphylococcal infections can be simple and quick. Resistant strains, however, sometimes require prolonged administration of one of the newer antibiotics for extended periods of time. Drainage of abscesses and surgical removal of infected tissue is sometimes required. Although it deserves our respect, the staph germ is not a terrible menace to most of us, for we are usually resistant.

Control of the spread of the virulent strains of staphylococcus is difficult and often discouraging, particularly if it happens to invade a hospital where many patients have decreased resistance to infection. Careful handwashing is of primary importance. Meticulous and careful disposal or disinfection of contaminated bedlinen, clothing, and eating utensils is essential. Complete isolation and elimination of unnecessary hospital personnel and visitors is often necessary.

One menace which still causes problems is staph FOOD POISONING. Severe vomiting and diarrhea, occuring within a few hours after eating contaminated food, are caused by a potent toxin which is produced by staphylococcus growing in the food. When foods such as creamed casseroles and potato salad containing mayonnaise are left out of the refrigerator overnight after having been inoculated with the germ by a careless food handler, the stage is set for an outbreak of food poisoning.

All those who handle food should keep their hands scrupulously clean and should carefully avoid any possibility of contaminating food by coughing or sneezing, or from infected skin. Always refrigerate leftovers, or throw them out.

Spread by Food and Water

Bacteria may enter the body through the mouth and live there or pass into the intestines, where they thrive. The large bowel is inhabited by a teeming "inner universe of bacteria." We excrete over 100 trillion bacteria with each bowel movement; at least half of the feces is made up of bacteria. The bowels of breast-fed infants have large numbers of friendly Lactobacillus, similar to the organism which changes milk to yogurt. Bottle-fed infants have mostly coliform bacteria, which can be irritating. Other organisms may produce potent chemicals by putrefaction. Our bowel wall, lymphatics, and liver have a well-developed series of enzymatic defenses to detoxify these chemicals. Most of us have immune mechanisms which protect us from infection, but some infants with low immunity can develop serious diarrhea from strains of coliform bacteria which do not harm older children and adults.

The significance of the intestinal microorganisms on human health is poorly understood. It is known that animals raised in a germ-free environment develop more muscle than those living with germs, and that adding antibiotics to livestock feed stimulates increased meat production, presumably because the antibiotic suppresses the bowel bacteria.

Under some conditions, bacteria in the intestine produce useful B vitamins, and under other conditions, they may destroy vitamins. Major shifts in the bacterial population of the bowel are brought about by the type of food available. Foods containing sugar encourage gas-producing bacteria. The milk sugar "lactose" encourages the Lactobacillus. Antibiotic treatment profoundly alters the intestinal bacterial population. Many of the "good" bacteria are destroyed by antibiotics, while those remaining are resistant to the drug. Disease-producing germs may in this way become the predominant organisms. On occasions, often after treatment with antibiotics, the bacterial flora is largely replaced by yeast. Lactobacillus (yogurt) can be given with milk and usually will take back over from the other organisms.

When the intestines are inflamed (enteritis) due to virus "flu" or diarrhea infections, intestinal bacteria can secondarily infect the intestinal mucosa and cause delayed healing. In an attack of appendicitis, the bacteria may escape into the peritoneal cavity causing an infection—peritonitis.

In girls and women, bowel bacteria from the nearby rectum can create vaginal irritation and infection. Most bladder infections in girls and women come from bowel bacteria on the vulva which reach the bladder through the urethra (see Chapter 11).

The most dangerous disease bacteria which enter the body through the intestinal tract are cholera, shigella, and salmonella. They can cause fever, cramps, diarrhea, and dehydration.

Spread by Air and Hand

Airborne infections are contracted by breathing in bacteria. The hairs and mucus in the nose filter out most inhaled bacteria, trapping them so that the white cells can destroy them. Staphylococci sometimes live in the nasal area, as do other potentially dangerous organisms such as the pneumococcus and the beta-hemolytic streptococcus. Newborn infants, as well as individuals with poor resistance to disease, are susceptible to infection, which may spread to other parts of the body from the nose. Bacteria which usually enter the body by the airborne route include the streptococcus, pneumococcus, hemophilus influenza, pertussis (whooping cough), meningococcus, diphtheria organisms, and tuberculosis germs.

BACTERIA AND ILLNESS: BY THE ALPHABET

Anthrax

Anthrax spores can be found in soil, animal hides (such as on bongo drums), and new wool. The spores can infect both animals and people though a scratch, leading to fatal disease if untreated. Infections start as a local sore on the skin.

Bacterial Venereal Diseases

A large number of infections—bacterial, viral, fungal, and parasitic —can be passed from person to person through sexual contact. The bacterial venereal diseases are gonorrhea and syphilis (see pages 289 and 291).

Beta Streptococcus

The beta-hemolytic streptococcus excretes over twenty damaging toxins and enzymes and is the cause of an impressive list of diseases:

1. Erysipelas—an infection which spreads rapidly in the deep skin.
2. Puerperal fever—an infection of the uterus after delivery.
3. Sepsis—a blood stream infection.
4. Wound infections—not infrequent in children.
5. Strep throat, which frequently extends to the ears and mastoids as well as occasionally to the brain.
6. Scarlet fever—which is a strep throat or wound infection with a rash from strep toxin.
7. Peritonsillar abscesses.
8. Strep impetigo, a blistery, crusty, rapidly spreading skin lesion similar to staph impetigo.
9. Ear, sinus, or brain infections secondary to strep throat.

The major complications of infection from beta-hemolytic streptococcus are caused by an immune reaction in the body of susceptible persons. They may develop:

10. Rheumatic fever.
11. Rheumatic heart disease.
12. Glomerulonephritis.
13. Chorea (a brain reaction of nervousness which has been called the St. Vitus Dance).

Of course, most people who have B strep infections do not develop any of these nasty complications. There is probably a genetic factor which predisposes some to hypersensitivity complications.

Streptococcal infections are frequently resistant to treatment and recur quickly when medication is stopped too soon. Although the organism is very sensitive to penicillin, this drug does not always work. It is speculated that beta strep may possibly form a resistant spore-like state in the tissue. Sometimes strep survive because they happen to be near a germ which produces an enzyme, called penicillinase, which destroys penicillin. Not infrequently, beta strep recurs from small abscesses deep in the tonsils where pencillin cannot penetrate. The most common source of reinfection, however, is the original source—that is, an untreated carrier of the disease. This may be another child or an adult. Adults who have built up a significant immunity have only about a fifth as much strep infection as do children. However, parents with no symptoms can become carriers and continue to re-infect their children. One in twenty people may carry streptococci.

One major reason for recurrences of B strep infections is failure to follow a complete program of medication. People find that the penicillin relieves the symptoms of strep throat within a day, so they neglect to continue the medication. It takes at least ten days of treatment to eliminate the disease and to prevent recurrence.

Other strep, in addition to the bad beta strep, can cause disease. The green strep, which usually inhabits the mouth, can cause infection of the heart valves, although this occurs rarely except in cases of congenital heart disease.

Botulism

The botulism organism, while not a cause of direct infection in humans, produces toxin which can lead to nerve paralysis and death. The muscles rather quickly become limp and the victim becomes so weak he cannot breathe and suffocates without artificial respiration. Spores of botulism may grow in meats but the most common source of this disease is home canned vegetables which have not been heat-processed long enough to kill all of the botulism spores. Whenever canning at home, be sure to find out in advance what temperature and time are necessary to ensure complete sterility.

The botulism organism grows in the bowels of some small infants, and its toxin may cause the infants to be limp, have a weak cry, and have trouble breathing.

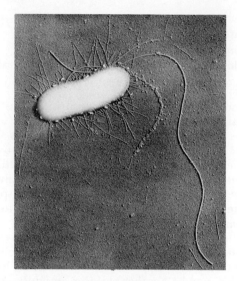

FIGURE 51   *Electron microscope photograph of a single bowel bacteria that swims by moving arm-like fibers called cilia. You would have to line 10,000 of these germs end to end to make a line one centimeter long.*

Brucellosis (Undulant Fever)

The germ of brucellosis infects cattle, goats, dogs, and, occasionally, people. It is found in unpasteurized milk from infected animals or can be caught by direct contact with infected animals. Around one half of one percent of American cattle carry the infection. Most infections occur without symptoms, but the disease is chronic and can be debilitating. Symptoms include night fevers, nervousness, swollen glands, hepatitis, and joint pain. Doctors diagnose brucella infection by blood tests, skin tests, and culture.

Diphtheria

The diphtheria bacillus has killed hundreds of thousands of people. It excretes an extremely potent toxin which damages the lining of the throat, causing a thick grayish membrane which can kill by obstructing the throat—choking the individual to death. The lymph glands in the throat swell, and the breath develops a peculiar odor. The toxin can damage the heart and nerves.

Proper immunization will prevent this disease. Epidemics still occur in the United States because of laziness or ignorance about keeping up immunizations. Many adolescents and adults have inadequate levels of diphtheria antibodies and are susceptible to the disease. They should receive booster injections of diphtheria toxoid every ten years.

Gas Gangrene

The spore-forming germs of gas gangrene are found in the intestinal tracts of people and animals, and they get into the soil from feces. In human and animal body tissues, they excrete tissue-killing toxins and often produce a gas, causing gas gangrene. Thorough cleansing of all deep penetrating wounds is essential in order to prevent this extremely serious infection.

Gonorrhea

Gonorrhea is principally a disease of the mucous membrane linings of the male and female reproductive organs, but it can invade and infect other areas of the body, including the tissues of the eyes, nose, throat, and rectum; or it can spread by the bloodstream to the joints, the heart, or other areas. It is transmitted by sexual contact.

In the male, gonorrhea usually begins with burning on urination, accompanied by a pus-like discharge from the penis. Untreated gonorrhea in men can lead to serious prostate and bladder problems in later life. The disease is often difficult to detect in women, because its symptoms are usually mild and sometimes even nonexistent. Gonorrhea can be carried for many years in women who have a chronic low-grade infection. The disease can travel to the female internal reproductive organs, where severe infection and sometimes sterility will be the outcome.

An infant born of a mother with gonorrhea may develop the infection in the eyes, with resulting blindness. Most states now require that preventive medication (usually silver nitrate drops) be put into the eyes of all newborns to kill any possible gonococci.

Although gonorrhea usually responds to antibiotics, resistant strains of the germ have developed. Early treatment is essential in order to prevent the development of complications. Prevention of the spread of the disease can be accomplished best by immediate reporting of all possible contacts so they may receive treatment before transmitting the infection to others. The careful use of condoms (rubbers) during sexual intercourse is reasonably effective in preventing the disease.

Hemophilus Influenza

This fastidious "blood-loving" germ is capable of causing severe damage to those without adequate immunity. It can exist in the nasopharynx in a carrier state and infects susceptible youngsters in a variety of ways. One symptom is SEVERE CROUP, with the sudden onset of a swelling above the vocal cords which can block breathing. The organism can invade the blood stream, and is a major cause of meningitis in youngsters. Small children are generally susceptible to the organism. Older individuals become increasingly immune.

Leptospirosis (Weil's Disease)

Leptospira occur throughout the world, causing a variety of diseases in rats, dogs, rodents, cattle, swine, and humans. People are infected from accidental ingestion of water (swimming, bathing, drinking) contaminated from animal urine. Children are most frequently infected from dog urine. Weil's disease causes fever, yellow skin and eyes, an influenza-like illness, and, occasionally, meningitis.

Meningococcus

The meningococcus resides in the nasopharynx, and, depending on the individual's immunity, is either killed, remains in a carrier state, or invades the bloodstream. It can kill in a matter of hours, or it can lodge in the brain, causing MENINGITIS—which can also be fatal. It tends to hit children and young adults who live close together. Its spread can be reduced by reduction in crowding and by good ventilation.

Plague

Bubonic plague, or the "black death," has killed millions of people. It is not merely a tragedy of ancient history. In fact, sporadic cases and deaths still occur in California. The organism is found in many rodents, and can become epidemic in rats. It is spread by fleas which bite infected rodents and then people. The lymph glands swell, and later, bleeding occurs in the skin, turning it black—hence the term, "black death." It can cause pneumonia and become air borne.

When bubonic plague is untreated, up to ninety percent of its victims may die. The organism is primarily carried by the ground squirrel and its fleas. Antibiotics are effective for treatment. Rat and flea control can keep the disease in check.

Pneumococcus

The pneumococcus, a bad actor, is a cousin of the streptococcus. Like strep, it lives in the nose or throat of some people in the carrier state without making them sick. But if a virus disturbs the body's defenses, the pneumococcus grows with abandon. It causes severe EAR INFECTIONS (otitis media) in children as well as SINUS INFECTIONS and PNEUMONIA, and can invade the bloodstream, where it travels to the brain causing MENINGITIS. In 1940, prior to the use of antibiotics, pneumococcus infection was a leading cause of death in the United States. Severe damage or death still occurs in a few unlucky infants, children, or older people with impaired immunity. The organism can be identified quickly and can be killed with penicillin.

Rat Bite Fever

Where there is garbage, or inviting bowls of pet food left outside, there are rats. A rat bite may infect an individual with the spirochete spirillum minus, causing a local sore, swollen glands, rashes, and a relapsing fever.

Soil Bacteria

Most soil bacteria are harmless to man and are essential for plant growth, but there are four dangerous soil germs which form highly resistant spores, allowing them to survive for long periods of time in extremes of temperature. These bacteria cause tetanus, gas gangrene, botulism, and anthrax.

Spirochetes

Spirochetes are thin, swimming, corkscrew-like organisms which can infect man through a wide variety of entry points. The most important diseases in this group are: syphilis, Weil's disease, and rat-bite fever.

Syphilis

Untreated syphilis is a devastating disease which persists throughout life, causing a wide variety of symptoms. In its final forms it leads to nearly complete destruction of many body tissues, including the liver, heart, and brain.

The first sign of syphilis is marked by the appearance of a painless ulcer or sore, called a chancre, usually on the penis or vulva of the infected person. The organism can be seen under the microscope in fluid taken from the chancre, or diagnosis can be made by testing for antibody in the blood. Later a generalized rash may appear on the body.

Congenital syphilis is acquired by the infant of a syphilitic mother due to passage of the organism into the baby's circulation during fetal life. Severe and permanent developmental defects, including mental retardation, can be caused by congenital syphilis. For this reason, all pregnant women should have a blood test for syphilis in an early stage of pregnancy. If a possible contact with the disease has occurred during the later stages of pregnancy, the test should be repeated prior to delivery.

With early and adequate treatment, complete cure is usually possible. As with gonorrhea, early case finding and prevention is essential.

Tetanus Bacillus

The spores of tetanus are especially widespread where horse and cow manure have been deposited. When inoculated into a deep wound, the organisms grow and excrete a nerve toxin which cause the muscles to go into spasm so that the victim may be unable to walk or swallow. The infection, which can come from a very small infected sore, often leads to death. It can be prevented by adequate tetanus immunization. A booster injection of tetanus toxoid should be given if it has been over five years since the last one, and if the wound is a puncture wound or dirty.

Tuberculosis

Tuberculosis is a "heavy," waxy, coated germ which is excreted in infected sputum or urine or cow's milk. It can cause a chronic infection of the lungs, kidneys, lymph glands, bone, or brain. In recent years, the use of tuberculin tests and chest x-rays to diagnose the disease early, followed by antibiotic treatment, has permitted the closure of T.B. hospitals in the United States. The organisms may yet appear, however, from someone infected forty or fifty years ago. The organisms can live in old sputum for days. They are resistant even to strong antiseptics, but are susceptible to boiling water.

Most often, T.B. is diagnosed in a "well" child or adult with no symptoms by a positive tuberculin skin test or by an x-ray of the chest indicating past exposure. Children with a positive tuberculin skin test, even if not ill, should be treated with antibiotics. This preventive approach has almost eliminated the dread tuberculous meningitis.

If something happens to the resistance of an infected individual, the T.B. may become active years later. A few develop progressive tuberculosis. This is a subtle and treacherous disease which still deserves attention and respect.

The lymph nodes in the neck which drain the tonsils can become infected with tuberculosis. This may result from drinking unpasteurized milk from a cow that has T.B. of the udder. (*Never drink unpasteurized milk*—it may also carry beta strep infections, diphtheria, or typhoid.)

There are milder forms of tuberculosis caused by germs which infect animals, birds, and reptiles, and, in turn, people. Separate skin tests show the presence of these forms.

There are two types of T.B. skin tests. The *tine test* involves making four little puncture holes in the superficial layer of forearm skin. The dots may turn red for a day; but, if any of the four spots are still red after forty-eight hours, one should return to the doctor for a reading. The *P.P.D. Test* for tuberculosis exposure is given with a small needle into the skin of the forearm, and is read in forty-eight hours. A positive skin test usually means past exposure to T.B. It does not necessarily mean that there is any real T.B. disease—but it might. A positive test could mean, instead, that the individual has been exposed and has cured himself, or that he has a non-disease-producing strain of tuberculosis. Sometimes the doctor will want to do additional tests to see if the tuberculin test might be a false positive caused by a different organism, such as histoplasmosis.

Tularemia (Rabbit Fever)

Tularemia is caused by a relative of the plague bacillus. Although primarily a disease of wild rabbits and squirrels, it can spread to people through insect bites or from skinning infected game. At first, a local red bump ulcerates. Then the germs spread to the lymph glands and cause fever, headache, and vomiting.

Typhoid and Paratyphoid

Typhoid and paratyphoid are caused by species of salmonella bacteria. The organism lives in the bowel but can survive in water. It spreads where sanitation is poor and water supplies are unchlorinated. It exists in human carriers (often in the gall bladder), and may get on their fingers from stool and urine. Careless washing after going to the toilet leaves organisms under the fingernails. If the individual handles food, the organisms get into the food.

Typhoid invades through the bowel wall and spreads throughout the body, causing fever in from three to forty days after exposure. Only half of the victims develop diarrhea.

Typhoid immunizations partially protect the individual against future exposure. Antibiotic treatment helps, but often does not completely kill the germs. Up to five percent of individuals may become carriers after the infection. Antibiotic-resistant strains brought back by tourists who have travelled in foreign countries threaten to spread the disease in the United States.

A milder diarrhea and food poisoning are caused by many other salmonella species, including paratyphoid. Widespread among animals and man, they are excreted in urine and feces. Food exposed to mice and rat or fly excretions may become contaminated. They can contaminate milk, shellfish, eggs, coconut, meats, and pets (turtles, dogs, cats). They often occur in chicken and turkey. Like typhoid, the organism is difficult to eradicate from the intestinal tract, and carriers who handle food will spread the disease.

Water Bacteria

The "water bugs," pseudomonas and proteus, are water bacteria which grow profusely anywhere that moisture can be found. They occur commonly in the bowel, and although not highly infectious, can occasionally cause bladder infections. Open skin wounds, especially burns, may become infected, since antibiotics which kill all other bacteria often do not affect these two tough organisms. Most strains are susceptible to newer antibiotics.

Whooping Cough

The whooping cough bacillus, pertussis, is similar to hemophilus. It is transmitted by airborne droplets from coughing or sneezing and grows on the bronchial lining. It does not invade like strep but sets the stage for severe secondary infection. After a two-week incubation period, there is an onset of mild coughing and sneezing. Later, a spasmotic explosive cough is followed by a whoop of air on inspiration. Infants still die from this disease, which is preventable by early administration of D.P.T. vaccine—the P stands for pertussis.

IN-BETWEEN GERMS (MINI BACTERIA!)

In between viruses and bacteria are a relatively newly recognized group of germs which cause a lot of diseases. Although they are larger than viruses, like them, they are small enough to live inside our cells. These in-between germs are unlike viruses in that they are treatable with anti-biotics. Unfortunately, they do not aways respond terribly well to our bacterial fighting antibodies, so infections often persist and recur in spite of antibiotics. They probably cause a variety of minor diseases, such as sore throat, conjunctivitis, and colds and flu-like symptoms, as well as the following significant diseases. Meet your "In-Between" mini bacteria:

Atypical Pneumonia Germ

This germ, known as mycoplasma, probably makes all of us sick at one time or another. They are most well known as the cause of atypical pneumonia, a disease with little or no fever and not much illness, yet a chest full of pneumonia that can persist for weeks. Mycoplasma also are known to cause tonsillitis and urinary tract infection.

Lymphogranuloma Venerum Germ

This germ, a chlamydiae (a WHAT?!), causes a venereal disease, starting three to twenty days after intercourse with an infected partner. There are swollen glands around the groin and rectum as well as rashes, fever, joint pains, and eye infections.

Psittacosis

This Parrot Fever germ is a disease of birds which spreads to man by inhalation of infected dust from bird feces. After an incubation period of ten days, there are fever and respiratory symptoms which can mimic atypical pneumonia or influenza. Since the illness may be fatal, anti-biotics are usually needed for treatment.

Rickettsiae

Rickettsiae are "mini-bacteria" which infect insects such as mites, fleas, lice, and ticks. Even the bugs have bugs! The insects seem to get along with them, but rickettsial infections can make people quite ill. These small bacteria have caused large troubles, killing hundreds of thousands of people with TYPHUS. Smaller numbers of people are made ill by ticks carrying ROCKY MOUNTAIN SPOTTED FEVER. Symptoms of these infections are similar: headache, fever (flu-like, lasting up to three weeks), fatigue, and skin rash. Antibiotics are helpful in treating rickettsial infections. Before antibiotics, deaths were common. Control of the insects is the best way of prevention. The organisms can remain alive

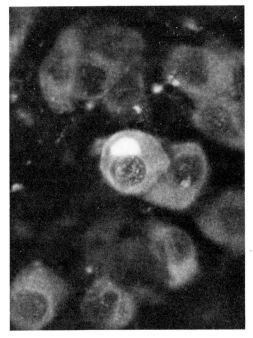

FIGURE 52   *The half moon white spot inside the cell in the center of the electron microphotograph is a group of mini-bacteria called chlamydia. The cell was scraped from the inside of an eyelid.*

for months in dried insect feces. Human infection comes from bug bites, from rubbing insect feces into the scratched skin, or from inhaling the dust of feces which contain the organisms.

Trachoma

Trachoma is caused by a chlamydiae which blinds over twenty million and infects four hundred million people throughout the world. It occurs in areas of low sanitation in Africa and Asia, and in some American Indian reservations. The infection starts with pus in the eyes and may, if untreated, progress to scar the cornea, causing blindness.

Symptoms and Conditions Caused by In-Between Germs

It might look as though we have listed organisms that only rarely cause disease in the United States. The ones above are nasty actors and have therefore been studied more intensely than the less well known ones that probably commonly infect us. Actually most of us have suffered, and most of our children will suffer, from the mycoplasma germ that causes atypical pneumonia. There are, undoubtedly, many strains and varieties of all of these mini-bacteria which cause low grade infections in many of us. Certainly they can cause a wide variety of symptoms, disease and conditions as you can see in the following list:

Blindness	Fatigue	Pneumonia
Bronchitis	Fever	Rashes
Chronic cough	Headache	Tonsilitis
"Colds"	Influenza-like symptoms	Urinary tract infections
Cystitis	Joint pains	
Eye infection	Lymph gland swelling	

17

VIRAL DISEASES:
THE "INCURABLE" CAUSES

From colds to measles to chicken pox, mankind is beset with organisms which cause disease and misery and do not respond to any medical treatment. Antibiotics, especially including penicillin, are of no help. Each of us has to utilize our own immunity and resistance to fight off the "incurable" viruses. Still, once you understand, there are steps you can take and things you can do to prevent complications. Viruses are so small that you can't see them with your eye, but they are as real as you and I. They have been well photographed through electron microscopes, so we can begin to take their measure. Join us in a look at these almost molecular sized pests.

WHAT ARE VIRUSES?

Viruses, the smallest sized particles of life, live inside cells of all sorts. Inside these unwilling hosts, the viruses multiply and manufacture a coat made out of the cell's protein. This covering protects the virus and enables it to survive outside the cell. Viruses are so small that some strains can even infect bacteria. In order to realize how small a virus is, compare it to the Staphylococcus bacteria. This bacteria is 1/25,000th of an inch in diameter, and yet it is 50,000 times bigger than a polio virus. If a Staphylococcus bacteria were as big as this page, a virus would cover a spot less than the size of the period at the end of this sentence.

Viruses are made of complex molecules called R.N.A. and D.N.A., which are also the basic substances of our chromosomes, the same substance that carries our inherited tendencies and directs the chemical reactions inside the cell. Viruses are made up of "gene-like" material without a cell. All they need is a cell to live in. Viruses may even have the equivalent of "sexual" mating in that they may combine and reproduce "children" different than the parents. Bacterial viruses can even transfer a gene from one bacteria to another, giving the bacteria a new combination of genes.

How Do You Get a Virus Infection?

Viruses multiply in great numbers and spread in many ways. The spread of measles is direct, from person to person by cough, kiss, or sneeze. The virus of infectious hepatitis is sometimes spread in food and drink contaminated by urine or stool, which probably gets into the food from under the cook's fingernails. Animal bites transmit rabies; and bugs such as mosquitos can transmit yellow fever. People excrete viruses in urine, stools, or saliva just prior to becoming obviously ill, during an illness, and *often for a considerable length of time after an illness*. The contagious period usually starts just before the fever and *is almost over when the fever has gone*. However, in some people, contagion can continue a long time. Individuals who become carriers excrete viruses chronically. Care in handwashing and disposal of stool and urine helps reduce infections.

How Can You Fight a Virus Infection?

Even viruses out of the body are hard to kill. In order to purify water, for example, it is necessary to use high levels of chlorine. Viruses *will wash off with soap and water,* and they are killed by boiling. Because the virus lives inside the cell and uses the cell's metabolic mechanism, it is unlikely that an effective chemical agent will be found soon that will damage the virus without damaging the cell. As there are thousands of different viruses with different structures and properties, it is unlikely that humanity will be spared from all viral infections in the near future, if ever.

Doctors use two valuable methods to fight viral infection: vaccination with a live but weakened virus, and the use of strong immune serum from individuals previously infected by the virus. Antibiotics do not kill viruses, so scientists are experimenting with various chemicals in an effort to find cures for viral infections. So far, there has been little practical progress with antiviral chemicals, although one drug does provide partial temporary protection to an individual exposed to smallpox.

Vaccination with live, weakened virus stimulates antibodies against the disease. This immunizing or antibody-producing mechanism helps explain the success of Sabin polio vaccine and of measles and smallpox vaccines. Our cells are not damaged significantly by the artificially developed weak virus, and the body responds with antibodies which protect against the stronger or virulent virus strains encountered in the future. Every effort is made to make certain that a vaccine is safe. It is certainly safer than the disease it protects against. But people are different, and it is always possible that a vaccine will make some individual ill. Put in balance, those who do get somewhat ill from viral vaccines would undoubtedly be *gravely ill* if they did not get the vaccine and did get the disease. It is better to have even a severe reaction from vaccination than to get smallpox.

Viral infections occur more often in infants and children than in adults, because antibodies are developed only after contact with a virus. The sheer number of viruses explains why children are ill so often. It is unlikely that your physician will try to determine the specific cause of every viral infection, because to do so is a slow and expensive process and the disease is over by the time the virus is identified.

Many infections are not apparent, since individual resistance to viruses varies greatly. One person may not feel the effect of a virus which makes another seriously ill. Fortunately, our immune system enables most of us to live in reasonably good health while supporting hundreds of different viruses in cells.

VIRUSES YOU SHOULD KNOW

Adenoviruses

The common adenoviruses, so named because they were first found in human adenoids, may cause epidemics of illness. The thirty-one known strains spread by direct contact and by droplets of saliva in the air but also by hands or food contaminated by bowel movements. The virus is present in the stool for two months after an illness in phenomenal numbers: 1/5th of a teaspoon of stool may have 10,000,000 infective doses! Adenovirus infections may cause:

No illness	Bronchitis
Sore throat	Rash
Pink eye (conjunctivitis)	Diarrhea
Fever	

Chicken Pox

The chicken pox virus is one of the most highly contagious diseases of childhood. The virus is spread both by direct contact and by droplets in the air. The incubation period is usually twelve to sixteen days.

The disease is characterized by pox on the skin, raised pimple-like bumps about the size of a large match head which develop a greyish "dew drop" translucent blister on top. This is usually scratched off, leaving a crater at the top of the pimple. Cases can occur with only one or two pox, while others have thousands of pox with clusters and crops appearing over a four day period. They usually begin on the chest and back but soon appear on the face, in the hair, in the mouth, and finally on the extremities. There is little fever in some cases, while others run fever to 105° for the four days during the eruption of the rash. The fever should subside after the fourth or fifth day and the pox then becomes dry. The crusted scabs may take as long as a week to disappear.

Complications are rare. Bacterial infection (strep or staph) may occur in the open pox. Pox can occur in the mouth or vagina, and are frequently thicker in the diaper area. Itching can be severe. Call your doctor if cough or headache are prominent or if boils, pus, or much redness appear on or around the pox. Adults are more likely than children to develop complications such as pneumonia, and should consult a doctor if high fever occurs. Pregnant women who have not had chicken pox should carefully avoid exposure to the disease, as it may infect the unborn baby. People on cortisone or other immuno-suppressive drugs (for nephritis, leukemia, transplants, etc.) should avoid exposure, as chicken pox may be extremely serious or fatal. Researchers are working on a live vaccine.

Keep cool and rested. Don't overdress or stay under a lot of covers. Cut the fingernails short. Frequent cool baths or showers are good. Your doctor may advise you to wash daily with an antiseptic soap in order to keep strep and staph germs from the skin. Sometimes, relief from itching can be obtained with over-the-counter preparations. Ask your druggist. If there are pox around the mouth or vagina, use an antibiotic ointment you can buy across-the-counter. Ask your druggist. Your doctor can pre-scribe oral medication for the itch if it is severe. Other suggestions offered by pediatrician Henry Richanbach:

- Use a small paint brush to apply plain calomine lotion.
- A laundry or corn starch bath twice a day is very soothing. Argo or Linit starch from the grocery store are fine. WARNING: This makes the tub very slippery; help the child in and out or he may fall.
- Give the child a bowl of cornstarch with cotton balls for dabbing on the pox. It gives them something to do with their hands when itching is severe.

Colds

What most people call "a cold" is often an infection caused by viruses, such as adenoviruses, echo virus, or even early measles or mumps. Scientists have, however, isolated a family of simple common cold viruses called Rhinoviruses. We know that the average adult suffers from the common cold one to three times a year, the average school child four to five times a year, and the preschooler five to six times a year. Some ninety *Rhinoviruses* ("nose" virus) found in the upper respiratory tract are evidently responsible for most of these "colds." The small cold viruses irritate the nose, the throat, and, occasionally, the vocal cords. The incubation period is only two to four days, and the illness lasts a week, although residual symptoms may persist up to three weeks. The swelling of membranes and lowered local resistance may predispose to secondary bacterial infections of the ears, sinuses, and bronchial tubes.

Resistance to colds is a puzzle. Nasal membranes produce local antibodies specifically for each virus. Only half of a group of volunteers deliberately exposed to cold virus could be infected with the virus; yet many of the resistant volunteers caught the same cold virus at later times.

Most people who get a cold are resistant to another Rhinovirus cold for a few weeks. Resistance may have something to do with the special virus resistance factor, interferon. The Rhinovirus colds are spread by droplet infection, as was noted by such ancients as Ben Franklin, who advised against travelling in a coach with someone who had a cold or "you would surely catch it."

A common fallacy is that newborn infants are immune to colds. Any immunity they have would have been passed on from mother, yet mother is also susceptible to colds. In fact, infants develop complications from virus infections, and they should be protected from exposure to sick people by every possible means. *Colds always come from people,* not from drafts, teething, cold feet, or outside air. However, Dr. A. S. Hashim contends that cold feet can trigger a cold if the child happens to be harboring a virus, by causing changes in the mucous membranes of the nose. Well, maybe?

At present, there is no way to cut down the number of colds except to practice good hygiene, provide a proper diet, adequate rest, and plenty of exercise. Avoid unnecessary indoor contacts with others known to have a cold. No satisfactory immunizations are yet available. Home remedies, such as chest rubs, medicated vapors, mustard plaster, and so forth are of little value.

Cool mist humidifiers keep a cough loose and are helpful, especially for croup, but such additions as tincture of benzoin or sprays are of no benefit. Most respiratory infections have been shown to be due to viruses and do not respond to antibiotic therapy such as penicillin, sulfa, and the other antibiotics.

Home Treatment of "Colds"

We asked pediatrician William Misbach to give you the instructions he gives his patients on home treatment for colds. He made the following suggestions:

1. The younger the child, the more alert you should be to call the doctor. In older children, call whenever fever (above 101°F) is present for over twenty-four hours.
2. When fever is present, diet should be primarily fruit juices, carbonated drinks, clear broth, and water. Small amounts of candy given several times a day help supply nourishment to a sick child. It is often best to let your child decide what foods or liquids he receives. When the temperature stays down, gradually return to a normal diet.
3. The sick child belongs in bed. Sometimes a couch or big chair is satisfactory. Running about the house will tire a child who is already weakened by infection. Activity should be resumed slowly *after* the temperature has remained normal for a day or two.

Pediatrician Glen Griffin doesn't think it is realistic to keep a child in bed unless he is sick enough to stay there voluntarily. I guess it is a matter of how sick is sick. As you can see, the harder a disease is to treat, the greater the disagreements between doctors. This is probably a good index of our frustration—to say nothing of mother's!

Does Vitamin C Prevent or Cure Colds?

It has been claimed that the regular ingestion of 1,000 mgm of Vitamin C plus using 4,000 mgm daily at the onset of colds reduces the incidence of colds by 45%. In a controlled study on the use of large doses of Vitamin C, researchers at the University of Toronto found an insignificant difference of 9% in the incidence of colds between those who used Vitamin C and those who didn't. Insignificant, that is, unless you might be one of the 9%—in which case, it could be chance, or maybe an outside possibility, that you individually benefit from extra Vitamin C, in spite of the statistics. Another study indicated that in most cases 200 mgm of Vitamin C is just as effective as 1,000 mgm. I have always thought it interesting that for years we have used 1,000 mgm doses of Vitamin C to treat bladder infections by acidifying the urine. Vitamin C is an acid, ascorbic acid, and at 1,000 mgm doses most of it ends up in the bladder where it can, by dint of its acidity, suppress bacterial growth. In other words, most of it is "peed out" in the urine. Because of the huge amount of vitamins many Americans take I'll bet that our sewage is about the most nutritious stuff on earth!

However, I don't know of any real harm from huge doses of Vitamin C. And in one study it seemed to improve resistance to "illness" in that fewer days work were lost by a group on large doses of Vitamin C compared with a group not on large doses of Vitamin C. Various researchers have stressed that their findings have not provided a clear answer to the controversy. One thing can be said, at least Vitamin C is, or should be, relatively cheap and harmless. Harmless that is unless you are allergic to the artificial food additive they use to color and flavor the pills! But who knows, maybe it really does help some people.

Is It Really a Cold?

If Vitamin C hasn't helped, and you have trouble keeping him in bed, and you are frustrated by chronic colds, perhaps you will want to think of the approach suggested by Dr. William Crook.

Frustrated mothers complain, "Johnny has one infection right after another. I just can't keep him well. No matter what I do, he's forever catching a cold. Even when he doesn't have a cold, he coughs at night or sniffs his nose. I wish I could give him a vitamin or something which would build up his resistance."

If this sounds like your child, he's probably allergic. Respiratory tract allergy often masquerades as a "cold" because the symptoms are so similar. Many children with persistent, recurrent respiratory symptoms are mistakenly treated for infection, and the underlying allergic cause is overlooked. Suspect allergy if your child:

1. Has more than his share of infections.
2. Has a runny, sneezing, and itching nose.
3. Has a chronic night cough.
4. Coughs when exerted and periodically has "bronchitis" or "pneumonia."
5. Coughs and sneezes, when other family members do not "catch" the cold.

Colds and Superstitions

Sometimes rest, fluids, aspirin, Vitamin C, allergy treatments, and tincture of time don't work. At least not soon enough to satisfy most of humanity. Perhaps we shouldn't be so skeptical. Dr. Merritt Low says that,

What you *think* may help prevent or cure a cold, sometimes does.

And for at least 3,000 years, people have been trying to cope with the common cold with faith, superstition, and hope. The American Lung Association collected some beloved remedies and time-honored rituals which they submitted to modern researchers for criticisms:

"Wrap a piece of flannel around your throat at the first sign of scratchiness." The cold germ will have a good laugh. The flannel is only a substitute for the teddy bear you clutched as a baby.

"Take a laxative to get rid of the cold germs." The cold virus won't be budged even if you may have to move.

"Get under a pile of blankets, and sweat." This is supposed to flush out the poisons produced by the infections. It hasn't been proved. Anyway, it's pleasanter to drink liquids, and you accomplish the same purpose—if you accomplish it at all.

"Feed a cold and starve a fever." Oh, come on. What do you do if you have a cold *and* a fever?[1]

Cold Sore Viruses

There are many known herpes viruses, of which the "cold sore" virus, herpes-simplex, is the best known. It causes a blistery lesion, the cold sore, usually at the junction of the lip and skin. The virus seems to stay in an inactive state almost forever, so that cold sores may recur many times.

Herpetic stomatitis, due to cold sore virus, type I, causes ulcers throughout the mouth, with fever—often lasting for two weeks. It occurs most often in small children who have not developed immunity from earlier infections. The incubation period is three to five days. Herpes on the eyelids or in the eye may indicate an *infection of the cornea,* which can lead to scarring and to permanent visual problems. On rare occasions, the virus can infect the brain. Patients with eczema may develop the infection in their damaged skin.

What Can You Do About Cold Sores?

Cold sores are untouched by antibiotics. Local inflammation may subside a bit if they are treated with Mercurochrome or iodine, but this is probably due to the destruction of bacteria which grow in the open sore. Most treatments are questionable. An experimental treatment uses a dye to penetrate the herpes sore, followed by irradiation with fluorescent light. In some people, relief can be obtained by multiple small pox vaccinations. Ether dabbed on a cold sore is said to be helpful.

Genital cold sores are caused by Herpes virus, type I or II. Newborns can contract the virus in the birth canal and develop generalized disease. Most people are never ill with either virus, although they live on us for life. Some studies indicate that there may be a relationship between the virus of Herpes II and cancer of the cervix.

Cytomegalic inclusion disease is so named because of the "large" bodies "included" in infected cells. The inclusion bodies are made up of viruses which resemble Herpes I virus. They evidently infect most of the human population without symptoms. Intrauterine infection of the fetus can result in damage to an unborn infant. It is suspected that they may be spread venereally, and evidence points to this virus as a major cause of retarded children (estimated to cause over 3,000 cases a year). Research is progressing toward an effective vaccine for this disease.

Coxsackie Viruses

Almost all of us have suffered from various coxsackie virus infections many times, for there are twenty-nine known strains of this common virus. Like polio viruses, they are found in the mouth and stools. These viruses are resistant to seventy percent alcohol and to most antiseptics. They usually infect humans during the summer and fall with a wide variety of disease symptoms. The incubation period is from two to nine days. Coxsackie viruses may cause nonspecific viral fevers easily confused with many other generalized viral diseases. Newborn infants may develop quite serious illnesses due to coxsackie viruses. In rare cases, the infection can settle in the heart and its membranes. Antibiotics are of no help. Among diseases caused by coxsackie viruses are:

- Herpangina—an illness with fever, headache, and sore ulcers on the back of the throat. It can be accompanied by vomiting and stomachache lasting from one to four days. The typical case is easily recognized, but atypical cases may mimic streptococcal throat infections.

- Pleurodynia—characterized by severe chest or abdominal pain lasting for a few days; it may then recur during the next two weeks. Most individuals have fever, and, occasionally, severe headaches.

- Aseptic meningitis—accompanied by headache, fever, vomiting, abdominal pain, and stiff neck—occasionally with temporary paralysis, although recovery from the paralysis is usually complete.

- "Common colds"—some varieties are caused by coxsackie viruses.

• Hand, foot, and mouth disease—characterized by a rash on the hands and feet and ulcers in the mouth; may be due to at least five different varieties of coxsackie viruses.

Echovirus

Although Echoviruses infect almost all of us, they usually do not make most adults sick, although children frequently suffer from such infections.

Over thirty types of Echoviruses have been found in the throat and intestinal tract. They are similar to coxsackie virus in that they can cause illness with a wide range of symptoms. The incidence of infection is far greater in children than in adults, due to the fact that antibodies to the viruses are formed as children grow older. *Febrile summer illness* with rash is common. One variety of Echoviruses, Echo 16, has produced the *slapped cheek fever,* with a rash on the face so red that it looks as if the face were just slapped. Some Echo viruses produce *common colds* and others produce *diarrhea* in infants. Echo 4 may cause *vaginitis* and *cervicitis.* Echo *aseptic meningitis* can occur.

It is important to note that most Echo viral infections do not make most people very sick. One reported outbreak of an Echo virus epidemic infected over 3,000 persons in a town of 20,000 population, but only twenty-seven contracted aseptic meningitis. Intestinal viral infections tend to become epidemic among children in crowded or unsanitary conditions.

Echoviruses are not only numerous, they are versatile and complex. To appreciate the difficulty in diagnosing the cause of an infection, look at the following list of conditions that can be caused by various echoviruses:

No illness	Diarrhea
Aseptic meningitis	Fever
Cervicitis	Rashes
Common colds	Vaginitis
Conjunctivitis (pink eye)	

Hepatitis Virus

There are two types of infectious hepatitis viruses. A and B. Although severe hepatitis causes jaundice, or yellow skin and eyes, with dark urine and pale stools, most cases of hepatitis are characterized by fever, loss of appetite, vomiting, and aches and pains. This is one of the infectious diseases where the adults become sicker than children, who rarely develop jaundice.

Type A hepatitis is usually transmitted in food and water contaminated from the urine or stool of an infected person. Symptoms start from two to six weeks after exposure. The virus is excreted in the stool and urine for weeks. Spread of type A hepatitis can be prevented by proper disposal of stool and urine and by careful handwashing, especially of food handlers. Gamma globulin given during the incubation period or prior to traveling in areas where hepatitis is common will prevent severe disease. A hepatitis B vaccine is being developed.

Serum hepatitis is caused by the type B virus, usually by injection under the skin or by blood transfusion. It may also be spread by close contact, such as kissing or intercourse. The virus reproduces in amazing quantity in the liver and blood. Symptoms do not start for two to five months after exposure, and are similar to type A hepatitis. Some people carry the virus in their blood all their lives. It is a tough virus, very resistant to chemical disinfectants and even to short periods of boiling. Ordinary gamma globulin does not protect against type B hepatitis, but a new anti-B gamma globulin is being developed, and research is producing a vaccine to prevent the disease.

Hepatitis can be from many other causes such as mononucleosis, yellow fever, syphilis, and some chemicals. Jaundice can also be caused by many other conditions and deserves a thorough medical work-up.

Infectious Mononucleosis

The diagnosis of infectious mononucleosis is enough to cause panic and intestinal spasms in many people. Actually, it is rarely as bad as most people fear. In fact, it occurs quite often in young children with little or no apparent illness. And it undoubtedly occurs quite often in an atypical form that is undiagnosed—the disease is called the great masquerader because it can cause so many types of illness. The typical infectious mono disease is described by pediatrician Leo Bell.

Infectious mononucleosis, which has been called "kissing disease," "mono," and "glandular fever," is a self-limited disease which runs its own course to its conclusion. It is caused by the "EB" Herpes virus which causes a large special mononuclear white blood cell to appear in the blood. After about ten days a special antibody is formed and can be measured in a blood test to help diagnose the disease. The course of mono is usually characterized by very sore throat with a white coating (membrane) on the tonsils. Other symptoms include fatigue, swollen glands in the neck, arms and groin, and a temperature lasting two weeks or more. Symptoms may recur over a period of three weeks to three months. Frequently the spleen becomes enlarged, and occasionally there is a rash. Occasionally the liver is enlarged and the urine turns dark from mono hepatitis. In the past it has been considered a disease of adolescents, but actually it occurs at any age. It is contagious, but not highly so. When a sore throat is present, the individual is probably contagious, but some must carry the disease without symptoms. It can be spread in saliva. A large number of children with no history of the disease have antibodies to the virus.

Rare complications include neurological and heart problems. If the spleen is enlarged it may rupture if there is a blow on the upper abdomen.

Treatment for this disease, like those for all virus diseases, is practically nonexistent, and only the symptoms may be alleviated as they arise. If throat cultures demonstrate bacterial complication, then appropriate antibiotics may be prescribed. Strenuous exercise, especially contact sports, should be stopped until all symptoms disappear and the doctor gives his O.K. A short course of cortisone may make the patient subjectively better if he is markedly ill with the disease, but it probably does not alter the course of the disease and is rarely recommended. *Adequate rest* is really the only treatment.

I suspect that there are many other viruses that can cause a mononucleosis-like disease. Then, because mono can hit so many areas in the body (even the breasts or the intestinal tract), it is often suspected when other viruses are causing the disease. The picture is complicated even more in that mono evidently can reduce some people's resistance, especially to beta strep infections, and a strep throat will occur along with the mono.

Allergy can cause symptoms that mimic infectious mononucleosis. These include fatigue, headache, and enlarged lymph glands. I had a patient who developed marked swelling of the lymph glands in the neck in a matter of minutes following a skin test for dust. Desensitization to dust cured her recurrent attacks of mononucleosis-like disease.

Influenza

The influenza virus is unique in that there are enzymes on the surface of the viral particle that dissolve the protective mucous covering of the membranes of the nose and throat. Thus this airborne virus can penetrate the cells of the respiratory tract quickly, and the incubation period is only one or two days. It causes a sudden onset of chills, aches, and fever, with a dry sore throat and a hacky cough. The fever usually subsides after five days, but in some it may recur. Muscle aches may follow, and in children, there is occasionally vomiting and diarrhea. The disease occurs in epidemics every two to three years. There are over thirty known strains of influenza virus, and each has the ability to produce new strains.

In 1918, with the upheaval of World War I, a world wide epidemic of influenza made swine and humans ill and killed millions of people—almost six people out of every thousand. Many of these deaths were untreatable at that time, as no antibiotics existed. In 1976, a small epidemic of around 1,000 cases struck Fort Dix, New Jersey, with one influenza death. Antibodies in the blood of people who survived the swine flu in 1918 reacted with the Fort Dix virus, making it possible that it was the same deadly strain of influenza that caused the epidemic of 1918. Alarmed scientists talked the government into backing a massive swine-influenza immunization program because of their fear that severe primary influenza might cause a very high death rate. Strangely enough, however, only a few new cases were reported anywhere in the world during the 1976-1977 season.

Immunizations for influenza may be indicated for the aged and for some children with chronic diseases. However, the immunity doesn't last long; it is ineffective against new strains of the virus; and protection from one strain usually doesn't protect against another strain. Children frequently react to the vaccine with enough chills and fever to make immunization unwelcome if not unwise. A new and better vaccine may be developed soon.

The patient should stay in bed during the acute phase of influenza and rest at least two to three days after the fever has subsided. Frequent small drinks of juice, pop, soups, tea, and so on should be encouraged. The appetite is usually poor, and there is little to be gained by trying to force foods. Aspirin, in the dose of one grain per year of age (one adult aspirin for a five-year-old, two for a ten-year-old), every four hours may be helpful for fever and pain. If the fever doesn't respond to aspirin, your doctor may have other suggestions. Cough is often persistent and distressing. A humidifier or steamer helps moisten the dry throat membranes. Cough suppressants may be needed, especially at night, in order to allow for adequate rest.

Complications of influenza are usually caused by bacterial infection, which may be combatted by antibiotics prescribed by your physician. These include ear infections, bronchitis, pneumonia, and sinusitis. Call your doctor if there is earache, cough that persists beyond the usual four to five days or that becomes productive of green or yellow sputum, if there is severe headache, foul breath, or swollen lymph glands, if there is not enough fluid intake, or if the urine output becomes small.

If Your Child Has Influenza, Should He Be Seen by His Doctor?

People often lump a wide variety of diseases under the term "flu." There is no vaccine against the "flu" or "colds." Not every case of fever and chills and cold symptoms is influenza. Pediatricians occasionally see children with strep throat or pneumonia misdiagnosed at home as "the flu." So should your child be seen in case he has influenza? This brings out differing advice from our contributors. Dr. A. S. Hashim states:

> By and large, yes. The child will be examined, to make sure there are no bacterial complications. The doctor will treat the symptoms, but you certainly don't need an antibiotic unless there is bacterial infection present, such as an ear infection or tonsillitis. This is one of the important reasons your doctor should see the child with the flu.
>
> Is there any other reason he should see your child? Yes, and it is an important one. The flu symptoms can mimic many diseases. You may not be able to differentiate between flu with respiratory symptoms and pneumonia, or between vomiting caused by flu and appendicitis, or between fever and headache of the flu and meningitis. Such dreaded

examples do happen, so don't be lulled into the belief that since the flu is hitting everybody, your child has nothing but the flu.

But Dr. Thomas J. Conway disagrees:

By and large, no. Proper communication over the telephone between a health-educated mother and the child's personal physician will usually make it unnecessary to see the doctor for influenza.

So take your choice, parents. You know your own child. If you know your doctor and he knows you, maybe it can be handled by telephone only. Read the material on how to get the most out of your doctor by telephone on page 110. If the doctor wants to see your child, he may have good reasons that are not covered in our simplified lists. If you don't know the doctor or if he doesn't know you, you probably should have the child seen. Influenza virus infections may cause:

- Little or no illness in some people
- Bronchitis
- Chills and fever
- Dry hacky cough
- Earaches
- Muscle aches
- Sore throat
- Vomiting and diarrhea in children

Measles

Measles, red measles, or "old fashioned ten-day measles" virus enters through the mouth or nose and multiplies in the mucus membranes. The virus is spread by droplets from the nose and mouth. It is highly contagious, and causes severe disease. Following an incubation period of ten days, there are "cold symptoms," increasing cough, red eyes, a rash on the inside of the cheeks, and high fever, and skin rash.

The bronchitis of measles predisposes to pneumonia. Secondary bacterial ear infections are common. More serious for the few who get it is a brain infection, measles encephalitis, which can cause severe damage and retardation. Measles infection may cause:

- No illness
- Bronchitis
- Cold symptoms
- Cough
- Fever
- Earaches
- Encephalomyelitis
- Pink eye (conjunctivitis)
- Rash

Immunization with live measles vaccine will prevent the disease in most children and should be given to all infants at fifteen months of age.

Mumps

Mumps is a viral infection usually recognized from swelling of the salivary glands in front of the ears. The virus invades many tissues in the body, and can cause fever, headache, stomachache, and vomiting. After an incubation period of 17 to 21 days, "cold" symptoms start, with headache and fever a day or two, before the salivary glands swell. Usually the disease lasts a week, but it can go six weeks, spreading to the brain, pancreas, and ovaries. The testicles are infected in about 20% of men, but this rarely results in sterility.

Ovary and pancreas infections cause stomachaches but with no after-effects. Brain infection, with meningitis, causing severe headache, is common, and in rare instances, a hearing loss in one ear may result. Even more rare are swollen joints or breasts from mumps. Many people are infected but not ill, yet they develop antibodies and resistance to mumps. The virus is found in the saliva, but evidently it is not highly contagious.

There is no treatment except aspirin, fluids, and rest—which should be continued at least three days after the swelling is down, for the disease may move to another part of the body. A mumps virus vaccine is used, but how long it will last it is not known. Some physicians believe that it should be given to toddlers to prevent the rare hearing loss. Others believe that it should not be given until puberty, when the disease is usually more severe. Let your physician help make this decision. Mumps infection may cause:

- No illness
- Cold symptoms
- Earache
- Fever
- Headache
- Hearing loss
- Stomachache
- Swollen breasts
- Swollen joints
- Swollen ovaries
- Swollen testicles
- Vomiting

Para-influenza and Respiratory Syncytial Viruses

The four strains of para-influenza viruses and their close relative, the R.S. virus, have infected almost all of us. Our immune systems do not work very well against these nasty viruses: The same strain of the virus can re-infect us, although with less severity, on succeeding occasions. The same strain can cause an infant to have bronchiolitis, and later, a respiratory illness with fever, when he is a child, and a cold when he is an adult. Type IV can also cause an illness with fatigue as the major symptom. Preliminary research on a vaccine against the R.S. virus looks encouraging. Para I and R.S. virus infections may cause:

- No symptoms
- Bronchiolitis
- Bronchitis
- Colds
- Croup
- Fatigue

Poliomyelitis

The poliomyelitis virus causes crippling spinal cord paralysis. President Franklin Roosevelt was the best-known victim of this disease, which was common and dreaded until the early 1960s, when the live Sabin Polio vaccine first became available. Three strains or types of polio viruses have been identified, and infection with one strain does not provide protection against the others. Polio virus can invade the body either through the tonsils or bowels. If it reaches the spinal cord, paralysis may result. However, this occurs in only a small portion of those infected. Most people have infections with no symptoms at all, some have mild illness, and paralysis occurs in only a few. The virus reproduces in the intestine, and is usually spread by fecal contamination on the hands and from there to food. It can also infect from respiratory secretions.

The Sabin oral vaccine is almost 100% effective in protecting against poliomyelitis. In order to assure immunity against all three types of polioviruses, children must receive at least five properly spaced doses of the Sabin vaccine. Poliomyelitis may cause:

- No symptoms
- Constipation
- Drowsiness
- Fever
- Nausea and vomiting

- Headache
- Paralysis
- Sore throat
- Stiff neck and back

Roseola

Roseola is a strange disease, a common cause of an acute rash in childhood. It is frequently confused with one of the "measles." We asked experienced pediatrician Sid Rosin to describe roseola for you.

Whenever a child is reported to have had measles three or four times, it is this disease that has been responsible for one of the episodes. The cause of Roseola is not known, although it is presumed to be a virus. It is not readily communicable, and although outbreaks in children have been reported, they are definitely rare.

Roseola usually strikes in the first two years of life, but it may be seen in older children. Fever, usually over 103°, is the only complaint. Fevers remain for three days, during which time the child is well except perhaps for a lowered appetite. Occasionally, a mild respiratory infection may be noted. The well-being of the child is in marked contrast to the high fever, and roseola is one of the few situations when this occurs in childhood. The fever is usually controlled with aspirin and body sponges. After three days, the fever drops to normal, at which time the child sometimes becomes much more irritable. After twenty-four hours without fever, a generalized fine, flat, pink rash of the trunk is noted, sometimes spreading behind the ears and on the face and extremities. By that time, the irritability has reached a peak, and occasionally it is so marked that it is thought to be due to mild encephalitis. The rash lasts about two days, after which the child is back to normal. Complications are rare, but there is a respiratory infection, and one may have otitis media or sinusitis. Although

uncommon, convulsions have been reported at the time of the high
fever. All treatment is symptomatic, directed against the fever. Avoid
antibiotics unless respiratory complications are present. There is no
prevention, and the incubation period, if there is one, is not known.
There is no need of the additional trauma of hospitalization.

It may or may not be helpful to you to know that a measley rash
means a flat, small, pink, scattered, insignificant rash. Such rashes are
usually caused by a large variety of viral infections. Small children tend
to have these rashes with infections more often than older children and
adults. If there are symptoms or signs such as red throat, cough, runny
nose or foul breath, you should suspect that the disease is not Roseola.
When convulsions do occur with Roseola they are unique to the disease
and usually are not febrile convulsions. This means you don't have to
worry as much about the child having febrile convulsions later on with
different infections.

Rubella

Typical Rubella or "three-day measles" has an incubation period of
two to three weeks. Often, there are mild cold symptoms and a low-grade
fever for a day or two before a rash appears. The lymph glands behind and
below the ears and on the back of the neck swell and may be tender. The
rash on the face and trunk consists of flat or slightly raised rose spots $\frac{1}{8}$
to $\frac{1}{4}$ inch in diameter. They fade out in about three days. Only 50% of
Rubella victims develop a rash. Swollen tender joints (which persist for
a week or two) occur in over 30% of individuals over eighteen years old.
It is difficult to diagnose Rubella accurately except in the typical case.
Atypical cases may require a later blood test for verification. Many other
viral diseases can mimic Rubella.

Rubella is usually a harmless disease for children and adults, but it
is catastrophic for the fetus. The pregnant mother may not be very sick,
but the developing baby can become mentally retarded, deaf, or suffer
heart damage. Rubella results in fifty percent abnormalities in the first
month of pregnancy, and fifteen percent abnormalities in the third
month. Twenty percent die at birth, and even if the baby is normal at
birth, the virus infection may persist chronically for a year or more,
sometimes causing growth failure.

Every woman of child-bearing age should be tested to see if she is
immune to Rubella. If not, she should be given the vaccine at a time
when she is neither pregnant or likely to become pregnant for three
months.

There is no special treatment available for Rubella. Immunization
of preadolescent and adolescent girls is certainly indicated. Immunization of children who may be around unprotected pregnant women is
probably justified. Pregnant women should have a blood test; and, if not
immune, should be vaccinated immediately after delivery. Some advocate
a premarital Rubella test, just as a premarital test for syphilis is re-

quired—both are designed to protect the unborn baby. Rubella infection may cause:

- No illness
- Cold symptoms
- Low grade fever
- Rash
- Severe damage or death to the fetus in pregnant mothers
- Swollen glands
- Swollen joints

Are Mass Rubella Vaccination Programs Worthwhile?

Everyone would like to have dependable facts and scientifically accurate advice, especially about disease and health. Because of this desire, it is emotionally satisfying to accept the words of health authorities and follow their advice. Generally, the medical establishment produces good advice. But not always. We often disagree among ourselves—perhaps more often than most of the public realizes—because the final answers are not yet in. This is certainly the case when it comes to the Rubella vaccination program. In this *Medical Manual* we believe that parents should be made aware that disagreements exist, so we asked pediatrician Robert Burnett to discuss the controversy about mass Rubella vaccination programs.

Rubella is a tragedy for the fetus, for the parents, and for society. However, Rubella for young children is a harmless disease with extremely rare complications. It has been assumed that if children were protected against Rubella by vaccination, there would be fewer epidemics and pregnant women would be protected from exposure. Government public health officials began a mass antirubella experiment in 1970, giving boys and girls who faced no risk from the disease a vaccine whose duration of effectiveness is uncertain. The result may be a generation of youngsters who, by their child-bearing years, will be totally susceptible to Rubella.

It is too early to assess the results of the experiment. Regardless of what happens in the next few years, we will have to know what happens in the next twenty years to subjects who received the vaccine in their early childhood. Meanwhile, there have been epidemics among the teenagers and young adults in communities where the children have been immunized.

Some pediatricians prefer to give the vaccine to teenage girls whom they know are not pregnant and for whom they have run a blood test to detect immunity to Rubella. This is usually the only sure way of ascertaining immunity, for many viruses cause a rash indistinguishable from Rubella.

Requiring a Rubella immunity blood test at the time of application for a marriage license would certainly be a forward step and should be encouraged nationally. Such a course will not affect pregnancies that occur prior to marriage, so these women should have Rubella testing, and then should be given the vaccine immediately after delivery to reduce future risks. This approach is not as easy as experimenting with the young age group, but often easy solutions are valueless. This may be the case with Rubella vaccine.

Rubella usually occurs in epidemics on a six to nine year cycle. The last epidemic occurred in 1964 and resulted in 20,000 damaged infants. Since then there have been sporadic local epidemics, but the failure of the predicted epidemic of 1970 to 1973 to appear is thought by some to indicate success from the mass vaccination program. On the other hand it has since been found that within a few years after rubella vaccination that twenty-five percent of the children have no detectable antibodies. This may mean that repeated booster shots will be needed or that we could end up with an adult population susceptible to rubella because they were protected from the disease as children. Meanwhile what should be done about rubella vaccination? Dr. Burnett advises:

All women, whether or not they have a history of having had Rubella, should have a blood test in order to determine if they are immune to Rubella *prior to becoming pregnant.* If exposed to Rubella when pregnant, it is imperative to be tested within a week after exposure. If the first test is negative, then the testing should be repeated a few weeks later; and if it is positive, this proves Rubella infection. Proven Rubella infection in the first three months of pregnancy is indication for consideration of abortion.

Smallpox

Smallpox is a serious disease with a significant fatality rate. Outbreaks appeared in Europe in 1972 and 1973, and still occur in Africa and Asia. The virus can remain infective for a long time on clothes and in dust. With modern air travel, the disease can move about rapidly. Past vaccination programs and careful screening at ports of entry have helped keep the disease out of America.

World Health Organizations specialists claimed, in December of 1974, that "smallpox will vanish in the next six months." At that time, there were fewer than 1,000 cases of smallpox in all of India, while tens of thousands of health workers concentrated on spotting new outbreaks. Early in 1977, the W.H.O. announced the elimination of smallpox. No new cases had been reported in months. Then a few cases occurred in Africa where the unsettled political situation and refugee problems in Ethiopia made it impossible for the W.H.O. to complete its task of eliminating small pox. If this is ever accomplished and turns out to be permanent, it will represent a giant step in preventive medicine and a major achievement. Meanwhile, the disease exists.

The virus enters the bloodstream from the respiratory tract, and after incubating twelve days, the patient develops fever. After a few days, the patient develops a pox rash which is usually more wide spread than that of chicken pox and which lasts longer, with pus on the top of the pox. Mild smallpox may only kill 1% of the victims, while severe strains may kill 40%.

Vaccination with a similar but milder disease, cowpox or vaccinia, creates some immunity to smallpox. The first vaccination result is an ulcer the size of a quarter surrounded by a large red area. Fever usually starts around the fifth day and lasts up to five days. The material which drains from the ulcer is as contagious as the vaccine itself.

Most experts, including the United States Public Health Service, now recommend against routine smallpox vaccine because they see the rare complications which occasionally result from smallpox vaccine. The vaccine can spread into skin sores such as eczema or open abrasions, resulting in a nasty case of generalized cowpox. No one should be vaccinated if he has eczema or open skin sores, or if he is around anyone else with such skin lesions, particularly eczema. The vaccine should not be given to anyone who hasn't had a good physical examination and history. Rare instances of low immunity, hidden cancer, or a patient on drugs for the treatment of cancer make some individuals extremely susceptible to vaccinia. Every year, out of four to six million primary vaccinations done in the United States, around two hundred people become seriously ill, and some die of the vaccine. Many pediatricians like Merritt Low, advise, "The risk from vaccination is greater in the U.S.A. now than the risk of smallpox. Eradication of the disease in the rest of the world is in the offing. Why vaccinate? It's a greater folly to do it than not to do it."

Others, however, feel that it is unwise to stop a proven successful program against smallpox. Health authorities in many other countries still insist on verified smallpox vaccination before allowing anyone into their country. Some physicians continue to urge smallpox vaccination as a prudent and proven protection. I suggest you ask your own doctor for advice about this.

Warts

Warts are caused by a papovirus that take over skin cells and make them grow to suit the virus. Each infected cell bulges with virus particles —under the electron microscope a cell looks like a large sack full of marbles. These viral particles are infective and are spread by close contact. They seem to infect the skin easier where there is friction or abrasion, for example, on the palms of children swinging from the playground bars or on the soles of the feet from the shower floor. On the soles, they are called plantar warts, and the pressure of walking forces them into the tissue, causing a callus. In most other areas the swollen cells of the warts grow up from their base in the skin as raised small irregular bumps called warts.

Antibodies develop to the wart virus, and in most children the warts spontaneously drop off within a few months to a few years. Some people, perhaps because of low immunity to this particular virus, have more trouble with warts than others. Warts can cosmetically disfigure, and plantar warts can become painful to walk on.

Treatment of warts is notoriously unreliable. All sorts of superstitions prevail, but given enough time warts usually go away anyway. Most medical treatments involve killing the wart by heat, chemicals, or freezing. But sometimes it is like pulling weeds in the garden. Others come back up with the next rain. A leading dermatologist has observed that warts have made more people mad at more doctors than any other skin disease known.

Insect Viruses That Can Infect Man

Over 250 viruses infect insects (evidently without making them ill, although we didn't inquire) and can be transmitted to man or animal by the bug's bite.

Viral encephalitis or brain inflammation from a mosquito virus causes severe headache, a stiff neck, fever, chills, vomiting, and muscle aches.

Colorado tick fever, transmitted by the bite of the tick Dermacentor andersoni, causes severe pain in the extremities, headache, vomiting, and two separate episodes of fever.

GENERAL FACTS ABOUT VIRAL DISEASES

1. Viral diseases are not suppressed or "helped" by antibiotics (only symptoms can sometimes be treated.)
2. Almost everyone suffers many viral diseases while growing up.
3. Not everyone suffers equally; some have such light cases that they cannot be diagnosed, while others can become seriously ill with the same virus.
4. Some viral diseases are highly contagious and can be spread by infected individuals before and after they are clinically ill with the disease. (Contagion is mostly associated with the fever and rash.)
5. Most viral diseases are spread by droplet infection from the mouth, or from feces or urine getting on fingers and from there into food.
6. Most virus particles are resistant to antiseptics, but can be killed by sunshine or washed away with soap and water.
7. There may be specific problems with some of these diseases that require a visit to the physician (usually telephone advice suffices).
8. Viral disease appears to lower resistance, opening the body to secondary bacterial infections that can and often do benefit from a physician's attention, prescriptions, and advice.
9. Many children with these common childhood diseases have rashes. Full-blown typical rashes help in the diagnosis. However, atypical rashes are not uncommon, and similar rashes may occur with other viral, bacterial, or allergic diseases. The same viral disease causes more rashes in children than in adults.

10. A major diagnostic tool for the physician is simply the knowledge of what is "going around" and to what your child has been exposed.
11. Vaccines against diseases that don't make most of us ill, yet cause catastrophic damage to some infants, are being developed. For example, if current research develops a good vaccine against cytomegalic inclusion disease and if its use in adults becomes widespread, it is estimated that it might prevent 3,000 infants a year from becoming retarded.

18

ODD DISEASES:
MOLDS, YEASTS,
AND PROTOZOA

Are you moldy? If you aren't, you probably have been or will be. The all-pervasive fungi usually manage to infect everyone sooner or later. Common bread molds are the kinds we see most often. Most fungi are too selective to grow on or in people, but their spores in the dirt or air make good use of conditions wherever they land. They grow wherever they can. Occasionally, they land on us, or get into our skin on a thorn, or are breathed into our lungs. They rarely make us sick, but they do make us uncomfortable. Individuals with low resistance because of illness or suppressed immunity are far more likely to become ill; but, ill or not, all humans are, on occasions, the soil for microscopic gardens of mold. The most common infection in people is athlete's foot. Other common fungal infections, histoplasmosis and coccidiomycosis, cause severe hypersensitive (allergic) reactions, and the body responds by surrounding the fungus with granulomas (proud flesh) or even abscesses. A third type of problem is experienced by large numbers of individuals who are hypersensitive to mold spores which they breathe. The allergic reactions can cause eczema, asthma, and "hay fever."

ATHLETE'S FOOT

This common infection of the moist skin in the toe webs causes small blisters to appear in the skin, which then peels. The nails may also be infected and become thick, brittle, and yellow. Secondary bacterial infection frequently occurs in the open skin, with resulting soreness and redness which can progress to pus formation or even to blood poisoning.

A similar looking and therefore confusing condition can result from allergy to shoes (see Chapter 14). The body also occasionally responds to athlete's foot with an allergic reaction which causes tiny itching blisters on the sides of the fingers.

Treatment of athlete's foot starts with good hygiene, clean dry feet, fresh clean socks, and dry shoes. Ointments, which tend to keep the skin moist, may be self-defeating, since the fungus grows best in moist skin. The same applies to foot powders which absorb moisture and become pastes when put on too thickly. Regardless of the agent used, the toes should have a prolonged dry "aired out" period every day. Once the athlete's foot medication suppresses the fungus, the skin heals. Many over-the-counter preparations work well. The liquid preparations, which one can air dry on the skin thoroughly before putting on socks, are preferable. However, the fungal spores are still in the skin, and, like weeds in the garden, they keep coming back. Therefore, it is best to treat for several weeks after the lesions have healed so that the skin containing the spores will slough off, avoiding recurrent infection.

RINGWORM

Fungus infections on the skin or scalp are usually circular, expanding lesions with flat, scaly centers and raised edges. One variety causes brownish red scaling patches on the arms, trunk, and neck. They can be confused with many other skin conditions. Skin scrapings for microscopic examinations or culture may be required for diagnosis. Some strains will respond to over-the-counter athlete's foot preparations.

Ringworm of the scalp is a disease of children which, if untreated, finally heals when puberty starts. The puberty effect is probably due to changes that occur in adolescent skin, increasing its resistance. Different species of the fungus produce different types of disease. Some look like bacterial infection. This is complicated by the fact that secondary bacterial infections of scalp ringworm lesions do occur. The hair breaks off or falls out, leaving bald spots. Cultures and microscopic examinations are frequently required for diagnosis; treatment is not always simple or easy. Oral fungal antibiotics often have to be given for a prolonged length of time. The disease is contagious to other children.

YEAST

The yeast *Candida* usually lives on our mucus membranes. The low immunity and tender skin of infants predisposes them to thrush, white plaques of yeast in the mouth that don't scrub off easily. Yeast can cause a very resistant diaper rash. Some women develop yeast vaginitis, especially after antibiotics, with itching and a cottage cheese-type discharge.

Your physician can prescribe medications, but treatment is often prolonged. Fingernail infections can occur, especially at the nail root.

BIRD AND SOIL FUNGI

Dirt contaminated by pigeon feces frequently contains an encapsulated yeast-like organism called cryptococcus. It can cause bronchitis if inhaled, and in rare cases may cause chronic meningitis. To control, avoid pigeon dung.

There is a good chance that you may have had the curious disease histoplasmosis, called "pigeon fever" by some. It is caused by inhaling the spores of a soil fungus that grows in areas contaminated by bird or bat dung. A whole troop of boy scouts was infected after cleaning up an old park where starlings had roosted. Widespread in the middle-west and east, the disease is frequently confused with tuberculosis, for it leaves calcified scars in the lungs. Some cases have "flu-like" symptoms of fever, fatigue, cough, and chest pains. Severe cases cause weight loss and protracted illness. Most people have such a mild illness that it is not recognized until later, when an x-ray shows spots on the lung and the skin test is positive. Infected soil and bird feces can be treated by spraying with formaldehyde.

Symptoms of "valley fever" are cough associated with fever and flu-like aches, followed by a hive-like skin rash which may be due to coccidioidomycosis. This disease, which may last for a month or so, is caused by tiny fungus spores inhaled from dust in the desert valley areas of the southwest United States. Almost all who live in areas such as the San Joaquin Valley of California, and some who pass through, are infected, and some have symptoms of "Valley Fever." Most people who inhale the fungus spores are naturally resistant and do not become ill.

THE MIDGETS THAT MAKE YOU SICK: PROTOZOA

The human body is made up of some one hundred billions of cells. Yet this phenomenal organization of cells can be made ill or even destroyed by a pugnacious animal with only a single cell called a protozoa. Most of them will have nothing to do with us. Others live on and in us. In the process, they may make us sick.

Chronic diarrhea is the major symptom of intestinal protozoa. It is more likely to be severe in children, although adults can be quite ill too, with bloody mucus, cramps, foul stools, and weight loss. Many people carry protozoa with no symptoms, yet spread the organisms by cysts passed in the bowel movements which contaminate food or water. These diseases are more likely to occur where hygiene is very poor. One protozoa, Giardia, looks like an animated pear with whips under the microscope. Most people infected with Amoeba have no symptoms, but still have small ulcers in the lower bowel.

A tender itchy burning of the urethra and prostate in the male and the vagina in the female can be caused by a fast-moving flagellated protozoa called Trichomonas. It doesn't survive well in weak acid, so vinegar douches help in control of infection (Two teaspoons of vinegar per quart of water).

Malaria is the most important and prevalent blood protozoa. It infects one hundred million people and kills around a million people in the world every year. It is spread by the blood-sucking Anopheles mosquito and lives inside red blood cells. It grows and periodically ruptures the blood cells, causing episodes of fever and chills and anemia. Untreated infections can last for years. Control of mosquitoes in temperate climates by insecticides such as D.D.T. and other methods has virtually eliminated the disease from all but tropical areas. Nets, repellents, screens, and drugs help protect man from mosquitoes and malaria.

"Flu-like" symptoms can be caused in people infected with the protozoa Toxoplasma. It is caught by eating raw or undercooked meat, or possibly from food contaminated with cat feces containing Toxoplasma. Most human Toxoplasma infections are so mild that they are undiagnosed, if noticed at all. Some people, however, get an infectious mononucleosis-like disease or prolonged fever. In rare cases, if a pregnant mother catches the disease, her fetus can become infected and may be born with the infection, leading to blindness and brain damage.

An occasional cat may get the disease from eating rodents or birds, and will pass the cysts in the feces. The cysts are resistant to disinfectants, and can live a long time in soil or sandboxes where cats bury their feces. One may avoid the disease by thorough cooking of food, careful disposal of cat litter, and spraying for flies. Pregnant women should avoid close contact with cats, although only about one in two hundred stray cats has been found to have the disease.

How to avoid the midget that makes you sick:

1. Good sanitation with modern sewage disposal.
2. Care in handling and thorough cooking of food.
3. Sanitary water supply.
4. Good vaginal hygiene.
5. Avoiding cat feces, especially during pregnancy.
6. Avoidance and control of mosquitoes and flies.
7. Use of malaria suppressive drugs in some areas.

19

WORMS

As children, most of us, with appropriate shudders, gleefully sang into squeamish ears, "the worms crawl in, the worms crawl out. . . ." And as children, at least half of us in the United States have had pinworms at one time or another. In areas in Appalachia, I found ninety percent of the children with roundworms. You should read this section on worms not so much for the shudders as for the prevention.

Almost all animals and fish carry parasite worms. Most of the worms that infect man are roundworms. Worms lay eggs in profusion, 200,000 per day for the roundworm Ascaris. Some worms depend on an insect for dissemination; others go through larvae stages in the dirt—the hook worm, for example; and others depend on feces to mouth transmission by way of water, food, or fingers. There are other shapes of worms, of course, as well as other methods of transmission, which are discussed below. Worms come in many different sizes: The size is unrelated to the damage a worm may do.

INTESTINAL WORMS

Pinworms are one centimeter (about one-fourth an inch) long and one-half millimeter thick. They look like a short piece of white thread that wiggles. The egg-laden female migrates out of the anus and lays its eggs in the skin in that general area. The child scratches, gets the eggs under the fingernails, and from there they are transported into the mouth. In girls, it may enter the urethra or vagina to deposit the eggs, leading to urinary infections and severe itching. The eggs are tough and can last a considerable time outside the body. They have been reported in house dust and can be inhaled, can lodge in the mucus of the nose, and can be swallowed. They can contaminate fingernails, clothes, bedding, and toilet seats.

In spite of lurid tales about fits and nervousness, the chief problem caused by pinworms remains the itch and the occasional urinary tract infection. The adult worms only live one month, but their eggs can last much longer. To avoid re-infection, children should wear tight-fitting pants and should have closely clipped and frequently scrubbed nails. One can remove the eggs from household objects by vacuuming, by washing in soap and water, or by soaking things in ammonia.

Round worms or *Ascaris* were referred to by ancient Greeks as ἐλμίνς στρογγύλη which must mean "those damned worms." They reach up to 49 centimeters (22 inches) in length. One female may produce 27 million eggs and lay 200,000 daily. The eggs become infective after a period in moist shady soil—when ingested, they hatch in the intestine. The larvae penetrate the intestine and are carried by the blood into the lungs, where they finally break through the capillaries, are coughed up and swallowed again, and pass into the small intestine, where they finally grow into adult worms. Worm eggs remain infective in the soil for months, often around the child's play area, which can be contaminated by stool. If this won't get you to wash your hands, nothing will! Control is by proper disposal of feces.

Both the larvae and the adult worms produce symptoms. The larvae which reach the lung are larger than the capillaries they lodge in and which they finally break through. Massive infection can lead to a form of pneumonia. The adult worms live in the small intestine.

If a host has a high fever, the large adult worms may migrate through the rectum, mouth, or nose. On occasion, they block the appendix or the bile ducts.

Doctors can make a diagnosis of roundworm by finding microscopic eggs in feces or by detecting passage of the worms. In ridding a person of these worms, one must take care not to stir the worms up and induce migration.

The key to prevention of Ascaris infection is proper sanitation. Parents must teach children to use toilets, not the ground. Contaminated soil should be deeply spaded. In countries where human feces is used for fertilizer, Ascaris eggs get on vegetables and on ground fruit such as strawberries. Those who want to go all the way back to nature by way of organic gardening and recycling should consider that they may become part of the Ascaris's recycling.

Dog and cat roundworm can come from pets. Don't let toddlers play around dog or cat dung, for they may become infected with *Toxocara canis,* the dog round worm, or *Toxocara cati,* the cat round worm. The eggs hatch in the child's intestine, but become trapped in the liver or other organs (even the brain or eye), where they cause various symptoms such as fever, large liver, and cough. The name of this disease is *viscerial laval migrans*. Dogs and cats should be dewormed and their feces should be carefully controlled.

TAPEWORMS

Fish tapeworm infections in men come from eating raw or poorly cooked fresh water fish infected by the larvae. The larvae hook into the small intestine and grow up to thirty feet in length. They may pass a million eggs a day into the feces. The eggs reach fresh water, where they are eaten by small shrimp in which they hatch as larvae. The little shrimps in turn become food for fish; when the fish becomes food for man, the cycle is complete. This organism is found in some lakes in the United States from the midwest to Florida.

The dwarf tapeworm is only four centimeters (1.6 inches) long. It is the most common tapeworm in the southern United States. It infects children who ingest the eggs from feces, and produces abdominal pain, convulsions, and dizziness. The eggs are found in the feces. The infection passes directly from child to child.

The pork tapeworm passes eggs in the feces which contaminate food eaten by hogs or by man. The eggs hatch, allowing the larvae to penetrate the intestine, from where the bloodstream carries them to lodge in muscles or in the brain. If infected pork meat is consumed by man, the larvae attach to the small intestine, where they grow into adult worms. There they cause only vague symptoms. Larvae in the tissues, however, create tissue reactions which eventually calcify the larvae in a cyst. Cysts in the brain may cause epileptic fits. Prevention of the pork tapeworm infection includes thorough cooking (or freezing) or fresh or pickled pork.

Uncooked beef may give you a beef tapeworm that can reach twenty-five yards in length. Symptoms may include diarrhea and abdominal discomfort, but frequently there are no symptoms. The eggs are passed in human feces. If they contaminate grazing land and are ingested by cattle, they hatch larvae that penetrate the intestine and lodge as cysts in the muscle. The little spots in the muscle are called "beef measles" by ranchers. Man is in turn infected by eating raw beef.

Wash your hands thoroughly after handling dog feces, or you may catch Echinococcus, a worm cyst that comes from the tapeworms of dogs and other animals. Eggs passed in animal feces are ingested by grazing animals. The larvae penetrate the intestine and form large cysts. Dogs then eat the bodies of the infected hosts and in turn become infected with the larvae. Man, as well as other animals, can become infected from accidental ingestion of contaminated feces and may develop a larvae echinococcus cyst in the liver, brain, or other organs.

Trichinosis is caused by a worm in raw or uncooked pork. Whipworm is a small three to five centimeter coiled worm that lives in the lower bowel. Infection is from eggs ingested with contaminated soil.

Don't let the children eat dirty food or defecate on the ground. Hookworm is caught in the South by walking barefoot in moist soil contaminated by human feces. They enter the skin, go to the lungs, are coughed up, and finally set up housekeeping in the bowel where they can cause anemia.

SUMMARY

Those damned worms can be avoided. It is obvious that most of them are worth avoiding, both from the standpoint of aesthetics and health. The rules are not too complex:

1. Watch for children scratching their behinds and suspect and get after the pin worms early.
2. Train children to use toilets and not the ground for bowel movements.
3. Wear shoes where worms are prevalent or where sanitation is poor.
4. Do not allow toddlers to play in areas where there may be dog and cat feces in the dirt.
5. Avoid mosquitoes.
6. Don't eat raw fish, beef, or pork.
7. Wash your hands well if you have dog feces on them and train your children to do likewise.
8. Avoid ground contaminated with dog, cat, or human feces.

20

STINGING, BITING, AND PESKY INSECTS[1]

By Claude Frazier, M.D., Allergist

There are over half a million varieties of arthropods, including insects, spiders, ticks, scorpions, and mites. The twelve-inch Atlas moth of India is of less importance to us than the 1/250th of an inch mite Demodex, which lives in our skin. Some insects are friends, some are enemies, and some, like the pollinating honey-gathering bees, are both.

BUG BITES AND STINGS

It is not always possible to tell what bug caused what lesion. Frequently, insect-caused skin sores look similar to skin lesions caused by virus infection, contact dermatitis, eczema, acne, impetigo, and burns. Intense itching is caused by biting midges, blackflies, mosquitoes, chiggers, and fleas. Pain is caused by bees, wasps, hornets, yellow jackets, caterpillars, fire ants, wheel bugs, and scorpions. Use the following tips to avoid insect stings:

- Wear shoes when outdoors.
- Avoid gardening, garbage, and orchard areas.
- Do not wear scented toiletries; the odors attract insects.
- Do not wear: bright colors, flowery prints, jewelry, wool, suede, and leather-like material; these attract insects.
- Do not eat watermelon, popsicles, or ice cream, and so forth out of doors.
- Keep window and door screens in good repair.
- Don't flail at bees; cover your eyes with your hands and get away.
- If there is an insect in the car, pull over, open the door and windows, and get out.

A thousand ways cut short our days
None are exempt from death
A honey bee by stinging me
Did stop my mortal breath

From a New England grave stone, 1814

ALLERGY TO STINGING INSECTS

If you are allergic to insect stings, they can be very dangerous. More Americans die each year from allergic reactions to insect stings than from snake bites. If you have the following symptoms, you may be allergic:

1. An increasing amount of reaction with each succeeding sting.
2. Swelling from a sting that extends beyond two joints (except for fingers and toes).
3. General allergic reactions:
   a. Slight reactions: generalized itching, hives, fatigue, and anxiety.
   b. Moderate reactions: swollen areas away from the sting, a tight feeling in the chest, wheezing, dizziness, nausea, vomiting, stomach pain.
   c. Severe anaphylactic reactions—any of the above, plus: labored breathing, difficulty in swallowing, hoarseness or thick speech, marked weakness, confusion, feeling of impending disaster.
   d. Shock reaction: grey or blue skin color, collapse, unconsciousness.
4. Toxic reactions—with multiple stings, you may suffer: swelling, headache, stomach pain, vomiting, diarrhea, fever, drowsiness, fainting, unconsciousness, spasms, or convulsions.
5. Delayed reactions: As long as two weeks following sting, serum sickness may occur, with fever, swollen glands, headache, hives, and swollen tender joints.

If you have any of the above symptoms, consult your doctor. After emergency treatment, he may wish to have you desensitized to the insect venom by repeated small injections. He will probably have you carry an emergency kit when you are in areas where stings may occur. You should wear a "medi-alert" "dog tag" or carry a Life Card telling what insect allergies you have. In case of a sting:

1. Scrape the stinger off with your fingernail or a knife. *Do not squeeze it* with tweezers or your fingers, for it may inject more venom into the skin.
2. Wash with soap and water and daub with antiseptic.
3. Cool with wet packs or ice.
4. Local warm soaks with Burrow's solution or epsom salts may help after a few hours.

First Aid for Allergy to Insect Stings

If there is no sting emergency kit available, if there is a history of allergy, or if the patient shows the signs and symptoms of allergy, do the following *while* you are on the way to the doctor:

1. Keep the area cold with ice or wet packs.
2. Put a tourniquet above the sting site; loosen it every fifteen minutes (see page 65).
3. Give oxygen if pale or blue.
4. Give mouth to mouth resuscitation if breathing ceases.
5. Lay the victim down and cover the body with blankets to treat shock.

If there is an emergency kit available, the above instructions are still valid, but first:

1. If it is a severe reaction, give 0.2cc of adrenalin at once as instructed in the kit.
   To give the adrenalin shot:
   a. Wipe the skin with alcohol.
   b. Remove needle cover.
   c. Push needle all the way in.
   d. Push plunger.
   e. Massage area.
2. In any case, give the following by mouth at once:
   a. Antihistamine
   b. Ephedrine
   c. Phenobarbital
3. If there is no adrenalin but if there is an anti-asthma inhaler available, have the victim take two deep breaths every ten minutes if the reaction is severe.

The doctor will give medications in the vein or muscle and will treat shock and respiratory difficulties.

Insect sting kits may be prescribed by your doctor. For some individuals, more items may be included than in the two commercially available kits (Hollister-Stier Laboratories and the Nelco Insect Sting Kit). The kits may contain instructions on how to use it, injectable epinephrine (either preloaded syringes or sealed ampules of epinephrine with sterile syringes), alcohol swabs, a tourniquet, and chewable antihistamine tablets.

ANT STINGS

Most ant stings or bites are insignificant, but two varieties of ants cause problems. Harvester ants form low mounds in sandy soil, are a centimeter long, and will bite if disturbed. They are found throughout the central and southwestern United States. Small fire ants live in two-inch-high mounds and "bubble out" when the nest is disturbed. Within seconds, they can produce thousands of stings. They are primarily located in the southeastern portion of the United States.

Ants hold the skin with their mouth while inserting their stinger. The bite produces small hive-like bumps which later blister and drain, leaving pustules which last many days and are followed by persistent lumps in the skin. Sensitive individuals may die of anaphylactic shock. Follow the first aid treatment given earlier for allergy to insect stings.

SCORPIONS

In the tropics, scorpions are so lethal they are called "public enemy number one." In Arizona, scorpions kill more people than rattlesnakes and spiders together. Most species in the United States, however, are only mildly poisonous. Their sting causes only local burning, swelling, and discoloration.

The sting of the dangerous species causes a *sharp pain followed by a local numb "pins-and-needles" sensation* which rapidly spreads. There is no local swelling or discoloration. If not treated soon, the nose and mouth begin to itch, speech becomes impaired, and generalized muscle spasms and pain occur, along with vomiting, wetting the pants, and frothing at the mouth. Death by convulsions follows. If the patient survives the first three hours, he usually survives the twenty-four to forty-eight hours of symptoms.

First Aid for Scorpion Sting

1. Start with a tourniquet above the area.
2. Cold or ice packs for the entire extremity.
   Remove the tourniquet five minutes after immersing the entire stung extremity in crushed ice or in a tub of ice water to slow down absorption of the venom. Leave the extremity in cold water at least two hours and do not remove it or attempt to warm it. Keep the rest of the body warm to prevent chilling. Antihistamines are of some help. Get the patient to the doctor at once. If the scorpion can be safely captured, take it, too. Specific antivenom is sometimes available.

In scorpion areas, it is unwise to have sand boxes for children, as scorpions may move into the sand. Use of insecticides to kill all insects in the area will help, and oiling areas near homes may discourage the "public enemy number one."

FLEAS

Some people are very sensitive to flea bites and develop hive-like bumps. Fleas of all varieties (human, cat, dog, etc.) bite people. They are selective, often biting only one person while sparing another. In the western United States, fleas can carry bubonic plague germs from wild rodents to humans.

Flea repellents are moderately effective. Tick and chigger repellents work best on clothes. Diethyltoluamide is the most satisfactory repellent, and is particularly effective against rodent fleas. A dust containing five percent malathion or ten percent methoxychlor is safe for dogs and cats. A dust containing one percent lindane can be used on dogs over eight weeks of age, but should not be used on cats or puppies.

Vacuuming infested rooms and spraying floors, carpets, and furniture is helpful. Rat fleas may be reduced by reduction of rats—eliminate the rats' food and shelter by ratproofing buildings and food supplies, including garbage. Outdoor yards and areas around the house may have to be sprayed with an insecticide.

VENOMOUS SPIDERS

Venomous spiders have always given people the creeps, although only seventeen out of forty thousand species of spiders cause severe reactions. The most misunderstood spiders, poor things, are tarantulas. Their bite is only as painful as a pin prick and has about the same effect. The thing about spiders that bothers me is their extreme "women's liberation"—the females often eat the small males after mating. Most spiders do not have strong enough fangs to penetrate human skin. Reactions from spider bites usually are due to local infection from bacteria introduced with the bite. If there is significant venom, the longer the spider hangs on, the worse it is. The most severe reactions in the United States are due to the Black Widow and the Brown Recluse spider.

Black Widow Spiders

This shiny black shoe-button-shaped spider has a red hour-glass marking on the underside of the abdomen. It grows to a body size of over

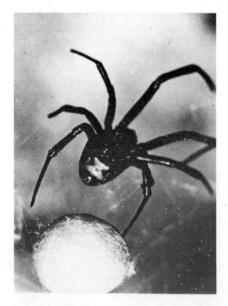

FIGURE 53   *The underside of the shiny black widow spider, showing the characteristic red hour-glass mark.*

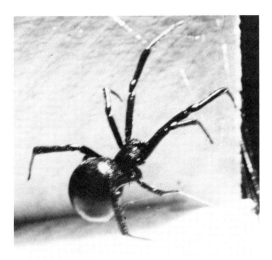

FIGURE 54 *The black widow spider from the back, characterized by a globular shiny black body. (The white spot is camera light reflection.)*

half an inch, and spins a coarse, strong, irregular web in rock piles, debris, basements, garages, and privies throughout the United States.

The pinprick bite is followed by some local pain, redness, and swelling. Bites on the lower extremities cause stomach muscle pain; bites on the upper extremities cause shoulder and neck muscle pain. Pains peak in three hours, and may last up to two days. There may be vomiting, shock, swollen eyelids, restlessness, and grunting. Contrary to popular belief, most victims do recover promptly and there are no after effects. If bitten again, the reaction is usually the same as after the first bite. Fatalities are very rare.

Brown Recluse Spider

This yellow brown spider has a dark violin-shaped mark on its back, starting at its head. They spin irregular webs in closets and attics. They are found in the midwest, south, and southwestern areas of the United States.

There is mild stinging at the bite area, followed with some redness, which fades as a blister forms. In from two to eight hours, there is mild to severe pain. On the second day, there may be chills, weakness, joint pains, vomiting, and a rash. Bleeding problems and anemia may develop. After three to four days, a firm violet star-shaped area develops which depresses in one to two weeks, leaving an unsightly scar. On occasion, skin grafts are required.

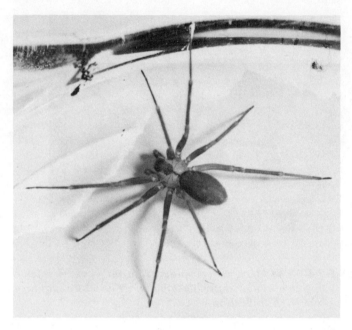

FIGURE 55   *The brown recluse spider has a distinctive dark violin-shaped marking on its back.*

First Aid for Spider Bites

Ice pack the bite area at once. If possible, bring the spider with you when you go for treatments, which may include antivenom if available. Wash all bite areas with soap and water and apply antiseptics and cold compresses. Bed rest may be advisable. Call your doctor, who may prescribe antihistamines and other treatments to reduce the serious symptoms.

How to Avoid Spider Bites
- Wear gloves when working in vines or rock piles.
- Keep flies out of privies to reduce the number of Black Widows.
- Remove webs with broom handles and crush spiders.
- Collect and burn egg sacs with caution—the black widow will bite then.
- Spray with D.D.T., Chlordane, or Lindane.

FLYING, BITING INSECTS

Biting insects cause local trouble, but they can also cause generalized allergic reactions, including generalized itching and hives on the skin or in joints, swelling, headaches, dizziness, or lethargy. Such biting insects include:

- Mosquito—water breeding; bite usually in the evening.
- Black fly—active during the day around water; painful bite.
- Deer fly—aggressive, fast, and persistent.
- Horse fly—slow, hard-biting, blood suckers.

Some of the bites can be avoided by the use of a hat, long sleeves, insect repellent, and good screens or nets. Insect sprays will control them around a house. Fly and flea bites can carry infections and occasionally may cause a local boil.

MOSQUITOES

Parts of the world have been made almost uninhabitable by mosquitoes. They have attacked mankind throughout the ages and even now help kill one million people each year. The female adult sucks blood through a tube after cutting through the skin and inserting saliva to dilute the blood. The saliva causes the welt, and may create allergy. In some individuals, the bites cause blisters and scarring or allergic skin hemorrhage.

Mosquitoes can spread viral and parasitic diseases, such as malaria, dengue, yellow fever, and equinine encephalitis.

They are attracted to some people more than to others, and are greatly attracted by sweat. Screening, insecticides, clothing, repellents, and avoiding mosquito areas are helpful measures. The most effective way of reducing the mosquito population is to reduce their breeding areas by eliminating potential areas of larval breeding water.

CREEPING, CRAWLING, HOPPING, AND BITING BUGS

Ticks

Ticks have six (larval stage) or eight crab-like legs sticking out from a "leather pouch" shaped body. Their small head has curved teeth that attach with a cement-like secretion in the skin. Once attached, they feed for three to five days before dropping off. Try to get them off with the head intact.

Removing Ticks
1. Put a drop of ether, gasoline, kerosene, or benzene on the head of the tick at the skin surface.
2. Wait a full fifteen to twenty minutes so the tick will loosen its grip voluntarily.
3. Then, with forceps or tweezers, seize the tick gently at the skin surface and pull it off. Avoid squeezing the body, as this may squeeze more toxin into the blood stream. If the head is left in the skin, a chronic local sore may occur.

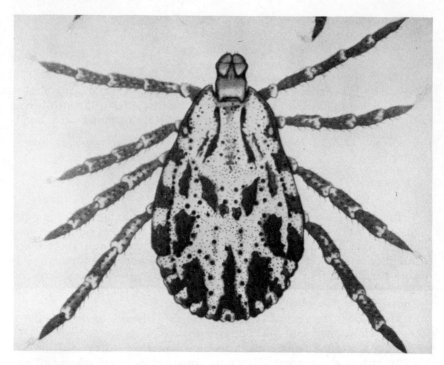

FIGURE 56   *Rocky Mountain male wood tick (Demacentor andersoni), averages one-fourth inch long.*

Tick bite paralysis can occur from several species of ticks, including the American dog tick, which secretes a nerve toxin into the wound. Children are affected most often, and may have a period of irritability and loss of appetite for a day preceding the paralysis.

How to Avoid Ticks
The best method of preventing tick bites is to stay out of infested areas during the spring and summer. To determine infested areas, drag a piece of white flannel over the ground and vegetation and check it for ticks. Wear high boots or wear your socks outside the pants. All-purpose repellents are effective against ticks. Dogs bring ticks into buildings. Treat the dogs regularly if you are in a tick area. Every three days, lightly apply derris powder with a rotenone content of at least three percent; or use a dip, via tub or brush, with one ounce of neutral soap and two ounces of derris powder in one gallon of tepid water, every six days. Do not get the dip or powder into the dog's eyes.

Mites

Chiggers are just one of some 1,600 varieties of mites. Mites can transfer to man from rodents, cats, birds, cockroaches, kangaroos, and wallabies. They can get on us from materials such as grass, hay and

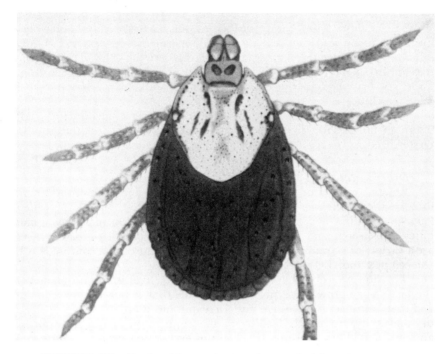

FIGURE 57   *Rocky Mountain female wood tick (Demacentor andersoni), averages up to one-half inch long.*

wheat, cheese covering, copra, and dried fruits. They are so small that they are usually missed—but their presence is made known by the itch they cause.

Chiggers

Chiggers live on low branches and grass. Once on the skin, they run until they meet some obstacle (belt, collar, skin folds), where they attach. They remain attached for two to four days of feeding and then drop off. The first sign is small flat red spots with the pin-point mite in the center. This develops into an itchy bump, often with a small clear blister on the top, within three to twenty-four hours. On the stomach, legs, and genitalia, the lesions become purple, and the foreskin, penis, or scrotum may swell. Scratching often starts secondary infection. The sores heal slowly. Treatment aimed at the chiggers is of no help, as they have usually dropped off.

1. Keep fingernails clipped.
2. Take starch baths.
3. Use U.S.P. calamine lotion.
4. Soak in Burow's or Domeboro solutions.
5. Take antihistamines by mouth.

Scabies

The scabies mite, barely visible to the naked eye, occurs where hygiene is poor, and can last a long time as the "seven year itch." The mite burrows under the skin, usually starting between the fingers (or the toes in infants), where the rash looks like eczema and can lead to impetigo. Eggs laid in the burrows hatch out and new generations of mites continue.

Successful treatments are possible, using several medications. All family members should be treated, and garments and bed clothes should be sterilized.

Other Mites

Related mites can occur in animals and can infect man, although usually the infections are of short duration. Dog scabies is called "mange." Poultry and bird mites, rat and rodent mites, straw and grain mites, mushroom and cheese mites—all can infect man. Usually, there are a variety of skin lesions which itch intensely and can be confused with chicken pox and allergic reactions.

The minute worm-shaped mite (Demodex) lives in the oil glands of the face. They grow more profusely on skin that is not washed enough and that is subject to excessive use of creams and powders. The skin feels dry and itchy, frequently leading to the application of more ointments and less soap. They can infest the roots of eyelashes, causing burning and stinging. Occasionally, the eyelashes fall out. Several treatments are available. Once under control, washing daily with soap and water maintains the improvement.

Body Lice

These minute dirty-white colored insects live in the seams of clothing, where they also glue their eggs. They come out to feed when their host is inactive. They move readily from person to person via clothing or bed linen, although they usually stay on an individual permanently, leaving only if fever or death occur. The eggs take two weeks to hatch, and the lice can live more than a week while waiting for a new victim. They can spread typhus and relapsing fever.

Head Lice

Head lice move rapidly and are hard to see. The eggs are cemented to the base of a hair on any part of the body, although they are rare in the pubic area. They resemble dandruff:

Crab Lice

These minute yellowish-grey crab-like insects attach to the skin and may remain for days. They are difficult to see and are easily transmitted from person to person, and from clothing, bedding, or toilet seats. Usually, they remain in the genital area, although they can migrate to the armpits, eyelashes, and eyebrows, or in rare cases, to the scalps of infants.

Lice bites: Itching rarely occurs in the first week of infestation, when sensitivity reaction seems to start. Marked infestations result in a tired irritable feeling, and a rash similar to rubella may develop. Live feces may be rubbed into the skin by the intense scratching, and can contribute to sensitivity or disease transmission. Small ulcers can occur on the legs, and eczema and thickened skin may develop from constant irritation.

Pubic lice cause variable itching, which may lead to local secondary infection. Individuals who are allergic to these insects may develop pea- to dime-sized bluish skin spots on the lower half of the body.

Treatment for Lice

Follow instructions carefully in using the various prescription treatments. Lice and eggs should be picked off of eyelashes and eyebrows with tweezers and fine-combed out of the hair. Keep medications out of the eyes. Bedding and clothes should be sterilized by boiling or by pressing with a hot iron. Hats and toilet articles may be infested. Rechecks should be made weekly for re-infestation.

Bed Bugs

Bed bugs are less than a centimeter in length, have a characteristic odor, live in crevices of walls and furniture, and come out intermittently at night for a ten to fifteen minute meal of human blood, obtained through a sharp proboscis. The bites, usually three in a row, become red, swollen, and itchy. Insecticide sprays should prevent bed bugs.

Kissing Bug

Similar to bed bugs. The painless bite results in either a firm lump, small blisters, a giant hive, or hemorrhagic bumps on the hands and feet, depending on the degree of sensitization. Insecticide sprays should control kissing bugs.

Wheel Bug

This monstrous looking bug with a cogwheel-like crest over its head usually bites hands disturbing the vegetation it regards as its own. The bites are quite painful.

Blister Beetles

Blister beetles contain a blistering agent released if the bug is touched or brushed even by clothes. If allowed to walk on the bare skin unbothered, it will not exude its blistering fluid.

Puss Caterpillar

Hives and intense burning pain result from handling this insect: Effects last up to six days. Numbness, swelling, and paralysis may occur. Baking soda compresses or crushed leaves of the garden *purslane* plant help relieve the pain.

PESKY INSECT PROBLEMS

Breathing Insect Dust

The dust and debris of dead insects become part of the surrounding air. Inhalation may cause hay fever or asthma in sensitized individuals. Known insects that cause these problems include the short-lived mayfly, the caddis fly, and aphids which die and become organic dust of a highly allergic nature.

Eating Insects in Food

Insects infest our food, especially cereals and grains, regardless of care taken in milling. They include the cockroach, weevils, moths, beetles, mites, and silverfish. Some are ground into the food and are then ingested with the food. Cockroaches contaminate food with their droppings. Allergic reaction to insect matter may create disease, as can bacterial and viral infections possibly carried by cockroaches. Cockroaches do some good though: They eat bedbugs!

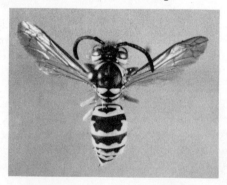

FIGURE 58   *Yellow jacket.*

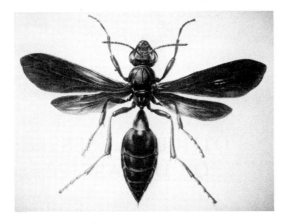

FIGURE 59   *Wasp.*

TABLE 11   *Features and habitats of venomous insects and arachnids.*

Insect	Distinctive features	Where found
Bumblebee	Large, glossy yellow-black, hairy, buzzes loudly	Nest in tree cavities, ground holes, flowers, and so forth.
Honey bee	Brown-black, barbed stinger	Nest in hives (domestic), tree trunks, flowers, and so forth.
Hornet	Black, yellow, white, heavy body	Football-shaped nest in trees, woods, flowers, and so forth.
Wasp	Red-brown, characteristic "wasp waist"	Elongated open-cell nest in doorways, eaves; enters buildings in winter; fruit, garbage.
Yellow jacket	Black-yellow stripes, heavy body, very aggressive	Enclosed nest in trees, bushes, ground holes: orchards, garbage picnics.

Arachnid	Distinctive features	Where found
Black widow spider	Shiny black, shoe-button shape, red hour glass marking on underside	Rocks, debris, basements, privies.
Brown recluse spider	Dorsal violin-shaped marking	Closets, attics.
Scorpion	Black or yellowish, crablike, one-half inch to eight inches long, segmented tail with stinger	Rocks, debris, dark places anywhere in house (nocturnal).

21

OTHER CAUSES
OF DISEASE

ANIMAL DISEASES CAUGHT BY MAN

We asked Dr. Richard L. Parker, a veterinarian and chief of the United States Veterinary Public Health Service, to tell us about animal diseases that can be caught by people. A lot of fables exist in this area, so we decided to demolish them by an expert's testimony. However, one fable I hang on to personally is that warts can be transmitted from animals to man. It is mentioned in an old veterinary dermatology textbook,[1] although Dr. Parker expressed skepticism about it. We adapted the following, with Dr. Parker's help.

Animal Bites

Animals bite over a million people each year, and the bites frequently became infected with bacteria. Early and thorough cleaning is important. If there is any question of rabies, you must check with your doctor. Rabies can occur in skunks, bats, foxes, raccoons, cows, horses, sheep, goats, monkeys, and ocelots as well as in dogs and cats. If there is a bite (usually from dogs, and most often German Shepherds), make certain that the dog has had its rabies shots and remains well for at least two weeks. Report bites to the police, especially unprovoked bites. Public health expert Dr. Paul Wehrle explains what you should do when there is a possibility of a bite by a rabid animal.

1. Wash the wound thoroughly and immediately with soap and water. Flush repeatedly. Cleansing should be repeated immediately under medical supervision as soon as possible if there is a possibility of rabies. This is the most important single step in rabies prevention.

2. Antirabies serum or vaccine may be needed; start an immediate effort to locate the animal. Notify the police.
3. Get a tetanus booster if required; check with your doctor.
4. Usually the wound is left open, but check with your doctor.
5. Local antibiotic ointment may be used to prevent bacterial infection in the wound.

Rattlesnake bites are covered in the chapter on first aid. Cat bites and scratches are unique in that they and the lymph glands above them can become infected with a virus causing cat-scatch fever. Look for red streaks and swollen glands.

Animal Infections That Can Infect Man

Worm infections	Red tide poisoning: clams
Beef tapeworm	*Fungal infections*
Cat roundworm	Histoplasmosis: bats and birds
Dog hookworm	Ringworm: cat, dog, horse
Dog roundworm	*Viral infecti*
Dog tapeworm	Cat scratch fever
Fish tapeworm	Hepatitis: oysters
Pork tapeworm	Monkey bite encephalitis
Pork trichinosis	Rabies
Protozoan disease	Ricketsial pox: mice
Toxoplasmosis: cat feces	Viral meningitis: mice and hamsters

Facts, Not Fables, About Animal Diseases

1. Dog hepatitis is not transmitted to man.
2. Canine distemper virus does not infect man.
3. Beef measles describes cysts in beef from tapeworm.
4. Chicken herpes is not caught by man.
5. Cat leukemia does not carry leukemia to man.
6. Hog cholera does not infect man.
7. Toxoplasmosis comes from ingesting undercooked beef or cat feces.
8. Rabies is not more frequent during the hot "dog days"—it's just that in hot weather that dogs pant and drool more, and some people confuse this with rabies.

ILLNESS: PHYSICAL CAUSES

Radiation

The specter of silent damage from radiation fallout—atom bombs, nuclear power generators, and x-rays—brings cold fear to many of us.

The fear factor, especially of atomic bombs, overshadows the good aspects of nuclear energy. As director of the Brookhaven National Laboratory, Dr. Lee Edward Farr monitered the follow-up of radiation damage from Hiroshima and Bikini. A professor of environmental health, Dr. Farr was awarded the prestigious Wisdom Award of Honor for his clear-headed work on the positive uses of atomic energy. He believes that the average citizen knows more about radiation exposure than is realized and explains that:

> The first principle of radiation protection is that "the amount of heat loss is inversely proportional to the square of the distance." If you are two feet away from the heat and move to four feet away, the heat will drop to one fourth as much. For instance: The light that permits you to read this page is a form of electromagnetic radiation. So is heat. If you move away from a light bulb or fire, the amount of heat you feel drops off sharply. So, one form of protection from over-exposure to radiation is distance: distance which is measurable, predictable, and understandable.
>
> The second principle of protection is to put a *wall* between you and the source of radiation, whether it is x-ray or a fire. X-ray equipment is encased in "walls" of lead, steel, or thick concrete in order to contain its penetrating radiation within a protected area. Further, x-ray, like sunlight, can be filtered to eliminate or reduce exposure. The radiologist uses filtering, focusing, and shielding devices to protect himself and the patient, to limit the exposure to the minimum quantity, and to sharpen the image. X-ray, then, is very much like the more common, everyday forms of radiation we live with, and is, by these principles, able to be controlled and regulated.

Dr. Farr points out that although excess radiation is harmful, so is excess heat and sunshine. Modern x-ray equipment used intelligently offers far less risk than that of missing an early diagnosis. Man has learned to deal with fire; we have to learn to deal with radiation. The most reassuring piece of information I know of is that if you get a full size chest x-ray every day of your life you receive less irradiation than if you live in Colorado. Cosmic rays at high altitude are as damaging as x-rays, yet Colorado citizens are no worse off from irradiation than those in Manhattan.

Noise

Noise is sound pollution. The sense of hearing is easily damaged, and in this noisy mechanized age all of us lose hearing as we age. The middle ear is protected from excess sound by two small muscles that can easily tire, especially at prolonged loud rock concerts. Then the nerves in the inner ear are unprotected, and hearing is permanently damaged. It is a pity that a lot of young "music" lovers will be partially deaf when they reach middle age.

Smog

Many types of smog damage people. Aside from burning eyes and congested nose, Dr. Paul Wehrle has shown that *even healthy people are affected by smog*. Smog has been shown to impair the performance of healthy high school cross-country runners and has been associated with excess cough and headache at the concentrations often seen in urban areas. Many other symptoms have been described, but clear proof is lacking for most conditions. Dr. Wehrle explains:

The prevention of health effects due to air pollution is not a simple matter. Personal air pollution by tobacco smoke can be prevented by individual action, but for the remainder, pollutants represent the by-products of an industrial and mechanized civilization. Motor vehicle exhaust pollution may be reduced substantially by controls such as the California Air Quality Standards and Motor Vehicle Exhaust Emission Requirements, but complete prevention of the motor vehicle exhaust problem may lie in other energy sources for power. Controls in selected cities and states may be needed in order to prevent the burning of high sulfur content fuels, thus reducing the sulfur pollution, and similarly, restrictions may be required on the lead content of gasolines in order to reduce the lead exposure problem. Substantial improvements are apparent in industry, and major improvements in air quality have been made in many cities during recent years. This has been accomplished by altering manufacturing processes, and by introducing various precipitators and other technical equipment in the smoke stacks to reclaim or at least to prevent discharge of noxious fumes and particles. For some industries, this has represented a substantial investment.

We can expect the struggle between the environmentalists and those promoting industrial development or fighting the energy crisis to become more intense during the years to come, since the energy crisis may require the use of lower grades of fuel containing sulfur and other contaminants. Unfortunately, our air resources, like the land area of the world, are not unlimited.

22

POISONOUS PLANTS

Each year, 12,000 children eat toxic plants. Some plants that you and I eat safely may be poison to particular individuals because of digestive problems, lack of enzymes, or allergy. The plants people eat have been selected out by generations of trial and error. Those who guessed wrong instructed the rest by their discomfort or demise. Some of the legends, such as calling tomatoes "poison apples," are incorrect for most. Yet tomatoes certainly are poison to some. Parts of plants we eat routinely are food, and other parts of the same plants are poisonous. The "green apple belly ache" is an example where even the age of the plant has an effect. Professor George D. Maragos, M.D., M.Sc., says:

> The average adult rarely realizes the hidden danger of his own sinister garden. Children, who are both indiscriminate and physically closer to the plants than we are, often eat most unpalatable things.
>
> Many well-known decorative plants and large numbers of wild plants are poisonous. Any part of a toxic plant—root, leaves, flowers, seeds or fruits—may poison a person if swallowed. Symptoms can appear as early as the first bite or as late as five days after ingestion.

How Do You Identify a Plant?

Because of space and the complexity of identification procedures, we have not included descriptions of the hundreds of poisonous plants. Sketches of some of the more common poisonous plants appear in this chapter (Figures 60 to 90 on pages 345 and 348). A botanical guide is available in the book *Human Poisoning from Native and Cultivated Plants* along with some photographs and sketches. But the most practical and commonly used method of identification is to take a leaf and blossom

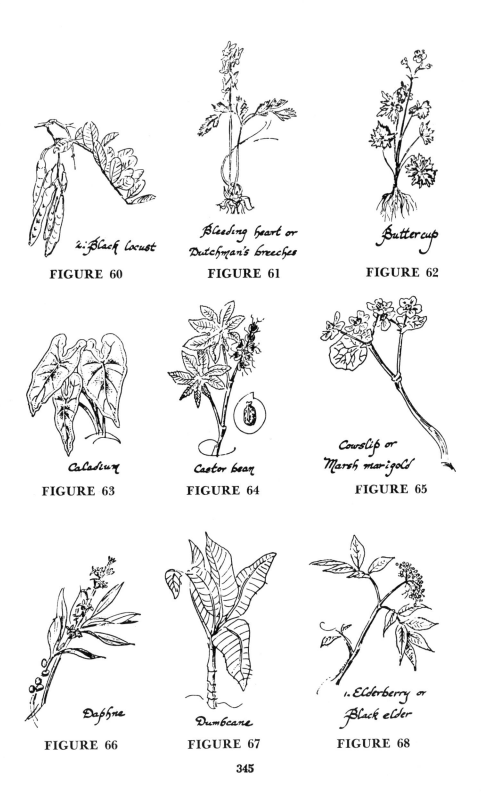

2. Black locust

FIGURE 60

Bleeding heart or
Dutchman's breeches

FIGURE 61

Buttercup

FIGURE 62

Caladium

FIGURE 63

Castor bean

FIGURE 64

Cowslip or
Marsh marigold

FIGURE 65

Daphne

FIGURE 66

Dumbcane

FIGURE 67

1. Elderberry or
Black elder

FIGURE 68

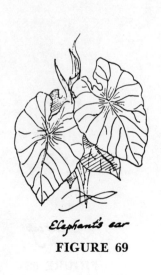

Elephant's ear

FIGURE 69

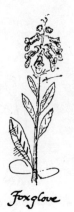

Foxglove

FIGURE 70

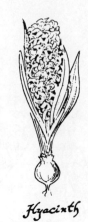

Hyacinth

FIGURE 71

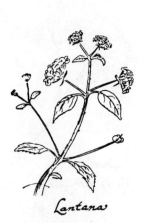

Lantana

FIGURE 72

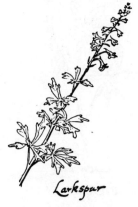

Larkspur

FIGURE 73

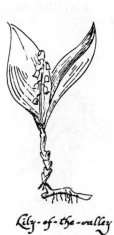

Lily-of-the-valley

FIGURE 74

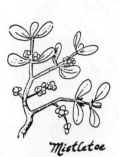

Mistletoe

FIGURE 75

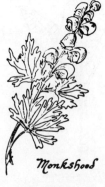

Monkshood

FIGURE 76

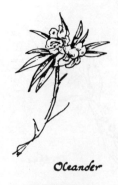

Oleander

FIGURE 77

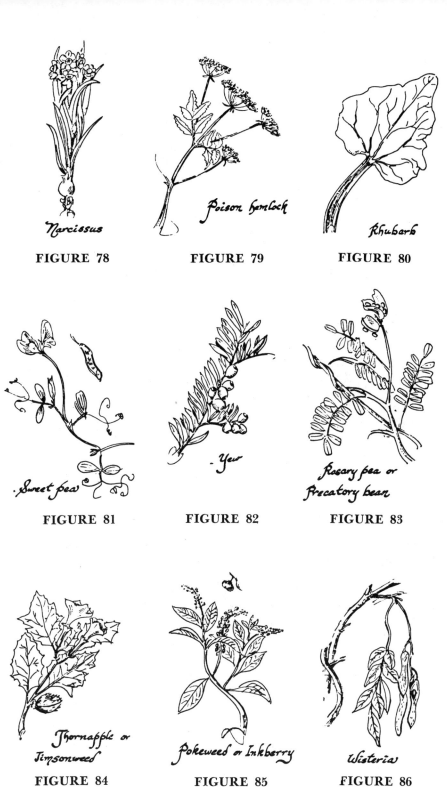

FIGURE 78   Narcissus

FIGURE 79   Poison hemlock

FIGURE 80   Rhubarb

FIGURE 81   Sweet pea

FIGURE 82   Yew

FIGURE 83   Rosary pea or Precatory bean

FIGURE 84   Thornapple or Jimsonweed

FIGURE 85   Pokeweed or Inkberry

FIGURE 86   Wisteria

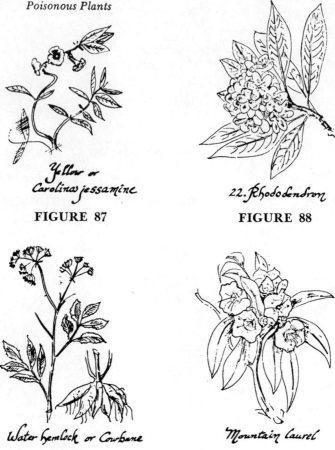

Yellow or
Carolina Jessamine
FIGURE 87

22. Rhododendron
FIGURE 88

Water Hemlock or Cowbane
FIGURE 89

Mountain Laurel
FIGURE 90

or berries from the plant in question to someone who knows: a gardener, a knowledgeable neighbor, or a plant nursery. Once identified you can then look up the plant either by one of its many common names in list I or its proper scientific name in list II on pages 366 to 380, to determine how poisonous the plant is and what sort of symptoms the poisoning may cause.

If you have plants in your yard or house, you should make certain that you have not planted a sinister garden. Get the names of your plants and look them up in the lists of poisonous plants. Keep in mind that it is impossible to tell whether or when your small child may take a bite from that nice but dangerous dieffenbachia in your hall, or try the berries from your daphne bush in the back yard. You can't muzzle the child, and he may or may not respond to mother's urgent plea of "Please, please, don't eat the daisies!" But daisies or not, if there is a question it is better to get the offending plant out of the stomach if you can.

FIRST AID FOR PLANT POISONING

1. Wash out the mouth.
2. Give a glass of milk at once to dilute the poison and protect the membranes.
3. If you can identify the plant, check the lists to see if it is potentially toxic.
4. If you cannot identify the plant, have someone take a part of the plant to a garden supply store while you *call your doctor* (he may have illustrations of poison plants) *or* your local *poison control center*. If there is a possibility that the plant may be poisonous:
   a. Give syrup of ipecac, obtainable from a pharmacy without prescription (three teaspoons every fifteen minutes for two doses) at once to induce vomiting. If syrup of ipecac is not available at home, get it from the nearest drug store, doctor's office, or hospital. If vomiting does not occur, gastric lavage may be performed.
   b. After vomiting has subsided, give half a cup of powdered activated charcoal mixed with about ¾ cup of water.
5. Note that symptoms of poisoning may be delayed, so don't wait for symptoms to appear before treating. Take the child to the doctor.
6. Your doctor may advise giving activated charcoal in water after the vomiting has subsided to help absorb the remaining plant poison.

POISONING FROM PLANTS

By Kenneth F. Lampe, Ph.D. and Mary Ann McCann

We asked Dr. Kenneth F. Lampe, professor of pharmacology and author of a physician's book on plant toxicity and dermatitis, with his research associate Mary Ann McCann, to outline the actual problems that can occur with various types of plant poisoning. What follows is a sobering description of serious and usually preventable illnesses.

Although there are hundreds of plant species growing in North America which contain toxic material thought to be harmful to animals and man, there are relatively few capable of producing serious human poisoning. Most cases of poisoning from plants occur in children under six and are usually due to the ingestion of house plants or those growing in the yard, or in a nearby park or playground. Thus, the risk of poisoning in young children may be greatly reduced if hazardous plants are eliminated from their immediate environment.

Unexplained Illness

It is not always possible for a parent to observe a child actually eating a poisonous plant. Quite often, the parents are unaware of the ingestion until the child displays symptoms of poisoning. These may vary with the type of toxic substances contained in the particular plant in-

gested. Ipecac should not be given to a comatose or convulsing child. If
the child has been vomiting profusely, it may not be necessary to give
syrup of ipecac, but the activated charcoal slurry should be given. Even
though it may be several hours since the child has eaten the toxic material, a portion of it may remain in the stomach. Harsh laxatives are not
recommended unless advised by the physician. They add to the child's
distress and produce an additional loss of body fluids which is dangerous
to a young child.

Types of Poisoning Produced by Plants

Vomiting and Diarrhea

Vomiting and diarrhea may be produced by many poisonous plants.
For some, it is the only consequence, but for others, it may be just a small
part of the overall toxicity of the plant. For example, the plants which
are toxic to the heart also produce some degree of irritation to the stomach and intestine. In this section, symptoms of various types of plant
poisoning will be given. Many of these symptoms do not occur in each
and every case of poisoning from a particular plant or class of plants.
Much depends on the amount ingested as well as the physical status and
age of the victim.

Sometimes poisoning may occur after the ingestion of a supposedly
nontoxic plant. These intoxications may be due to chemicals *on* the
plants (Group A).

(Insecticides), (Herbicides), (Liquid fertilizers)   [A]

Vomiting with Little or No Diarrhea

Plants of the amaryllis family and wisteria (Group B) contain substances which have a stimulating action on the vomiting center in the
brain. This will have an effect much like that of ipecac, and the toxic
material will be expelled from the stomach. Charcoal may be given to
absorb any remaining material.

Amaryllis, Wisteria   [B]

Irritant Plants

The majority of toxic plants contain irritants that produce their
action by damaging the mucus membranes, such as the lining of the
stomach and intestine. Depending on the type of toxic material contained in the plant, the symptoms may range from simple burning in

the mouth to severe vomiting and bloody diarrhea. In severe cases, this may result in death from dehydration or circulatory collapse. It is important to remember that a plant that may only produce a mild feeling of discomfort in an adult may cause serious poisoning in a young child.

Injury to the Mouth and Throat

There are many plants (Group C) that cause intense burning of the lips, mouth, and throat. The painful sensation produced by chewing these plants usually prevents the child from swallowing them and thereby causing damage to the stomach. Unfortunately, a large number of these are common house plants displayed within easy reach of infants and toddlers. The most hazardous of these is Dieffenbachia, as it may produce swelling of the throat, as well as intense pain.

> Caladium, Calla lily, Dieffenbachia, Elephant ear,
> Jack-in-the-pulpit, Monstera, Philodendron, Skunk cabbage   [C]

Irritation of the Mouth, Stomach, and Intestine

Other plants (Group D) contain stronger chemicals which produce irritation of the throat and mouth, even blistering and ulceration, and severe irritation of the stomach and bowel. The onset of pain is delayed from a few minutes to several hours after chewing the plant parts, so ingestion usually has taken place. This results in nausea, vomiting, and severe, often bloody, diarrhea. There is a great deal of abdominal distress. Salivation, sweating, and dilated pupils may occur, although dryness of the mouth and thirst have also been reported. Kidney damage may occur. Convulsions may precede death, but coma and respiratory paralysis are most prevalent.

> Anemone, Baneberry, Buttercups, Clematis, Daphne, Iris, Lords
> and ladies, Marsh marigold, May apple, Pokeweed, Rouge plant,
> Wicopy   [D]

Green plants only

Some of the plants in this group (Group E) are toxic only when the fruits, sprouts, or roots are green.

> Ground cherry, Jessamine, Irish potato   [E]

Varies with the season

Other plants in this group (Group F) vary in toxicity with the climate, season, and growing conditions.

Apple of Sodom, Chalice vine, Devil's apple, Nightshades   [F]

Manchineel tree poisoning (Group G)

Poisoning from the fruit of the Manchineel tree causes intestinal irritation about two hours after ingestion, followed by shock from fluid loss.

Manchineel tree   [G]

Yew poisoning (Group H)

Symptoms appear within an hour as dizziness, dry throat, and widely dilated pupils. These are followed by severe abdominal cramps, increased salivation, and vomiting. There is muscular weakness progressing to stupor and coma. A skin rash may appear, the face is pale, and the lips have a purplish discoloration. There are irregular heart beats and low blood pressure, shallow and slow breathing. Death is due to either respiratory or cardiac failure.

Yew   [H]

Delayed Abdominal Pain

Poisoning by another group (Group I) is usually from the fruits, berries, nuts, or seeds; however, all parts of these plants should be considered dangerous, as illness has been produced by the leaves and roots as well. Initially, they produce increased salivation, nausea, and vomiting. Both the stomach and intestine become highly inflamed and considerable abdominal pain is produced. This inflammation increases the absorption of the toxic material into the system. Headache, fever, and thirst are the usual signs of systemic involvement. Muscular weakness, incoordination, and anxiety are seen in severe poisoning. The pupils may be dilated and a face rash may appear. Paralysis or convulsions usually precede death.

Balsam pear, Blue cohosh, Buckeye,
Horsechestnut, English ivy, Golden dewdrop, Mock orange,
Monkey pod, Soapberry, Yam bean   [I]

Strangling and Vomiting

Another group of plants (Group J) cause symptoms two to six hours after ingestion, with intense burning and rawness of the mouth and throat, followed by a strangling sensation. The ability to speak is often lost. There is a feeling of nausea and considerable abdominal discomfort, followed by violent uncontrolled vomiting and diarrhea. Shock may develop as a result of fluid loss. Kidney damage has been reported in severe poisoning.

Autumn crocus, Glory lily   [J]

Delayed Abdominal Distension
Oxalic acid-containing plants (Group K) are digested very slowly. Only after massive ingestions do symptoms appear. In one or two days, the abdomen becomes distended, with severe cramping, which is followed by vomiting, and often by bloody diarrhea. Muscle spasms are rarely seen, but in severe cases permanent kidney damage may be produced.

Garden rhubarb, Garden sorrel, Virginia creeper   [K]

Castor Bean
Some of the most severe cases of plant poisoning are produced by the castor bean (Group L). Although all parts of the plant are toxic, the "bean" itself is most often ingested. The onset and severity of symptoms depends on the amount chewed and ingested. Beans swallowed whole rarely produce serious intoxication. The first sign of poisoning may appear within a few minutes or be delayed up to several days. Usually, a burning sensation precedes persistent vomiting and profuse diarrhea. The presence of blood in the vomitus and stool is an indication of hemorrhages in the stomach or intestines. These symptoms are followed by headache and dizziness. Later, signs of liver degeneration and kidney damage are evident. The mortality rate from castor bean ingestion is about 6%. The greatest chance for survival is among those victims with an early onset of vomiting.

Castor bean   [L]

Long-Delayed Symptoms
Another member of this group (Group M) is the rosary pea. Both the root and seed are poisonous. When ripe, the seeds have a bright red hard shell which seems resistant to the most vigorous chewing. Therefore, they are swallowed whole and pass through the digestive system without harm;

however, the green seed has a soft covering, and is so highly toxic that as little as one well-chewed seed has produced death in children. Symptoms develop from within a few hours to several days after ingestion. In addition to vomiting and diarrhea, the pupils are widely dilated, the pulse is rapid, and there is muscular weakness and twitching. The skin appears flushed, and hallucinations have occurred in some children. Kidney and liver damage has been reported, but the most serious effect is degeneration of the intestine. Survivors often have permanent visual defect as the result of hemorrhages in the retina. The black locust also acts similarly but less severely so; fatalities are rare and recovery is complete within two days.

Barbados nut, Black locust,
Coral plant, Crabs-eye, Physic nut,
Rosary pea, Sandbox Tree   [M]

Severe Diarrhea

There are a number of plants (Group N) that contain irritants producing a brief period of nausea and vomiting from 20 to 40 minutes after ingestion. This is followed by drastic and persistent diarrhea. Excessive fluid loss may lead to dehydration and shock. Of this group of miscellaneous plants, Tung nut is the most dangerous. They are often confused with pecans, and have produced serious poisonings in the southern United States.

Buckthorn, Candlenut, Celadine, Christmas candle,
Clusia, Dwarf poinciana, English holly, Golden shower,
Honeysuckle, Privet, Snowberry, Tung nut, Wood-
bine   [N]

Plants Toxic to the Heart and Circulatory System

Certain plants contain substances which exert a toxic action on the heart or circulatory system. Some of these substances have been isolated from the plant material and used in the therapy of many heart conditions and high blood pressure. Since most of these are highly toxic, their ingestion by a child or adult may result in acute poisoning. It is most important, therefore, to take the victim to a medical facility where equipment is available to monitor the heart and blood pressure, and where the proper medication may be given to counteract the action of the toxic material.

Digitalis-like compounds (Group O) irritate the mouth and stomach, causing vomiting, and, usually, diarrhea. There is headache; vision is sometimes affected, with objects appearing yellow or greenish; the pulse is slow. There may be cold sweats or fainting. Convulsions have preceded death in foxglove poisoning. The toxic action on the heart may take some hours to develop and then, in some cases, may persist for one to two weeks. Children have been poisoned by drinking the water from vases that have contained these plants.

```
Foxglove, Lily-of-the-valley, Oleander      [O]
```

Rapid Tingling

Any portion of plants of Group P cause symptoms which appear rapidly after ingestion as a tingling, burning sensation of the lips, tongue, and mouth followed by numbness. A similar reaction occurs in the throat, often with a feeling of constriction and difficulty with speech. Contrary to the irritant plants, there is no swelling or reddening of the tissues. The feeling of warmth and tingling may spread over the body, starting in the fingers and toes. Salivation is increased; nausea and vomiting may be seen. The poison is absorbed into the system quickly. The pulse will become slow and irregular. There may be blurred or double vision; and the pupils remain constricted until just prior to death. Breathing is slow and labored. The victim is weak, dizzy, and uncoordinated. This poisoning is a medical emergency: Death may occur within one hour.

```
Delphinium, Larkspur, Monkshood, Wolfbane      [P]
```

"Heart Attack" Pain

Alarming but rarely life-threatening symptoms are caused by this group (Group Q) of plants. There is a burning sensation and pain in the upper abdominal area, followed by increased salivation, nausea, and spasms of vomiting. There may be sweating, blurring of vision, and confusion. The pulse is slow, and there is a feeling of prostration due to a fall in blood pressure. An adult may describe these symptoms as "having a heart attack." Even in severe poisoning, recovery is usually complete in less than 24 hours.

```
Hellebore      [Q]
```

Honey Poisoning

Another group (Group R) causes a transitory burning in the mouth. A few hours later, there may be increased salivation, vomiting, diarrhea, and a tingling sensation in the skin. There is a feeling of intense drowsiness due to the fall in blood pressure. Coma may develop. Recovery is usually complete within 24 hours. Poisoning from these plants is usually associated with eating "wild honey" rather than ingesting the plant itself.

Azalea, Death camas, Lambkill, Mountain laurel, Rhododendron   [R]

Plants Having Other Systemic Effects (Group S)

Symptoms usually appear within one hour as increased salivation and violent vomiting. Occasionally, the vomitus may contain blood. The victim feels dizzy and thirsty and may exhibit confusion and delirium. Headache is common. The face is usually pale and the pulse rapid. Breathing is initially rapid, becoming progressively weaker. Pupils may be normal or slightly dilated. If a moderate amount is absorbed, there are muscular twitchings and convulsions. Large amounts produce paralysis and coma.

Cardinal flower, Fool's parsley, Golden chain, Lobelia, Kentucky coffee-tree, Indian tobacco, Mescal bean sophora, Poison hemlock, Tree tobacco, Wild tobacco   [S]
[T]

"Fever Plants" (Group U)

Belladonna-containing plants produce symptoms of widely dilated pupils, hot dry flushed skin, and a rapid pulse. Salivation is decreased; speaking and swallowing may be difficult. These alkaloids produce an elevated body temperature, face rash, and excitement, followed by headache, uncoordination, and confusion. Delirium, hallucinations, and psychotic behavior may develop. Convulsions occur in younger children. Recently, adolescents have ingested these plants because of their so-called hallucinogenic properties. Some of the intoxications produced were severe enough to require hospitalization.

Angel's trumpet, Deadly nightshade, Henbane, Jessamine, Jimson weed, Matrimony vine   [U]

Jessamine Poisoning

The Carolina yellow jessamine (Group V) produces headache, dizziness, dim or double vision, dilated pupils, and dry mouth. There are two alkaloids present in this plant, and, depending on the concentration of each alkaloid, in severe cases, the victim may display either profound muscular weakness, such as dropping eyelids or an inability to keep the mouth closed, or rigidity, such as a firmly locked jaw. Convulsions have occurred, as well as difficulty in breathing and loss of consciousness. In nonfatal cases, visual disturbances may last for several days.

Carolina yellow jessamine   [V]

Miscellaneous Toxic Plants (Groups W, X, and Y)

There are a number of plants that have produced either bizarre toxic effects associated with isolated or single instances of poisoning. For the most part, the material responsible for these poisonings has not been identified.

Weakness and Vomiting

Poisoning occurred in a number of preschool children from eating the green berries of the lantana plant. Symptoms began from 2-½ to 6 hours after ingestion and included a feeling of weakness and lethargy followed by vomiting. Diarrhea was present in only one case. The pupils were dilated and respiration slowed. There was one fatality preceded by coma.

Lantana   [W]

"Diabetes-like" Poisoning

A diabetic-like response was produced in a child after eating jet bead berries. Abdominal pain and vomiting occurred a few hours after ingestion. During the course of the next several hours, the child developed a fever and became comatose. Laboratory tests were normal prior to hospitalization, but later results were similar to those seen in cases of diabetic coma. The fever rose to 106°, and the child experienced convulsions, but responded to treatment and was essentially normal in two days.

Jet bead   [X]

Mistletoe Poisoning

The only documented fatality from the American mistletoe is that of a woman who drank a tea prepared from the berries. After two hours, she became nauseated and had severe abdominal cramping. This was followed by profuse vomiting, diarrhea, and frequent urination. Approximately 12 hours after the ingestion, she was taken to the hospital complaining of acute abdominal pain, and in a state of severe shock. She died within 15 minutes. American mistletoe should not be confused with the European mistletoe, which belongs to a different plant genus and contains substances toxic to the heart. No substances of this type have been found in American mistletoe.

American mistletoe   [Y]

Cyanide Poisoning from Plants (Group Z)

Poisoning from plants containing substances that are converted to cyanide by stomach acids are usually associated with preschool children who have eaten large amounts of the "pips" or the soft inner kernel portion of the stones from fruits of the various members of the genus *Prunus*. Symptoms are delayed several hours, and appear in the following sequence: vomiting, incoordination, weakness, difficulty in breathing, twitching, stupor, and coma. Convulsions may occur either prior to or following loss of consciousness. The lips and tongue may have bluish discoloration. Serious poisoning rarely occurs in older children or adults unless massive amounts of material have been ingested.

Apricot pits, Cherry pits, Choke cherry pits,
Hydrangea buds, Loquat pits, Manihot roots, Peach pits,
Plum pits, Wild cherry pits, Zamia roots   [Z]

Plants Toxic to the Nervous System

The principal toxic action of the plants covered in this section is on the nervous system. Although convulsions, tremors, and paralysis are seen in severe or fatal intoxications from plants covered elsewhere in this chapter, these are not the primary toxic effects from those plants, and, in the case of convulsions, may be secondary to damage produced to other systems.

Convulsants

Most intoxications occur from eating the root of the plants in Group AA. Symptoms appear from within 15 minutes to an hour after chewing and swallowing the root—nausea, salivation, vomiting, and tremors. This is rapidly followed by violent intermittent convulsions. Death can occur from respiratory failure. If the victim survives, there are usually no permanent effects and often no memory of the intoxication.

> Spotted cowbane, Water hemlock   [AA]

Intoxications are rare and symptoms preceding convulsions vary in Group BB.

> Carolina Allspice, Chinaberry, Herb teas,
> Moonseed, Pink root, Strychnine tree, "Tonics"   [BB]

Herb teas, tonics, and home remedies made from Arbor Vitae, White Cedar, Cypress, Juniper, and Tansy contain substances that produce convulsions only after several doses. A single large dose usually exerts only a cathartic action. Convulsions from eating the raw plants has not been reported.

Paralysis

A unique type of poisoning is produced from eating the berries of the Coyotillo plant, which grows in the parts of Southwestern United States and Mexico. The symptoms are delayed for several weeks after ingestion and begin as a progressive weakness in the ankles and legs. Limping is noted, and soon the victim is unable to walk. The paralysis spreads upward, and the entire trunk and arms are affected. Breathing is difficult, and there is weakness of the neck and facial muscles. Tests show a degenerative process in the nerves of the muscles. Recovery is slow, and the paralysis subsides first in the face, neck, and arms, gradually diminishing in the trunk, and, finally, in the legs. Recovery is essentially complete six months after ingestion of the fruit.

> Coyotillo   [CC]

Mushrooms and Toadstools

The identification of unknown mushrooms is difficult, so with any known mushroom ingestion, syrup of ipecac should be given at once. One group of mushrooms may cause symptoms as early as fifteen minutes after eaten: stomach cramps, excess saliva, and sweating. The Amanita muscaria mushroom (red cap with polka dot white spots) causes symptoms within two to three hours, with drowsiness followed by excitement and

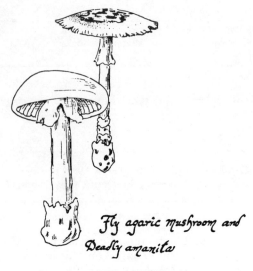

Fly agaric mushroom and Deadly amanita

FIGURE 91

hallucinations. Most other mushrooms cause vomiting, diarrhea, and stomach cramps.

The most serious of all mushroom poisons is from the deadly Amanita phalloides group. Fifty to ninety percent of people die from eating as little as one-third of the "death cap." Symptoms don't start until around twelve hours after ingestion. First, there are cramps with vomiting, and, sometimes, bloody diarrhea. This settles down, only to be followed by often fatal kidney and liver disease, with dark urine and yellow skin.

Most cases of serious intoxications and fatalities from plant ingestion are associated with mushrooms. *Unlike adult mushroom poisoning, where a misidentified species has been cooked prior to ingestion, intoxications in children are usually from eating raw mushrooms. Thus, many species considered edible when cooked may produce poisoning when eaten raw by a young child.* It is therefore extremely important that the ingestion of any raw "wild" mushroom be considered as a potential poisoning. The ipecac and charcoal emergency measures should be carried out immediately (see page 349). The child should be taken to the nearest medical facility. A specimen of the mushroom should be taken along for identification.

Mushroom intoxications vary with the species ingested. They may be broadly divided into two categories, depending on the time between ingestion and the appearance of symptoms: Mushrooms producing symptoms either immediately or within six hours of ingestion, and those in which the symptoms are delayed six hours or more. The most serious and potentially fatal poisonings occur with this latter group.

Mushrooms Producing Early Signs of Intoxication
Certain members of the species *Inocybe, Conocybe* and *Omphalotus* produce symptoms of poisoning within 15 minutes. Profuse sweating and

visual disturbances are experienced first. These are followed by drooling, watery eyes, and abdominal cramping. Vomiting and diarrhea do not always occur. The pulse is slow. There is an effective antidote for this type of intoxication, so medical attention should be sought without delay.

The initial symptoms from Amanita *muscaria* and *pantherina* intoxication usually appear within an hour as drowsiness, uncoordination, and general fatigue. The victim may sleep for a few hours and upon awakening be in a highly agitated state. This excitement is followed either by a state of delirium, such as is seen with high fevers in a young child, or by hallucinations which may be associated with fright and extreme anxiety. Medication may be given to terminate this psychosis if it is severe. Untreated, the victim will recover in several hours. The toxicity of these mushrooms may vary from location to location and even in the same area in different growing seasons. Consequently, they have been known occasionally to produce symptoms of intoxication similar to those associated with the *Inocybe* and *Conocybe* poisoning. It is therefore important that an accurate description of the symptoms be given to the physician so that the appropriate treatment is given.

A number of species of *Agaricus, Boletus, Cantherellus,* and so forth produce nausea, vomiting, and diarrhea within about two hours after ingestion. The severity of symptoms depends on the species as well as the amount ingested. This type of poisoning is often associated with eating so-called edible species raw. Some mushrooms (*Chlorophylum molybdites*) often grow in "fairy rings" in yards after rain and are quite attractive to children. If the vomiting and diarrhea are profuse, dehydration may occur.

Mushrooms Producing Delayed Symptoms

It has been estimated that about 95% of the fatalities from mushroom poisoning are the result of deadly *Amanita* intoxication. *Amanita phalloides, verna,* and *virosa* contain two types of toxins. The initial toxic effect occurs about 12 hours after ingestion. This is seen as nausea, vomiting, severe cramping, and watery diarrhea sometimes containing blood and mucus. These symptoms are usually successfully managed by preventing dehydration. The victim appears to recover, but in from 3 to 5 days, signs from the second toxin appear. If a small amount of material is absorbed, kidney damage may be the predominant feature; with intermediate amounts, both liver and kidney damage are seen. Large amounts produce extensive liver damage before the kidneys are affected. The brain is affected as a result of liver and kidney involvement. Despite glowing reports of a new miracle antidote, there is little scientific evidence that it is any more effective than the modern intensive medical management used for acute liver conditions. In Europe, the number of fatalities occurring as the result of Death Cap poisoning has been reduced 50% by employing such techniques.

Symptoms of poisoning from another mushroom, *Helevella esculenta,* usually appear from 6 to 8 hours after ingestion, but may be delayed up to two days. Headache and fatigue appear first, followed by general discomfort and a feeling of fullness in the stomach. Abdominal pain increases, accompanied by persistent vomiting. Diarrhea is rare. In about 2 to 3 days jaundice appears. The liver and spleen are enlarged, giving the abdomen a distended appearance. The jaundice subsides in a few days, and recovery is rapid. In extremely severe cases where liver damage is extensive, the brain is affected and coma precedes death. Poisoning from these mushrooms is rare in the United States, but some mild intoxications have been reported in the eastern states.

PLANTS PRODUCING RASHES AND INJURY TO THE SKIN

By Kenneth F. Lampe and Mary Ann McCann

By far the most prevalent and troublesome rash produced by plants is the "poison ivy" or allergic contact type dermatitis. This type of skin reaction occurs in individuals who have become sensitized to a chemical present in the plant. Thus, one must be exposed to the plant material on more than one occasion in order to develop the rash. Many different plant families contain species to which some individuals are sensitive; however, the *Toxicodendron* (*Rhus*) species (poison ivy, poison oak, etc.) contain a chemical to which the vast majority of the population may develop sensitivity. It is not necessary to have direct contact with the plant itself, as, quite often, one may be exposed to the chemical through contaminated pets, clothing, garden tools, toys, and so forth. Therefore, if exposure is known or suspected, all skin and other articles should be thoroughly washed. The appearance of itching, blisters, and vesicles is usually within one to two days after contact with the plant material, and the severity of the condition depends on the degree of exposure and the individual's sensitivity. About the most effective treatment during the acute stage is plain ice water compresses. Over-the-counter creams or ointments are often harmful, and may worsen the condition or prolong its duration. Severe cases should be treated by a physician.

Another type of contact dermatitis is produced by plants which contain irritant chemicals. This differs from the allergic reaction in that it appears within a few minutes to hours after plant exposure and is usually associated with a burning sensation, and with reddening and blistering of the skin. No prior exposure is required to produce this reaction, and everyone will respond in a similar manner to the particular irritant. Cleansing the exposed skin as soon as possible to remove the chemical may limit the severity of the injury. If the material should get into the eye or mouth, flush with water thoroughly and consult your physician immediately.

Many plants are capable of producing mechanical injury to the skin by means of their thorns, sharp leaf edges, and so forth. Usually, the only treatment required is to remove the embedded plant parts and keep the wound clean to prevent infection. After one encounter with plants of this type, children learn to avoid them.

There are two other types of rashes due to plants which may not be easily recognized as "plant dermatitis." The first is photo- or sunlight dermatitis. Certain plants contain a chemical which is absorbed into the skin and in itself produces no reaction unless the skin is exposed to sunlight or unusually strong artificial light. Then a rash appears, with reddening and vesicles. When the rash has subsided, there is a darkening of the particular area of the skin. This pigmentation, as it is called, may be permanent in severe cases. In the event of possible photodermatitis, avoid sunlight and consult a dermatologist. With the exception of ragweed oil, the photodermatitis produced by plants is not an allergic reaction and may occur in anyone with a sufficient amount of the chemical in their skin and exposure to high intensity light.

The second type of dermatitis often not recognized as being of plant origin is pollen dermatitis. This is an allergic or sensitivity reaction which occurs at the same time each year. The chemical in the pollen which produces the dermatitis is not the same allergen which causes respiratory allergies such as hay fever or asthma. The rash is over exposed areas of the skin such as the face, the V of the neck, the arms, and so forth. Individuals suffering from pollen dermatitis should be under the care of either a dermatologist or an allergist. (For lists of rash-producing plants, see page 382.)

PART FOUR

MEDICAL LISTS

This part contains lists of poisonous and rash-producing plants, of foods containing minerals, vitamins, and cholesterols, of foods for a gluten-free diet, of allergenic foods for elimination diets, and of additives to foods, drugs, and cosmetics. I suggest that you at least look over this section briefly to become more aware of the amount of information that is available.

You may well ask, "Why should I have these lists around, much less look at them?" One reason, although not too impressive at first, is that these lists contain a lot of information not usually accessible to parents. For that matter, some of this material has not previously been conveniently accessible to physicians. For most readers these lists will be of very little value except under special circumstances. With a little luck you will never have to study any of them. Yet to parents of young children, the lists of poisonous plants may be life-saving. These plant lists are hard to come by, and we are especially proud of ours, for they are the most complete, accurate, and practical lists we know of—they were prepared by two outstanding experts in the field of plant poisoning and draw from the entire spectrum of medical literature. Some of the information here is new to most of us. Just the lists of rash-producing plants alone are shocking. Although I knew that there were a lot of plants that can cause rashes in susceptible individuals, I was amazed at the number. If you have a sensitive skin, this list alone may be worth at least whatever a visit to the doctor or dermatologist will cost.

The lists of vitamins and minerals in foods can be of value to parents who are concerned about nutrition. The best way to ensure good nutrition is to eat a wide variety of good foods. However, many small children don't heed such advice. Here you can check and make certain that your child's diet at least has most of the basics. If you have the not-uncommon problem of iron deficiency anemia, you can find which foods are iron rich. If your child can't take cow's milk, you can determine whether he is getting enough calcium in his diet. And you can check the requirements and intake of other essential minerals as well as vitamins.

Then, of course, there are the special diets for those who are allergic: Those with chronic nasal congestion, wheezes and cough, puffy face and headaches, and eczema and welts, intestinal cramps and diarrhea. If there is a possibility that food allergy is the cause, you will find elimination diets here for some of the more common and difficult allergenic foods to avoid. Then there is the gluten-free diet for those who have diarrhea, weight loss, and other symptoms of gluten sensitivity.

Finally, there is the bewildering array of additives in foods, drugs, and cosmetics. Dr. Lockey says that the average American eats five pounds of such additives a year in a "normal" diet. For most of us this means little, but if you have a hyperactive child whose hyperactivity could be due to food additives, the diets may look less formidable than the problem with the child. And if you have hives and itching, wheezing and swelling, irritation and yelling caused by some of these additives, these lists may offer you a chance to do some detective work that can be as absorbing to you as if you were helping Sherlock Holmes.

So good luck. Let's hope you *don't* have to use these lists. But it can be reassuring to have them available if you do need them.

LISTS OF POISONOUS PLANTS

The long List I of common names of poisonous plants reflects the large number of names by which a single plant is known. The number following each common name refers you to the number in List II assigned to each of the 250 botanical names of poisonous plants (page 372ff). The botanical list tells you more about the plant, how toxic it is, what parts are toxic, and, if significantly toxic, refers you back to Chapter 22 where a description of the specific symptoms of poisoning can be appreciated.

These lists were prepared by Dr. Kenneth Lampe and his research associate Mary Ann McCann of the pharmacology department of the School of Medicine, University of Miami. I have added to it a few plants that are thought to be potentially poisonous or that have been reported as causes of poisoning in Europe but not in North America, and a few said by other workers in the field to have caused poisoning. It is better to be safe than sorry; if possibly poisonous, the plant is better out of than in the stomach. We have roughly estimated the toxicity of the plants from the books of Lampe and Fogerstrom, Hardin and Arena, and Kingsbury, although many factors, including the age and size of the child and the quantity consumed can affect the toxicity.[1]

List I—Common Names of Poisonous Plants

Numbers following these names refer to botanical name and description in List II pages 372–381. Some of these plants are illustrated in Chapter 22.

Ackee	40	Alocasia	21
Aconite	3	Amaryllis	22, 114
Acorns	188	American cherry laurel	186
Adonis, spring	11	American ivy	187
Akee	40	American mistletoe	176
Alder buck thorn	194	American yew	234
Allamanda, pink or purple	78	Anemone	24
Allamanda, yellow	19	Angel's trumpet	84
Almond	186	Apple of Peru	88

KEY TO LIST OF BOTANICAL NAMES
OF POISONOUS PLANTS

You may notice that a single plant in these lists may be listed under two entirely different groups of poisons in Chapter 22. This is because some plants produce one set of symptoms when they are green and a different set of symptoms when they are ripe.

■ ■   Dangerously Toxic

■   Serious Intoxication

□   Moderate Distress

?   Unknown Potential for Human Poisoning

☆   Plants Incorrectly Labeled Poisonous in Older Literature

PH   Nectar Makes Poisonous Honey

♣   Uncertain as to Part of Plant

[M]   Refers to the title letter for sections in Chapter 22 (pages 350–359) explaining the symptoms of poisoning by the plant, and other plants with the same toxic effects.

List II—Botanical Names of Poisonous Plants*

	Name	Type of Plant	Poisonous Part	Refer to:
1. ■	Abrus precatorius	vine, weed	chewed seed	[M]
2. ■	Aconitum columbianum	wild flower	all parts	
3. ■	Aconitum napellus	wild & cultiv. flower	all parts	[P]
4.	Actaea alba (= Actaea pachypoda)			
5.	Actaea arguta (= Actaea rubra)			
6. ■	Actaea pachypoda	wild & cultiv. flower	berry	
7. ■	Actaea rubra	wild & cultiv. flower	berry	
8. ■	Actaea spicata	cultivated flower	berry	
9. ■	Actaea species	wild & cultiv. flowers	berry	
10. ■	Adenium species	cultivated shrub	all parts	[P]
11. ?	Adonis vernalis	cultivated flower	❖	
12. □	Aesculus hippocastanum	tree	nut	[I]
13. □	Aesculus species	tree, shrub	nut	
14. □	Aethusa cynapium	weed	all parts	[S]
15. ■	Agrostemma githago	weed	seed	
16. ■	Aleurites fordii	tree	nut kernel	[N]
17. □	Aleurites moluccana	tree	nut kernel	[N]
18. ■	Aleurites trisperma	tree	nut kernel	
19. □	Allamanda cathartica	vine, shrub	sap, fruit	
20. □	Allium canadense	weed	bulb	
21. □	Alocasia species	house plant	leaf, stem	
22. □	Amaryllis species	cultivated flower	all parts	[B]
23. □	Anemone patens	cultivated flower	all parts	[D]
24. □	Anemone species	wild & cultiv. flowers	all parts	[D]
25. □	Anthurium species	house plant	all parts	
26. ?	Apocynum species	weed	❖	
27. □	Aralia species	shrub, tree	leaf	
28. ☆	Areca cathecu	palm tree	❖	
29. □	Arisaema draconium	wild flower	leaf	
30. □	Arisaema triphyllum	wild flower	leaf	[C]

* See pages 350–359.

List II—Botanical Names of Poisonous Plants (*Cont.*)

		Name	Type of Plant	Poisonous Part	Refer to:
31.	□	Argemone mexicana	weed	seed	[D]
32.	□	Arnica montana	cultivated flower	flower, root	[D]
32a.		Arum cornutum (see Suaromatum guttatum)		uncooked root	
33.	■	Arum maculatum	cultivated plant	all parts	[D]
34.	■	Arum palaestinum	cultivated flower	all parts	[D]
35.	■	Arum species	mostly cultivated	♣	
36.	?	Asclepias curassavica	weed	all parts	[F, U]
37.		Atropa belladonna	cultivated flower	♣	
38.	PH	Azalea species	cultivated shrub	seeds	[R]
39.	□	Baptisia species	wild & cultiv. flower	fruit	
40.		Blighia sapida	tree		
40a.		Brugmansia species (see Datura species)			
41.		Bulbocodium vernum (see Colchicum vernum)			
42.	□	Buxus sempervirens	evergreen shrub	leaves	[N]
43.	□	Caesalpinia gilliesii	shrub, house plant	seeds	[N]
44.	■	Caesalpinia pulcherrima	shrub, tree	seeds	[C]
45.	□	Caladium species	house plant (f. 65)	leaf	
46.	□	Calla palustris	wild flower	all parts	[D]
47.	■	Calotropis procera	shrub, small tree	all parts	[BB]
48.		Caltha palustris	wild flower (f. 67)	all parts	[D]
49.	?	Calycanthus fertilis	shrub	seeds	
50.	☆?	Calycanthus floridus	shrub	♣	
51.	?	Calycanthus occidentalis	shrub	seeds	
52.	?	Calycanthus species	shrubs	seeds	
53.	□	Cannabis species	weeds	marihuana source	[N]
54.	□	Cassia fistula	tree	seed	
55.	□	Cassia nodosa	tree	seed	[I]
56.	□	Caulophyllum thalictroides	wild flower	berry	
57.	?	Celastrus scandens	vine	seeds in quantity	[E, V, U]
58.	□	Cestrum diurnum	shrub	berry	[E, V, U]
59.	□	Cestrum nocturnum	shrub	berries in quantity	[E, V, U]
60.	□	Cestrum parqui	shrub	berries in quantity	

No.		Species	Type	Part(s)	Code
61.	□	Cestrum species	shrub	berry	[E]
62.	□	Chamaecyparis thyoides	evergreen tree	herbal teas	[BB]
63.	□	Chelidonium majus	cultivated flower	all parts	[N]
64.	■	Cicuta maculata	swamp weed	all parts	[AA]
65.	■	Cicuta species	swamp weeds	all parts	[AA]
66.	□	Clematis species	vine or shrub	all parts	[D]
67.	□	Clusia rosea	tree	sap	[N]
67a.		Cnidoscolus stimulosus (see Jatropha stimulosa)			
68.	■	Colchicum autumnale	cultivated flower	tuber, seed	[J]
69.	■	Colchicum speciosum	cultivated flower	tuber, seed	
70.	■	Colchicum vernum	cultivated flower	tuber, seed	
71.	■	Colchicum species	cultivated flowers	tuber, seed	
72.	□	Colocasia species	house plant	leaf	[C]
73.	■	Conium maculatum	weed	all parts	[S, T]
74.	■	Convallaria majalis	cultivated flower	all parts	[O]
75.	■	Coriaria myrtifolia	shrub	fruit	
76.	■	Coriaria species	shrubs	fruit	
77.	□	Crotalaria species	weeds	seeds in herbal tea	
78.	□	Cryptostegia grandiflora	vine, shrub	all parts	
79.	□	Cupressus species	evergreen trees	herbal teas	
80.	■	Cycas circinalis	palm-like shrub	root	[D]
81.	■	Cycas revoluta	palm-like shrub	root	[D]
81a.		Cytisus laburnum (see Laburnum anagyroides)			
82.	■	Daphne mezereum	shrub	fruit	[D]
83.	■	Daphne species	shrub	fruit	[D]
84.	□	Datura arborea	cultiv. small tree	seed, all parts	[U]
		(= Brugmansia arborea)			
85.	□	Datura candida	cultivated flower	seed, all parts	
86.	□	Datura inoxia	cultivated flower	seed, all parts	
87.	■	Datura metel	cultivated flower	seed, all parts	
88.	□	Datura strammonium	weed	seed, all parts	
89.	□	Datura suaveolens	cultivated shrub	seed, all parts	[U]
		(= Brugmansia arborea)			
89a.		Daubentonia species (see Glottidium species)			
90.	■	Delphinium ajacis	cultivated flower	all parts	[P]
91.	■	Delphinium species	wild & cultiv. flowers	all parts	[P]

List II—Botanical Names of Poisonous Plants (*Cont.*)

	Name	Type of Plant	Poisonous Part	Refer to:
92.	☐	Dicentra species	wild flowers	all parts	[C]
93.	☐	Dieffenbachia species	houseplants	leaf, stem	[O]
94.	■	Digitalis purpurea	cultivated flower	all parts	[D]
95.	☐	Dirca palustris	shrub	bark	
96.	■	Dolichos lablab	vine	uncooked bean	[I]
97.	☐	Duranta repens	shrub	fruit	
98.	☐	Echium plantagineum (= E. lycopis)	cultiv. flower, weed	herbal tea	
99.	■	Eriobotrya japonica	tree, shrub	seed kernels	[Z]
100.	?	Ervatamia coronaria (= Tabernaemontana divaricata)	tree, shrub	seeds	
101.	☐	Euonymus species	trees or shrubs	fruit, all parts	
102.	■	Euphorbia species	herbs, shrubs, trees some "cactus-like"	fruit, all parts	
103.	☐	Fagus sylvatica	tree	seeds	[V]
104.	■	Gelsemium sempervirens	vine	flowers	
105.	☐	Genista tinctoria	cultivated flower	seed	
106.	☐	Gloriosa rothchildiana	vine	tuber	[J]
107.	☐	Gloriosa superba	vine	tuber	
108.	☐	Glottidium species (= Sesbania and Daubentonia species)	weeds	seeds	
109.	☐	Gymnocladus dioica	tree	seed	[S]
110.	☐	Hedera helix	vine	berry, leaf	[I]
111.	☐	Hedysarum mackenzii	cultivated flower	seed	
112.	☐	Heliotropium species	weeds, cultiv. flowers	herbal teas	
113.	☐	Helleborus niger	cultiv. flower, houseplant	berry, all parts	[Q]
114.	☐	Hippeastrum species	cultiv. flower, houseplant	bulbs	
115.	☐	Hippomane mancinella	tree	fruit, dermatitis from all parts	
116.	■	Hura crepitans	tree	seed	[G]
117.	☐	Hyacinthus orientalis	cultivated flower	bulb	[M]

376

No.		Species	Growth form	Part / use	Ref.
118.	■	Hydrangea macrophylla	shrub	flower buds	[Z]
119.	□	Hyocyamus niger	weed	all parts	[F, U]
120.	□	Ilex aquifolium	tree	berry	[N]
120a.		Inga saman (see Samanea saman)			
121.	□	Ipomoea violacea	vine	hallucinogenic seed	[D]
122.	□	Iris germanica	cultivated flower	root	[D]
123.	□	Iris pseudoacorus	cultivated flower	root	[D]
124.	□	Iris species	cultivated flowers	roots	[M]
125.	■	Jatropha curcas	tree	seed	
126.	■	Jatropha gossypifolia	weed	seed	
127.	■	Jatropha hastata (= J. integerrima)	shrub	seed	
128.	■	Jatropha multifida	shrub to small tree	seed	[M]
129.	□	Jatropha stimulosa (= Cnidoscolus stimulosus)	weed	stinging needles	
130.		Juniperus sabina	evergreen shrub	herbal tea	[BB]
131.	PH	Kalmia angustifolia	shrub	—	[R]
132.	PH	Kalmia latifolia	shrub	—	[R]
133.		Karwinskia humboldtiana	shrub to small tree	seed	[CC]
134.	■	Laburnum anagyroides	tree	seed	[S]
135.	■	Lantana camara	weed, cultiv. flower	unripe berry	[W]
136.	■	Lathyrus species	vine	prolonged ingestion of seeds	
137.	PH	Leucothoe species	shrub	—	
138.	■	Ligustrum ovalifolium	shrub	berry	[N]
139.	■	Ligustrum vulgare	shrub	berry	[S]
140.	■	Ligustrum species	shrubs or small trees	berries	[S]
141.	■	Lobelia berlandieri	weed	all parts	[S]
142.	■	Lobelia cardinalis	wild & cultiv. flower	all parts	[S]
143.	■	Lobelia inflata	weed	all parts	
144.	■	Lobelia siphilitica	swamp wild flower	all parts	
145.	?	Lonicera periclymenum	vine	berry	[N]
146.	?	Lonicera tatarica	vine	berry	
147.	?	Lonicera xylosteum	vine	berry	
148.	□	Lophophora williamsii	cactus	all parts hallucinogenic	[N]

List II–Botanical Names of Poisonous Plants (*Cont.*)

		Name	Type of Plant	Poisonous Part	Refer to:
149.	☆	Lupinus species	cultivated flower	—	[U]
150.	☐	Lycium halimifolium	shrub	berry	[Z]
151.	**PH**	Lyonia species	shrubs	—	[Z]
152.	■	Manihot species	shrubs	uncooked root	[BB]
153.	■	Melia azedarach	tree	fruit	[BB]
154.	☐	Menispermum canadense	vine	fruit	
155.	☐	Mirabilis jalapa	cultivated flower	root, seed	[I]
156.	☐	Momordica charantia	weed vine	orange body of fruit	[C]
157.	☐	Monstera species	houseplants	leaf, stem	
158.	☐	Morus rubra	tree	unripe fruit, sap	
158a.		Mucuna deeringiana (see Stizolobium deeringianum)			
159.	☐	Myristica fragrans	tree	large quantity seed hallucinogenic	
160.	☐	Narcissus species	cultivated flowers	bulbs	[O]
161.	☐	Nerium indicum (= Nerium oleander)			[O]
162.	■	Nerium oleander	shrub	all parts	
163.	☆	Nicandra physalodes	weed	—	
164.	■	Nicotiana alata	cultivated flower	all parts	[T]
165.	■	Nicotiana attenuata	weed	all parts	[T]
166.	■	Nicotiana glauca	weed shrub, small tree	all parts	
167.	■	Nicotiana tabacum	cultivated tobacco	all parts	
168.	■	Nicotiana trigonophylla	weed	all parts	
169.	☆	Ochrosia elliptica	tree	—	[I]
170.	☐	Ornithogalum umbellatum	weed	flower, bulb	[N]
171.	☐	Pachyrhizus erosus	vine	seed	
172.	☐	Papaver somniferum	flower	opium source	[Y]
173.	☐	Pedilanthus tithymaloides	weed, cultiv. shrub	seed, milky juice	[E]
174.	**PH**	Pernettya species	shrubs	—	
175.	☐	Philodendron species	houseplant, vine	leaf	
176.	☐	Phoradendron flavescens (= P. serotinum)	parasitic plant on trees	berries in quantity, herbal tea	
177.	☐	Physalis species	decorative plant	unripe berries	

378

No.		Name	Type	Toxic part(s)	Ref.
178.	■	Phytolacca americana (= P. decandra)	weed	all parts except ripe berry	[D]
179.	PH	Pieris species	shrub to small tree	—	
180.	■	Pinus palustris	tree	turpentine	
180a.		Pithecellobium saman (see Samania saman)			
181.	□	Podophyllum peltatum	wild flower	all parts except ripe fruit	[D]
182.		Poinciana gilliesii (see Caesalpinia gilliesii)			
183.		Poinciana pulcherrima (see Caesalpinia pulcherrima)			
184.	□	Poncirus trifoliata	tree	fruit	[N]
185.	■	Pongamia pinnata	tree	seed, root	[I]
186.	□	Prunus species	shrubs and trees	seed kernels	[Z]
187.	□	Psedera quinquefolia	vine	fruit	[K, N]
188.	□	Quercus species	trees	acorns in quantity	
189.	■	Ranunculus acris	cultivated flower	all parts	
190.	■	Ranunculus bulbosus	cultivated flower	all parts	
191.	■	Ranunculus sceleratus	weed	all parts	
192.	■	Ranunculus species	wild & cultiv. flowers, weeds	all parts	[D]
193.	□	Rhamnus cathartica	tree	fruit, leaf	[N]
194.	□	Rhamnus frangula	tree	fruit, leaf	[K]
195.	□	Rhamnus species	trees and shrubs	fruit, leaves	[R]
196.	□	Rheum rhaponicum	cultivated garden plant	leaf in quantity	
197.	PH	Rhododendron species	shrubs	—	
198.	PH	Rhododendron macrophyllum	shrub	—	
199.	■	Rhodotypos kerriodes (= R. scandens, R. tetrapetala)	shrub	berry	[X]
200.	■	Ricinus communis	weed, cultivated ornamental	seed	[L]
201.	□	Rivea corymbosa	vine	hallucinogenic seed	[D]
202.	□	Rivina humilis	ornamental plant	all parts	[M]
203.	■	Robinia pseudoacacia	tree	bark, ? seed	[K]
204.	□	Rumex acetosa	weed	all parts	[K]
205.	□	Rumex species	weeds	all parts	
206.	□	Samanea saman	tree	seed	
207.	□	Sambucus specis	shrubs to small trees	unripe berries, sap	[I]

List II—Botanical Names of Poisonous Plants (*Cont.*)

	Name	Type of Plant	Poisonous Part	Refer to:
208.	□ Sapindus saponaria	tree	fruit	[I]
209.	Saponaria officinalis	weed	fruit	
210.	■ Sauromatum guttatum	cultivated flower	all parts	
211.	■ Scilla species	cultivated flowers	bulbs	
212.	□ Senecio species	weeds	herbal teas	
213.	Sesbania species (see Glottidium species)			
214.	□ Solandra species	vine	all parts except fruit	[E, F]
215.	□ Solanum aculeatissimum	weed	fruit	[F]
216.	■ Solanum carolinense	weed	fruit	[F]
217.	□ Solanum dulcamara	houseplant	fruit	[F]
218.	□ Solanum gracile	weed	unripe berry	[F]
219.	□ Solanum nigrum	weed, sometimes cultivated	unripe berry	[F]
	(= S. americanum)			
220.	□ Solanum pseudocapsicum	houseplant	fruit	[F]
221.	□ Solanum sodomeum	weed	fruit	
222.	□ Solanum tuberosum	vegetable	green colored skin, sprouts	[E]
223.	□ Sophora secundiflora	tree	seed	[E]
224.	□ Sophora tomentosa	tree	seed	[T]
225.	□ Spigelia marilandica	weed	all parts	[BB]
226.	☆ Strelitzia reginae	cultivated flower	—	
227.	□ Stizolobium deeringianum	vine	bean	
	(= Mucuna deeringiana)			
228.	■ Strychnos nux-vomica	tree	seed	[BB]
229.	□ Symphoricarpos albus	shrub	berry	[N]
	(= S. racemosus)			
230.	□ Symplocarpus foetidus	swamp plant	berry	[C]
230a.	Tabernaemontana divaricata (see Ervatamia coronaria)			
231.	■ Tanacetum vulgare	wild flower	herbal tea	
232.	■ Taxus baccata	tree	all parts, chewed seed	[BB]
233.	■ Taxus brevifolia	tree	all parts, chewed seed	
234.	■ Taxus canadensis	shrub	all parts, chewed seed	

380

		Species	Form	Toxic part	
235.	■	Taxus cuspidata	shrub or small tree	all parts, chewed seed	[H]
236.	■	Taxus species	shrubs or trees	all parts	
237.	■	Thevetia peruviana (= T. neriifolium)	small tree	all parts	
238.	■	Thuja occidentalis	tree	herbal tea	[F]
239.	■	Thuja orientalis	tree	herbal tea	
240.	□	Ulex species	shrubs	beans	
241.	■	Urechites lutea	vine or shrublike	all parts	[Q]
242.	□	Urginea maritima	cultivated flower	bulb	
243.	□	Veratrum californicum	wild flower	all parts	[B]
244.	□	Veratrum viride	wild flowers	all parts	
245.	□	Wisteria species	vines	seeds	[Z]
246.	□	Xanthosoma species	houseplants	leaf, uncooked root	[C]
247.	□	Zamia species	palm-like plant	uncooked root	
248.	□	Zantedeschia aethiopica	houseplant	all parts	[R]
249.	■	Zygadenus species	wild flowers	bulbs	
250.	■	Zygadenus venenosus	wild flower	bulb	

RASH-PRODUCING PLANTS

The following list of botanical and common names of rash-producing plants was compiled by Kenneth Lampe, Ph.D., and his research associate Mary Ann McCann. Each of these plants has caused a rash on someone, either by direct chemical action or allergy. This doesn't mean that you or your child will get a rash from handling these plants—but you might. If you have a family history of sensitive skin or skin allergy, you may wish to avoid planting an itchy garden. If you develop a rash from unknown causes, get your Sherlock Holmes cap and consider the 185 plants listed here.

Key: The number following the common names in List I refers to the number of the botanical name in List II.

LIST I
COMMON NAMES OF RASH-PRODUCING PLANTS

Agave, 6
Algae, fresh water 14
Algae, salt water 114
Algerian ivy 86
Ash 80
Australian silk oak 85
Balsam fir 1
Barberry bush 27
Beggar-ticks 7
Bermuda grass 52
Birdseye primrose 142
Black-eyed Susan 157
Black walnut 107
Bleeding heart 61
Bloodtwig dogwood 50
Blue gum 68
Boat lily 153
Box elder 2
Boxwood 29
Brazilian pepper tree 162
Brazil nut 28
Bulbous buttercup 150
Bull bay 116
Bull nettle 47
Burning bush 63
Buttercup 152
California blue bell 132
Candelabra cactus 69
Caper spurge 70
Carrot 60
Cashew nut 15
Castor plant 155
Celery 20
Century plant 16
Chevil, wild 19
Chrysanthemum 41
Cocklebur 185
Copper weed 123

Coral sumac 118
Cow parsley 19
Cow parsnip 92
Crab grass 65
Cresote bush 110
Crown flower 30
Crown of thorns 72
Cuckoo-pint 25
Cursed crowfoot 151
Daffodil 120
Dalmation chrysanthemum 33
Daphne 59
Dock 158
Dog fennel 28
Dog grass 8
Dumb cane 64
Eastern poison oak 171
Elm 176
English elm 176
English ivy 87
Eyebane 75
Feverfew 39
Fig 76
Fleabane daisy 67
Gailardia 81
Garlic 4
Gas plant 63
Giant hogweed 91
Grasses 8, 52, 65
Guayule 124
Hogweed, giant 91
Holly, Florida 162
Hop 96
Horse apple 115
Horse nettle 165
Hyacinth
Ivy, Algerian 86
Ivy, English 87

LIST II
BOTANICAL NAMES OF RASH-PRODUCING PLANTS

19 Anthriscus sylvestris
20 Apium graveolens
21 Argemone mexicana
22 Aristolochia elegans
23 Artemisia ludoviciana
24 Artemisia vulgaris
25 Arum maculatum
26 Asimina triloba
27 Berberis species
28 Bertholletia excelsa
29 Buxus sempervirens
30 Calotropis gigantea
31 Calotropis procera
32 Campsis radicans
33 Chrysanthemum cinerariaefolium
34 Chrysanthemum coccineum
35 Chrysanthemum leucanchemum
36 Chrysanthemum marshallicarneum
37 Chrysanthemum maximum
38 Chrysanthemum morifolium
39 Chrysanthemum parthenium
40 Chrysanthemum roseum
41 Chrysanthemum species
42 Citrus aurantifolia
43 Citrus aurantium
44 Citrus limonia
45 Citrus paradisi
46 Clematis species
47 Cnidoscolus stimulosus
48 Corchorus capsularis
49 Corchorus olitorius
50 Cornus sanguinea
51 Covillea glutinosus
52 Cynodon dactylon
53 Cypripedium acaule
54 Cypripedium calceolus
55 Cypripedium candidum
56 Cypripedium reginae
57 Cypripedium species
58 Daphne mezereum
59 Daphne species
60 Daucus carota
61 Dicentra spectabilis
62 Dichondra repens
63 Dictamnus albus
64 Dieffenbachia species
65 Digitaria sanguinalis
66 Dirca palustris
67 Erigeron canadensis
68 Eucalyptus globulus
69 Euphorbia lactea
70 Euphorbia lathyrus
71 Euphorbia marginatum
72 Euphorbia milii
73 Euphorbia pulcherrima
74 Euphorbia tirucalli
75 Euphorbia species
76 Ficus carica

77 Ficus pumila
78 Ficus repens
79 Franseria acanthicarpa
80 Fraxinus species
81 Gaillardia species
82 Geranium species
83 Ginkgo biloba
84 Grevillea banksii
85 Grevillea robusta
86 Hedera canariensis
87 Hedera helix
88 Helenium autumnale
89 Helenium microcephalum
90 Heracleum dulce
91 Heracleum mantegazzianum
92 Heracleum species
93 Hespernocnide species
94 Hippomane mancinella
95 Humulus lupulus
96 Humulus species
97 Hura crepitans
98 Hyacinthus orientalis
99 Hyacinthus species
100 Hydrangea species
101 Iva angustifolia
102 Iva xanthifolia
103 Jacaranda species
104 Jatropha stimulosa
105 Jatropha urens
106 Jatropha species
107 Juglans nigra
108 Lactuca sativa
109 Laportea canadensis
110 Larrea tridentata
111 Leptilon canadense
112 Libocedrus decurrens
113 Lycopersicon esculentum
114 Lyngbya majuscula
115 Maclura pomifera
116 Magnolia grandiflora
117 Mangifera indica
118 Metopium toxiferum
119 Narcissus jonquilla
120 Narcissus species
121 Nerium oleander
122 Oryza sativa
123 Oxytenia acerosa
124 Parthenium argentatum
125 Parthenium hysterophorus
126 Pastinaca sativa
127 Pastinaca urens
128 Phacelia crenulata
129 Phacelia grandiflora
130 Phacelia parryi
131 Phacelia viscida
132 Phacelia whitlavia
133 Philodendron cordatum
134 Philodendron oxycardium

135 Philodendron scandens-cardatum
136 Philodendron selloum
137 Philodendron speciosum
138 Philodendron species
139 Phoradendron flavescens
140 Populus species
141 Primula cortudoides
142 Primula farinosa
143 Primula obconica
144 Primula sieboldii
145 Prosopis juliflora
146 Psoralea carylifolia
147 Psoralea species
148 Pulsatilla patens
149 Ranunculus acris
150 Ranunculus bulbosus
151 Ranunculus sceleratus
152 Ranunculus species
153 Rhoeo discolor
154 Rhoeo spathacea
        Rhus species (see Toxicodendron)
155 Ricinus communis
156 Rosa odorata
157 Rudbeckia species
158 Rumex species
159 Ruta graveolens

160 Sarcobatus vermiculatus
161 Schinopsis lorentzii
162 Schinus terebinthfolius
163 Secale cereale
164 Setcreasea purpurea
165 Solanum carolinense
166 Syntherisma sanguinale
167 Tagetes minuta
168 Tanacetum vulgare
169 Tectona grandis
170 Toxicodendron diversilobum
171 Toxicodendron quercifolium
172 Toxicodendron radicans
173 Toxicodendron vernix
174 Toxicodendron species
175 Tulipa species
176 Ulmus species
177 Urtica californica
178 Urtica chamaedryoides
179 Urtica dioica
180 Urtica urens
181 Vitis vinifera
182 Wigandia caracasana
183 Xanthium spinosum
184 Xanthium strumarium
185 Xanthium species

LISTS OF MINERALS AND VITAMINS IN FOODS

The following lists are adapted from "Composition of Foods," Agriculture Handbook No. 456, Agricultural Research Service, United States Department of Agriculture. Their extensive list of nutritional components of 1,500 foods is available from the U.S. Government Printing Office, Washington, D.C. 20402 for $5.15.[24] Some approximations have been made in order to allow for simplifying the lists.

In all lists, the amount of the nutrient is measured in edible portions of 100 grams or 3⅓ ounces. The following symbols appear after some foods:

X = check other forms of the same food
# = an approximation
+ = a fortified food
! = contains a trace
R = raw
C = canned
CO = cooked
* = all of contents may not be released

MINERAL REQUIREMENTS

Calcium 0.4 to 1.4 grams (See page 386.)

Copper
    Average daily requirement: 0.15–10.0 mg.
    Sources: Liver, oysters, meat, fish, whole grains, nuts, legumes

Fluoride
  Average daily requirement: 0.5–1 mg.
  Sources: Water (in some areas), sea foods, other foods grown on soil containing fluoride
Iodine
  Average daily requirement for infants: 25–45 micrograms
  Children 1–10 years is 55–110 micrograms; 10–18 years is 125–150 micrograms.
  Sources: Iodized salt, sea foods, foods grown where there is iodine in the soil
Iron 6 to 18 milligrams (See page 388.)
Magnesium (See page 390.)
Zinc
  Average daily requirements: Unknown
  Sources: All foods

Calcium

The average daily requirement for calcium is 0.4–0.6 grams for infants, 0.7–1.0 grams for children under 10 years, and 1.2–1.4 grams for children over 10 years of age. Calcium is essential to bone growth. The best source is cow's milk. Because of problems with milk allergy or intolerance, some children may receive less than optimal calcium in the form of milk, and other sources such as soybean formulas or foods will have to be used.

It should be recognized that having a nutrient in a food does not necessarily mean that it will be absorbed. Some of the calcium in whole milk may combine with milk fat to form undigestible bulky chemical compounds that are passed in the stool. Oxalic acid in foods such as beet greens, rhubarb, spinach, and swiss chard will combine with calcium or magnesium, preventing their release. Oxalic acid in these vegetables may even combine with the calcium or magnesium content of other foods, actually depleting the amount of these minerals available to the body. The phosphorus in nuts, beans, and the outer layer of cereal grain may combine with some of their calcium, magnesium, or iron content and pass unabsorbed through the intestinal tract.

List of Foods Containing Calcium

Unless otherwise shown, cooked, ready-to-eat (3⅓ ounce) portions contain:

Above 200 mgm of calcium
  * Almonds
  Baby cereal, dry
  Carob flour
  Cheese
  Collards
  X Oat cereal shredded
  C Salmon, Pacific
  Sardines
  Seaweed
  Smelt

Above 100 mgm of calcium
  Bread, white with milk solids
X#* Bread, whole wheat
  Buckwheat
  Buttermilk
  Cream

  Dandelion greens
  Egg yolk
C Herring
  Ice cream
  Kale
CX Mackerel
  Milk, cow's
  Mustard greens
X Oat flakes
  Rennen products
  Scallops
  Soybeans
  Turnip greens

Above 50 mgm of calcium
  Beans, snap
  Beans, white

* Beet greens
Bran
Bread
Broccoli
* Chard
Clams
Cornbread
Egg, whole
Endive
Farina, quick cooking
Fishcake
Lobster
X Oats, puffed
Onions, green
Oysters
Peanuts
X Peas
Prunes, dehydrated
Raisins, uncooked
* Rhubarb
Rutabagas
Salmon, Atlantic
Shrimp
* Spinach
*X Walnuts, English
X Wheat, shredded

Above 25 mgm of calcium
Beans, red
Beans, lima
Breakfast cereals
Brussels sprouts
Cabbage
Cakes
Carrots
Cod
Cowpeas
Crab
Crackers, saltine and graham
Figs, raw
\# Flounder
Haddock
\# Lettuce
Lima beans
\# Loganberries
Milk, human
Perch
Oranges
Potato chips
Raisins, cooked
\# Raspberries
Squash
Sweet potato
Turnips

X Wheat, puffed

Above 10 mgm of calcium
Apricots
Asparagus
Bacon
Beets
Berries
X Bread, Italian
Cauliflower
Celery
Cherries
Chicken
Coconut
Cornflakes
Cucumbers
\# Grapefruit
Halibut
Ham
Kidneys
\# Lamb
Liver
\# Macaroni
\# Noodles
X\# Oatmeal
Orange juice
CX Peas
Pineapple and juice
Plums
Pumpkin
Rabbit
Rice
Tomato
Veal
X Wheat

Below 10 mgm of calcium
Apple juice
\# Beef, raw
Corn
Farina, regular
Heart
Hickory nuts
Hominy
Mackerel, cooked
Peaches
Pears
Pork
\#X Potato
Sausage
Tomato juice
Tuna
Turkey
X* Walnuts, black

Iron

The average daily iron requirements for infants is 6–15 milligrams; for children 1 to 3 years it is 15 mgm; for 3 to 12 years it is 10 mgm; and for 12 to 18 years it is 18 mgm. In presenting a list of "iron containing foods," we acknowledge that recognized nutritional experts still talk about "our present muddled views of iron in nutrition." This hasn't changed too much since the days when people assumed spinach is "a good food because it contains a lot of iron"—only to find later that much of its iron is unabsorbed by the body. Even egg yolk, an acknowledged source of iron, is being challenged as a good iron source; there is a question about whether its iron is released for utilization. Nonetheless, nutritionists point to the fact that an egg a day seems to work in improving nutrition and preventing anemia. This is aside from the question of its high cholesterol content. The nutritionists also report that the processing and grinding of wheat makes its iron more available than that from non-ground wheat. Furthermore, they have shown that foods cooked in iron utensils have more iron in them than those cooked in glass. The following list reflects our current state of knowledge.

List of Iron Containing Foods

Unless otherwise shown, cooked and ready to eat (3⅓ ounce) portions contain:

Above 50 mgm of iron
+ Baby cereals
   Fish flour (whole)

Above 10 mgm of iron
X Cocoa dry powders
+ Corn, flaked
   Liver
   Molasses, blackstrap
   Potato flour
X Syrup, sorghum
Soybean flours
   Wheat bran
Wheat germ

Above 4 mgm of iron
 * Almonds
X Apricots, dried
   Bran
   Buttermilk
X Chicken giblets
   Chickpeas
   Clams
+# Corn, puffed cereal
*? Egg yolk
X Fish flour, filets
Heart
   Kidneys
X Molasses
X+ Oats, puffed or flaked
   Oysters
   Peaches, dried
   Prunes, dried

   Sardines, Pacific canned
   Seaweed
#X Sugar, brown
 * Walnuts
#X Wheat, whole
X Wheat
X+ Wheat, cold cereals

Above 1 mgm of iron
X Apple, dried
   Artichokes
   Baby liver or beef with cereal
   Baby meat, strained
X Baby peas and beans
   Bacon
   Barley
   Beans
CX Beans, green, and wax
   Beef
   Brazil nuts
+X Bread, white, enriched
X Bread, wheat
   Brussels sprouts
   Buckwheat
Candy
   Chard
X Chicken
   Chocolate
X Cocoa milk powders
   Coconut
   Corn flour
   Corn flakes
   Corn bread

Cowpeas
X Crackers, graham
X Crackers, saltines
Dandelion greens
Dates
X Egg, whole
X Figs, dried
Fish
Frankfurters
Groundcherries
Kale
Lamb
Mustard greens
X Oat cereals
Peanuts
X Peas, canned
X Peas, split
Pickles
Popcorn
Pork
X Potatoes, French fries
X Potato chips
X Prunes
Rabbit
Raisins
+ Rice, puffed
# Rye flour
Sausage (lunchmeat)
Scallops
Syrup cane
Soybean
Spaghetti
Squash, acorn
Spinach
Squash, butternut
Squash, winter
Strawberries
Sweet potatoes
Tongue
Turkey
Turnip greens
Veal
Wheat flour
* Whole wheat

Over 0.5 mgm of iron
Apple juice
Asparagus
Avocados
X# Baby dinners
X Baby prunes with tapioca
X Baby vegetables
Bananas
X Beans, green and wax, boiled
Beets
Blackberries
Blueberries
X Bread: white, Italian and French,
unenriched

Broccoli
Carrots
Cauliflower
Cheeses
Collards
X Corn
Crab
X Crackers, whole wheat
Eggplant
+ Farina
X# Figs
Halibut
Lettuce
Lobster
Macaroni
Noodles
X Oatmeal
Onions
Parsnips
X Peas
Plums
X Potatoes, cooked
Raspberries
Rhubarb
+**X** Rice
Soups, bean
X Soybean milk
#**X** Spaghetti
Tomatoes
X Wheat flour
X Wheat, hot cereal

Under 0.5 mgm of iron
X Apple
Apricots
X Baby fruit
Beer
Cabbage
Celery
X Cereal, breakfast
Cherries
Cranberry juice
Cucumbers
Grapefruit
Lemon
! Milk, cow's
Milk, human (0.1 mgm)
Melons
Oranges
Peaches
Pineapple
X Rice

Under 0.5 Mgm of iron
X Soups
X Squash
X Sugar cane
Turnips

Magnesium

The average daily requirement of magnesium for infants is 40–70 milligrams; for children, 1–3 years is 100–150 mgm; for 3–12 years is 200–300 mgm; and for 12–18 years is 350–400 mgm. Magnesium has long been recognized as essential, but dietary information has been lacking. As more information is gathered, it appears that the magnesium content of the diet may prove to be of importance, so the following list is included in *The Parents' Medical Manual*.

List of Foods Containing Magnesium

Unless otherwise shown, cooked and ready to eat 3⅓ ounce portions contain:

Over 150 mgm of magnesium
  * Nuts
    Cottonseed flour
    Soybean
    Wheat cereal, bran and shredded

Over 100 mgm of magnesium
    Beet greens, raw
    Chocolate syrup
  X Molasses, blackstrap
    Oats
    Salt, dry
  X* Wheat flour, whole

Over 20 mgm of magnesium
    Beans
    Banana
  X Beets, raw
    Blackberry
    Breads
    Broccoli
    Brussels sprouts
    Buckwheat flour
    Carrots

    Celery
    Cheeses
    Chocolate milk
    Coconut
  X Corn
    Cornmeal (under 10)
    Crackers
    Dandelion greens
    Fish
  # Fowl
    Macaroni
  # Meat
  X Molasses
    Peaches, dried
    Peas
  # Potato
    Raisins, dry
    Raspberries, fresh
    Rice, brown
    Rye flour
  * Spinach
    Sweet potato
  X Wheat flour

LISTS OF ESSENTIAL VITAMINS

Vitamin A
  1,500 to 5,000 IU/day Vitamin A precursors (See page 391.)
Vitamin C
  35 to 60 mgm/day (See page 393.)
Vitamin D
  The average daily requirement is 400 IU. Sources: Sunshine or ultraviolet light on the skin. Fortified milk and margarine, fish liver oils.
Vitamin E
  The average daily requirement for infants is 5 IU; children 1–6 years 10 IU; 10–14 years 20 IU; 14–18 years 25 IU. Sources: Vegetable fats, seeds, nuts, eggs, leafy vegetables.
Vitamin K
  The average daily requirement is 1–2 mgm a day. Sources: Green leafy vegetables, soybeans, fish, and intestinal bacteria.

THE B COMPLEX VITAMINS

Vitamin B 1
> The average daily requirement for infants is 0.2–0.5 mgm; children 2–10 years 0.6–1.1 mgm; 10 years and older 1.2–1.5 mgm. Sources: Meat, milk, whole grain cereal, wheat germ, legumes, nuts. (See page 393.)

Vitamin B 2
> The average daily requirement for infants is 0.4–0.6 mgm; children 2–10 years 0.6–1.2 mgm; 10 years and over 1.3–1.5 mgm. Sources: Milk, fish, poultry, liver, whole grain and enriched cereals, green leafy vegetables, eggs, beans. (See page 393.)

Vitamin B 6
> The average daily requirements for infants is 0.2–0.4 mgm; children 1–10 years 0.5–1.2 mgm; 10–18 years 1.4–1.8 mgm. If abnormal metabolism exists, requirements may increase to 5–10 mgm. Sources: Meat, liver, kidney, whole grains, peanuts, soybeans.

Vitamin B 12
> The average daily requirements for infants is 1–2 micrograms; children 1–18 years 2–5 micrograms. Sources: Meat, sweetbreads, fish, eggs, milk, cheese.

Folic Acid Group
> The average daily requirements for infants is 1–2 micrograms; children 1–18 years 2–5 micrograms. Sources: Liver, green vegetables, nuts, cereal, cheese.

Niacin
> The average daily requirements for infants is 5–8 mgm; children 2–10 years 8–15 mgm; 15–20 years is 20 mgm. Sources: Meat, fish, poultry, liver, whole grain and enriched cereals, green vegetables, peanuts. (See page 393.)

Vitamin A

The average daily requirement of vitamin A for up to 1 year of age is 1,500 IU/day; for 1 to 12 year olds, 2,000 to 4,500 IU/day; for over 12-year-olds, 5,000 IU/day of vitamin A precursors. If pure vitamin A is taken, then 900 to 3,000 IU is adequate.

List of Foods Containing Vitamin A

Per 3⅓ ounce portions:

Over 10,000 U
X Apricots, dried
  Carrots
  Dandelion greens
  Liver
X Peppers, red

  Mustard greens
  Pumpkin, canned
  Spinach
  Sweet potatoes
  Turnip greens

Over 5,000 U
  Braunschweiger
  Chard
  Collards
\# Giblets
  Kale
  Liverwurst

Over 1,000 U
X Apricots
  Broccoli
  Butter
  Cheeses
  Chicken stewed with skin
  Crab
X Cream

Eggs
Melons
Onions, green
X Peaches, dried and fresh
X Plums, purple
Prunes
X Squash, winter
Swordfish
Whitefish

Over 500 U
Asparagus
Beet greens
Brussels sprouts
X Cherries, sour
X Cream substitutes
Halibut
Herring
X Ice cream
Kidney
Lettuce
Mackerel
Peaches, cooked
Peas
Peppers, sweet
Pork sausage
Rutabagas

Over 100 U
Avocados
Bananas
Beans, snap
Beans, lima
Cabbage
Celery
Cereals, breakfast
X Chicken

Cod
X Corn
X Corn breakfast cereals
Cowpeas
Frankfurters
Grapefruit, pink and red
Grapes
Ice milk
Loganberries
X Milk (skimmed has trace only)
Milk, human
Oranges
Oysters
Pickles
X Plums
Salmon
X Squash, summer
Tomatoes
Tuna

Over 40 U
Apple
Beef, patty
Berries
Fish
Cauliflower, raw
Cottage cheese, creamed
X Cherries, sweet
Chicken, lean
Dates
Noodles
Pineapple
Rhubarb
Soups, canned
Soybean milk
Strawberries
Yogurt

List of Foods Containing B Complex Vitamins
(Thiamine, Riboflavin, Niacin)

In portions of $3\frac{1}{3}$ ounces:

Good in all B complex vitamins
Almonds
Apple
Apricots
Baby dinners
Beets
Berries
+X Breads
Buttermilk
Cabbage
Candy
Carrots
Cauliflower
Celery
Chard
Cheese
Cherries
Cucumbers
Grapefruit
Lemon
Lettuce
Macaroni
Milk
Melons
Mustard greens
Oats
Oranges
Peas
Pineapple
Plums
Potato
Soybean
Spaghetti
Spinach
Squash

Sweet potato
Tomato
Turnips
Wines
Yogurt

High in some B complex vitamins
Asparagus
Avocados
+ Baby cereals
Bananas
Barley
Beans
Bran
Bread, enriched
Broccoli
Brussels sprouts
Chicken
Collards
Corn
Cowpeas
Crab
Egg
+ Farina
Fish
Heart
Kale
Kidneys
Liver meats
Nuts
Peanuts
Prunes
+ Rice
Walnuts
+ Wheat

Vitamin C

The average daily requirements for Vitamin C for infants is 35 mgm.; 1–12 years is 40 mgm.; 10–18 years is 40–60 mgm.

List of Foods Containing Vitamin C

In $3\frac{1}{3}$ ounce portions:

Over 1,000 mgm
R X Acerola (Barbados or
West Indian cherry)

Over 50 mgm
CO Broccoli
CO Brussels sprouts

R Cauliflower
CO Collards
R # Currants
R Guava
Kale
R X Lemons
R Limes

R # Oranges and juice
R Pawpaws
R Papayas
R Peppers, hot
R # Peppers, sweet
R Persimmons
Pimientos
R X Spinach
R X Strawberries
X Turnip greens
Watercress

Over 25 mgm
CO X Asparagus
C + Baby banana
R Beet greens
R Cabbage
CO Cauliflower
Cantaloupe
+ Cranberry juice
R Elderberries
R Grapefruit
CO Liver
R X Loganberries
R Lychee
R Mangos
CO Mustard greens
R X Onions, green
R Oysters, Pacific
R Radishes
C X Raspberries
CO Spinach
R CO Tomato
CO X Turnip greens

Over 10 mgm
X Apples, dried
R X Apricots (fresh and dehydrated)
C X Asparagus
R Avocados
C Baby liver and bacon
C Baby peas
C # Baby sweet potatoes
R Banana
CO X Beans, lima
CO X Beans, snap
R X Beets
R X Berries
C Cabbage
R Casaba Melon
R # Celery
CO Chard
R Cherries
R Clams
CO Cowpeas
R Cucumbers
CO Dandelion greens
R Endive

C Garbanzos
R X Lettuce, cos or romaine
C Limeade
R Muskmelons
CO Okra
CO Parsnips
CO Peas
R Pineapple
C Pineapple Juice
CO Potatoes, baked, fried, boiled
C Sauerkraut
CO Soybeans
C Spinach
CO Squash, summer
CO Squash, winter
C Strawberries
C Sweet potato
C Tomato
C Tomato juice
CO Turnips

Over 5 mgm
C X Beans, lima
CO X Beets
C X Berries
R X Carrots
CO Celery
CO C Corn
CO Giblets
C X Lemonade
R X Lettuce
C X Loganberries
R Milk, human
CO X Onions
R X Peaches
C Pickles
C X Pineapple
R X Plums
C Pumpkin
C X Raspberries
CO Rhubarb
C X Sweet potato

Over 2 mgm
R X Apples
C X Apricots
C X Beans, snap
C X Carrots
C Cherries
CO Crab
CO Eggplant
Grapes
X Haddock
CO # Heart
C Peaches
C X Plums
R Prunes
C X Soybeans

Trace or 1 mgm
   + Breads
   Milk, cow's
   Raisins

None
   Beef

Chicken
Corn flour
X Fish
Lamb
Rice
X Soybean milk
Soybean flour

CHOLESTEROL AND FAT[3,4]

The average American diet is high in cholesterol and saturated fats, which may, in some individuals, lead to the later complications of heart attacks and strokes. This is not meant to imply that everyone on such a diet will have problems. Our ability to handle such foods differs and there are undoubtedly some people who can eat all the cholesterol and saturated fats they desire without harm, while for some, even small amounts of these substances can cause problems early in life. And most people who consistently and vigorously exercise, don't overeat, and "burn up" fats probably need not be too concerned about such dietary intake. But in general, it is best to limit your intake of the high cholesterol foods in the following lists, and to substitute polyunsaturated fats for saturated fats as much as possible.

Saturated fats are usually of animal origin: animal fat, hydrogenated solid vegetable shortening, and coconut oil. Eliminate lard, suet, salt pork, bacon drippings, and vegetable shortenings, and avoid fatty meats. Refrigerate meat drippings and remove the hardened fat; gravies made from the remaining *meat juice are* allowable.

Polyunsaturated fats are usually of plant origin: safflower oil (excellent), corn oil (excellent), olive oil, peanut oil, and mayonnaise. These should be used in cooking and in dressings.

List of Foods Containing Cholesterol

In 100 gram (3⅓ ounce) portions

Very high cholesterol—above 100 mgm			
Animal hearts	231	Sponge cake	246
Animal kidneys	804	Sweetbreads	466
Brains	2,000	Turkey skin	127
Butter	250	Whipping cream	133
Caviar	300	Whole egg	504
Cheese souffle	167		
Crab imperial	140	*High Cholesterol—51 to 100 mgm*	
Cream puffs (custard)	144	Beef, lean	94
Egg yolk	1,480	Beef, fat	74
Ladyfingers	356	Cheese, cream	111
Lemon chiffon pie	169	Cheeses, general type	87–102
Liver	438	Cheese, Mozzarella	66
Lobster Newburg	182	Cheese, Neufchatel	76
Omelet with milk fat	411	Cheese, ricotta	51
Popovers	147	Cheese, American pasteurized	72
Roe, salmon, raw	360	Cheese, American spread	64
Sardines, canned	120	Chicken	87
Shrimp	150	Cookies, brownies	83
		Cornbread	70

Crab, deviled	102
Cream, table	66–85
Fish	60–94
Frankfurter	62
Lamb, lean	98
Lamb, fat	100
Lobster, meat	85
Noodles, dry	94
Pancakes	74
Pie, custard	105
Pie, lemon meringue	93
Pie, pumpkin	61
Pork	89
Potato salad with eggs	65
Rabbit	91
Salad dressing and mayonnaise	70
Sausage	62
Turkey, light meat	77
Turkey, dark meat	86
Turkey, skin	127
Veal	99
Waffles	60

Low Cholesterol—50 mgm and under

Beef stew	26
Beef (dried, chipped, creamed)	27
Beef pot pie	21
Bread, white or French	50
Bread pudding	64
Cake, chocolate	43
Cake, fruitcake	45
Cake, gingerbread	1
Cake, white	2
Cake, yellow	44
Cheese, hoop	50
Cheese, mozzarella	50
Cheese, sapsago	50
Cheese sauce	18
Cheese straws	32
Chicken fricassee	40
Chicken pot pie, homemade	31

Chicken pot pie, commercial	13
Chicken and noodles	40
Chop suey with meat	26
Chow mein	31
Chow mein, canned	12
Clams	50
Corn pudding	42
Cream, half and half	43
Fish, cod	50
Fish, flounder	50
Fish, halibut	50
Frog legs	50
Ice cream, regular	40
Ice cream, milk	20
Ice cream, soft serve	20
Macaroni and cheese	21
Margarine, one-third vegetable	50
Margarine, all vegetable	0
Milk, whole	14
Milk, low fat	6
Milk, canned, condensed	31
Milk, hot chocolate	14
Noodles, cooked	31
Oysters	50
Oyster stew	26
Pie, apple	0
Pie, peach	0
Potatoes au gratin	15
Potatoes, scalloped	6
Puddings, cooked	12
Puddings, rice	11
Rabbit	91
Salad dressing, mayonnaise-type	50
Salmon, canned	35
Spaghetti with meat balls	30
Tartar sauce	51
Turkey pot pie—homemade	31
Turkey pot pie—frozen	9
Welsh rarebit	31
White sauce	14
Yogurt	8

FOOD ALLERGY LISTS

Food allergies can cause symptoms varying from hives, swollen lips and ears, wheezing, eczema, fatigue, stuffy nose, swollen joints, diarrhea, cramps, headaches, hyperactivity, and emotional problems. Allergy is "the great masquerader." In a sense, foods, too, are great masqueraders. It is remarkable how many things contain an unsuspected common food, for example corn. The following list is of foods most commonly found to produce allergies.

Most food allergies come from eating the food; however, there are a number of people who react with a rash if the food touches their skin. This contact type of allergy is more common than many people realize. It becomes very hard to track down the cause, if it *is* food, because food substances are contained in a large number of items from envelope glue to toothpaste.

List of Foods Containing Wheat[5]

Key: *Some varieties of these foods can be obtained without wheat.

Beverages: Ale, beer*, cocomalt, coffee substitutes, gin, grain neutral spirits, malted milk, Ovaltine, Postum, whiskies.

Breads: Biscuits, corn*, crackers, gluten, graham, muffins, popovers, pretzels, pumpernickel, rolls, rye, soy, and white breads.

Cereals: All-bran, Apple Jacks, Bran, Cheerios, Corn, Crackles, Cream of Wheat, Farina, Grapenuts, Kix, Krumbles, Lucky Charms, Malted cereals, Muffets, Pep, Puffed Wheat, Rice Krispies, Raisin Bran, Shredded Wheat, Sugar Smacks, Team, Total, Triscuits, and Wheat Chex.

Flours: All-purpose cracked wheat, buckwheat, cake, corn, enriched entire wheat, gluten patent, graham, lima bean, pastry, phosphated durum flour, rice*, rye*, white, whole wheat, self-rising.

Others:

Bisques	Fowl rolled in flour	Puddings
Bologna	Gravies	Ravioli
Bouillon cubes	Griddle cakes	Rusk
Breaded foods	Hamburger	Salad dressing*
Cakes	Hot cakes	Sauces
Candies*	Ice cream cones	Semolina
Chili con carne*	Liverwurst	Some yeasts
Chocolate candy	Lunch meat	Soup alphabets
Chowders	Macaroni	Soup rings
Cooked meat dishes	Malt products	Spaghetti
Cookies*	Matzos	Swiss steak
Cream soups	Mayonnaise*	Synthetic pepper
Croquettes*	Meat rolled in flour	Thickening in ice creams
Custards	Meat soups	Waffles
Dumplings	Mostaccioli	Weiners
Fats used for frying	Most cooked sausages	Wheat cakes
Fish patties	Pancakes	Wheat germ
Fish rolled in flour	Pastry	Zwieback
Foods rolled in flour	Pies	

Foods and Contacts Containing Corn[6]

Adhesives:	Boxes (paper)
Envelopes	Breads
Stamps	Cakes
Stickers	Candy
Tapes	Canned (fruits, peas, string beans)
Ale	Capsules (fillers and gelatine)
Aspirin	Carbonated beverages
Bacon	Catsups
Baking mixes	Cheerios
Baking powders	Cheeses
Bath powders	Chewing (gum)
Batters for frying	Chili
Beers	Chop suey
Beets (Harvard)	Cookies
Beverages (carbonated)	Confectioner's sugar
Blanc mange	Corn flakes
Bleached wheat flours	Corn (fresh—cooking fumes)
Bologna	Corn soya
Bourbon and other whiskies	Corn Toasties

Cough syrups
Crackels
Cream O Soy
Cream pies
Cream puffs
Cups (paper)
Custards
Dates (confection)
Deep fat frying mixtures
Dentifrices
Envelopes (adhesive)
Excipients (or diluents in) :
  Capsules
  Lozenges
  Ointment
  Suppositories
  Tablets
  Vitamins
Flour (bleached)
Foods (fried)
French dressing
Fritos
Frostings
Frozen (fruits)
Fruits (canned, frozen)
Fruit juices
Fried foods
Frying fats
Gelatin capsules
Gelatin dessert
Gin
Glucose products
Graham crackers
Grape juice
Gravies
Grits
Gum (chewing)
Gummed:
  Envelopes
  Labels
  Stamps
  Stickers
Hams (cured, tenderized)
Harvard beets
Holiday type stickers
Ice cream
Ices
Inhalants:
  Bath powders
  Body powders
  Cooking fumes of fresh corn
  Popcorn
  Starch
  Starch from ironing starched clothing
Jams
Jellies
Jello
Kixs

Kremel
Linit
Liquors—ale, beer, gin, whiskey
Lozenges (filler)
Lunch meat (ham)
Meats:
  Bacon
  Bologna
  Cooked (with gravies)
  Ham (cured or tenderized)
  Lunch ham
  Sausages (cooked)
  Weiners (frankfurters)
Medications (tablet filler)
Milk (in paper cartons)
Mono-sodium glutamate
Mull-soy
Nabisco
Nescafe
Ointment (filler)
Oleomargarine
Pablum
Paper:
  Boxes
  Cups
  Plates
Pastries
Peanut butters
Peas (canned)
Pies (creamed)
Pills (tablet filler)
Plastic food wrappers coated with
  cornstarch
Plates (paper)
Popcorn
Post Toasties
Powdered sugar
Powders (bath and body)
Preserves
Puddings
Salt:
  A&P Four Seasons salt
  Salt cellars in restaurants
Salad dressings
Sandwich spreads
Sauces for:
  Sundaes
  Meats
  Fish
  Vegetables
Sausages (cooked or table ready)
Sherbets
Soap (Zest)
Soups:
  Creamed
  Thickened
  Vegetable
Soy bean milks

Stamps (adhesive)
Starch
Starch from ironing starched clothing
Stickers (adhesive)
String beans (canned, frozen)
Sugar (powdered)
Suppositories (filler)
Syrups (commercially prepared) :
  Cartose
  Cough
  Glucose
  Karo
  Medicated
  Puretose
  Sweetose
Tablets (filler or flavor)

Talcums
Tapes (adhesive)
Teas (instant)
Toothpaste—Craig-Martin & Bost
Tortillas
Vegetables:
  Canned
  Creamed
  Frozen
Vinegar (distilled)
Vitamins (filler)
Weiners
Whiskies
Yeasts
Zest (soap)

Foods and Contacts Containing Egg[7]

Key: *There are some brands free of egg.

Albumin
Agarol
Baking powders*
Batters for french frying
Bavarian cream
Boiled dressings
Bouillons
Breads
Breaded foods
Cake flours
Cakes
Candies (except hard)
Cocoa drinks (malted)
Coffee if cleared with egg
Consommés
Cookies*
Creamed pies
Croquettes
Custards
Dessert powders
Doughnuts
Dressings, Boiled
Dried eggs in prepared foods and
  dumplings
Dumplings
Egg albumin
Escalloped eggs
French fry batters
French toast
French tarte
Fritters
Frostings
Glazed rolls
Griddle cakes
Hamburger mix
Hollandaise sauce

Hot cakes
Ice Cream
Ices
Icings
Laxatives
Macaroons
Malted cocoa drinks:
  Ovaltine
  Ovomalt and others
Macaroni
Marshmallows
Meat jellies
Meat loaf
Meat molds and meringues
Noodles*
Omelets
Ovaltine
Ovomalt
Pancakes
Pancake flours
Pastes
Patties
Pretzels
Puddings
Rolls, glazed
Salad dressings
Sauces
Sausages
Sherbets
Souffles
Soups
  Noodle
  Mock turtle
  Consommés
Spaghetti*

Spanish creams
Tartar sauce
Timbales
Waffle mixes

Waffles
Whips
Wines (Many wines are cleared with
    egg white)

List of Milk and Milk Products[8]

Key: *Although all cheeses are to be considered as milk products, a patient not sensitive to milk may be found to be allergic to one or more cheeses. Therefore, consider each kind and brand of cheese as a potentially specific allergen.

Key: oNot all preparations of these contain milk. You must check this point! Kosher breads are milk free.

Au gratin dishes
oBaker's breads
Baking powder biscuits
Bavarian cream
Bisques
Blanc mange
Boiled salad dressings
Bologna
Butter
Buttermilk
Butter sauces
Breaded foods
Breads
Cakes
Candies (except hard or homemade)
Casein
Cereal blend
*Cheeses of every description
Chocolate or cocoa drinks or mixtures
Coffeemate
Chowders
Cookies
Coolwhip
Cream
Creamed foods
Cream sauces
Creamed soups
Curds
Custards
Doughnuts
Eggs (scrambled and escalloped dishes)
Foods fried in butter
    Fish
    Poultry
    Beef
    Pork
Foods prepared au gratin
Flour mixtures (prepared)
*Frankfurters
French dressing
Fritters
Gravies
o* Hamburgers
Hard sauces

Hash
Hot cakes
Ice creams
Junket
Lactalbumin
Mashed potatoes
Malted milk
Ovaltine
Ovomalt
Macaroni
Meat loaf
Cooked sausages
Milk chocolate
Milk:
    Condensed
    Dried
    Evaporated
    Fresh
    Goat's
    Malted
    Powdered
"Non-dairy" substitutes containing
    caseinate
Nougat
Oleomargarines
Omelets
Pie crust made with milk products
Popcorn
Popovers
Preem
Prepared flour mixtures:
    Biscuit
    Cake
    Cookies
    Doughnuts
    Muffins
    *Pancake
    Pie crust
    Waffles
Puddings
Rarebits
Salad dressings
Sherbets

Soda crackers	Timbales
Soufflés	Whey
*Soups	Waffles
Spanish cream	Wiener Schnitzel
Spumoni	Zweibach

Food, Drug, and Cosmetic Additives

Pioneer allergist Dr. Stephen Lockey has called attention to additives in foods, drugs, and cosmetics and their allergic effects in many people (see Chapter 15). Here we present his lists of types of foods, beverages, flavorings, and drugs to be avoided for a salycilate- and tartrazine-free diet. These different chemicals, contained in both natural and processed foods, cross-react and are a recognized cause of hives in some and a possible cause of hyperactivity in others. There is also a list of the types of food and materials containing the various food colorings.

Dr. Stephen D. Lockey, Sr., who first described allergic reactions due to FD&C Red No. 2 (Amaranth) in the Bulletin of the Lancaster General Hospital, September, 1948, and later published his observations on the sensitizing and cross-sensitizing properties of FD&C Yellow No. 5 (Tartrazine) in the September–October 1959 issue of the Annals of Allergy, has now compiled a list of drugs manufactured by American pharmaceutical firms that contain tartrazine. The list is a formidable one and quite valuable to persons clinically sensitive to aspirin, who cross react to tartrazine present (as a colorant) in many foods and drugs.

He has also compiled and published salicylate and benzoic acid Avoidance Diets plus updated elimination lists for individuals clinically sensitive to the following drugs: aspirin, barbiturates, penicillin, iodine, phenolphthalein, sulfonamides, tetracycline and mercury. In 1969, Dr. Lockey assigned all of his copyrighted drug elimination lists for distribution to the Allergy Foundation of Lancaster County, a volunteer non-profit tax-free organization devoted to the better scientific understanding, prevention and treatment of allergic diseases.

For price lists and further information write to: The Allergy Foundation of Lancaster County, Box 1424, Lancaster PA 17604.

Dr. Lockey's Basic Salicylate-Avoidance Diet[a]

Almonds	Dewberries	Peaches
Apples	Gooseberries	Pickles
Apricots	Grapes	Plums and prunes
Avocado	Green bell peppers	Raisins
Blackberries	Green peppers	Raspberries
Boysenberries	Melon	Strawberries
Cherries	Nectarines	Tomatoes
Cucumbers	Olives	White potato
Currants	Oranges	

*Bakery goods (except for plain bread)	Catsup
*Biscuits	*Cereals
*Butter	*Cheese
*Cake mixes	*Commercial mixes
*Cakes	Cloves
Candies—yellow and green	Cocoa mix

(continued on page 402)

*Coffee pastries
*Cooking fats
Corned beef
Frankfurters
*Frostings
Gum
Hot chocolate mix
*Ice milk
*Jam or jelly (commercial)
*Jello and gelatin
*Gingerbread
Mayonnaise
Meat processed with vinegar
*Muffins
Noodles
Oleomargarine
Prepared mustard
*Puddings
Salad dressings
*Sherbet
Tartar sauce
Tabasco
*Variety crackers
*Yogurt

Miscellaneous
*Lozenges
*Mint flavors
*Mouthwashes
Oil of Wintergreen
*Toothpaste and tooth powder

Beverages
All soft drinks
Beer
Birch beer
Cider and cider vinegar
Diet drinks and supplements
Gin and all distilled drinks (except
    vodka)
Powdered colored drinks
Wine and wine vinegar
All medicines containing aspirin or
    salicylates
Perfumes
Omit artificially flavored foods, drinks
    and drugs, particularly those that
    contain FD&C Dye Yellow No. 5—
    Tartrazine

a *Key:* *Check with the manufacturer's Consumer Service department for tartrazine or salicylate. If the product does not contain tartrazine or salicylate, it may be used.

List of Types of Foods and Materials Containing Various Food Colorings

This list is not all-inclusive and is subject to change.

Gelatin Desserts
FD&C Blue #1—triphenylmethane
    Yellow #5— (Tartrazine)
        pyrazolone
    Red #3— (Erythrosine) xanthene

Orange Skins
FD&C Citrus Red #2—monoazo

Maraschino Cherries
FD&C Red #3— (Erythrosine) xanthene

Sausage Casings
Orange B

Frozen Desserts (Ice Cream & Sherbets)
FD&C Blue #1—triphenylmethane
    Red #3— (Erythrosine) xanthene
    Yellow #5— (Tartrazine)
        pyrazolone

Carbonated Beverages
FD&C Blue #1—triphenylmethane
    Yellow #5— (Tartrazine)
        pyrazolone
    Red #3— (Erythrosine) xanthene

Dry Drink Powders
FD&C Blue #1—triphenylmethane
    Yellow #5— (Tartrazine)
        pyrazolone
    Red #3— (Erythrosine) xanthene

Bakery Products and Cereals
FD&C Blue #1—triphenylmethane
    Red #3—(Erythrosine) xanthene
    Yellow #5— (Tartrazine)
        pyrazolone

Spaghetti
FD&C Yellow #5— (Tartrazine)
        pyrazolone

Puddings
FD&C Red #3— (Erythrosine) xanthene
    Yellow #5— (Tartrazine)
        pyrazolone

Drug Solutions—Aqueous
FD&C Blue #1—triphenylmethane
    Red #3— (Erythrosine) xanthene
    Yellow #5— (Tartrazine)
        pyrazolone

Candy and Confectionery Products—
do not contain oils and fats
FD&C Blue #1—triphenylmethane
    Red #3—(Erythrosine) xanthene
    Yellow #5— (Tartrazine)
      pyrazolone

Candy and Confectionery Products—
oils and fats are ingredients
FD&C Lakes—chemically prepared from
    water-soluble FD&C colors.

Capsules
FD&C Blue #1—triphenylmethane
    Red #3—(Erythrosine) xanthene
    Yellow #5— (Tartrazine)
      pyrazolone

Ointments
FD&C Red 40 and its Lake
    D&C Blue #1—triphenylmethane Lake

Mouthwashes
FD&C Blue #1—triphenylmethane

    Red #3—(Erythrosine) xanthene
    Yellow #5— (Tartrazine)
      pyrazolone

Tablets
FD&C Blue #1—triphenylmethane
    Red #3—(Erythrosine) xanthene
    Yellow #5— (Tartrazine)
      pyrazolone
    Red 40

Hair-Waving Fluids
FD&C Yellow #5— (Tartrazine)
    pyrazolone

Hair Oils and Pomades
FD&C Lakes

Toothpaste
FD&C Red #3—(Erythrosine) xanthene
    Yellow #5— (Tartrazine)
      pyrazolone

Soaps
FD&C Lakes

GLUTEN DIET LIST

What is gliadin or gluten sensitivity? Patients who are sensitive to the gluten protein fraction of wheat, rye, and probably oats and barley, will develop intestinal disease. The symptoms vary, although most recognized victims have diarrhea with large bulky stools, cramps, and weight loss. A few have nausea and loss of appetite and even constipation. Malnutrition may develop with the fatigue and weakness of anemia, numbness and tingling of the fingers and toes from lack of vitamin B_{12}, cramps and bone pain from lack of calcium and vitamin D, bleeding from lack of vitamin K, and swollen feet from lack or loss of protein from the damaged bowel. Once diagnosed, the individual should avoid the offending grains the rest of his life. The damaging agent in the gluten is the polypeptid called *gliadin*. It is uncertain whether the disease is due to an enzyme deficiency or to an allergic reaction, but damage occurs to the lining of the upper intestine, hindering the absorption of foods and vitamins.

For a gluten-free diet:

1. Avoid foods containing wheat, rye or oats.
2. Well-cooked foods may be tolerated better than uncooked or partially cooked foods.
3. It may be of considerable aid to place the entire family on a low-wheat diet.

Foods Allowed

Amscol vanilla ice cream
Apple
Applesauce
Apricots
Arrowroot
Asparagus

Bakers yeast
Banana
Beef
Beets
Berries
Bread, gluten free

Broccoli
Broth, clear
Butter
Buttermilk
Carrots
Cheese
Chicken
Chutney (homemade)
Clear lollipops
Clear soups
Cocoa
Cocoa pops
Coffee
Cordials
Corn
Corn Flakes, Chex, Pops
Corn syrup
Cream of tartar
Custards
Eggs
Fats
Fish
Flour, gluten-free
Fritos
Fruit
Fruit juice
Gelatine
Glucose
Green beans
Gum drops
Hominy
Honey
Ice cream (homemade)
Icing sugar
Jams
Jelly
Kelloggs Sugar Frosties

Lamb
Liver
Lollipops, clear
Meringue (homemade)
Milk
Molasses
Nuts
Oatmeal
Oats, rolled
Olives
Peaches
Pears
Peas
Pineapple
Pork
Potatoes
Potato chips
Rice
Rice cereals (Bubbles, Krispies, Chex, Puffed)
Rice flour
Sago
Salad dressing (homemade)
Sodium bicarbonate
Soya bread (homemade)
Soya flour
Squash
Sugar
Sugar corn pops
Sweet potato
Swiss chard
Tea
Tapioca
Tomatoes
Turnip
Vegetables
Vinegar
Yams

Patients sensitive to gluten should avoid the following foods and should read all labels carefully.

Allbran
Ale
Baked beans (check contents)
Baking powder
Barley
Beer
Bouillon
Bran flakes
Bread
Candy bars
Canned soups
Cake, commercial
Cakes
Cake decorations
Chili con carne
Chocolate

Chutney
Commercial foods (check contents)
Corn bread
Corn flour
Cream of vegetables
Cream of wheat
Creamed vegetables
Doughnuts
Dumplings
Farex
Farina
Fish, canned
Fish paste
Flour
Frankfurters
Grapenut flakes

Gravies
Ham
Ice cream (check contents)
Ice cream cones
Licorice
Lunch meats
Macaroni
Malted milk
Margarines
Marzipan
Meat, canned
Meats cooked with stuffing
Meat loaf
Meat paste
Melba toast
Miracle whip
Muffins
Mustard
Noodles
Ovaltime
Pancakes
Pastry
Postum
Pretzels
Puddings

Puffed wheat
Puréed baby foods
Relishes, thickened
Rolls
Rye bread
Salad dressing
Sauces, thickened
Sausages
Semolina
Soups (check labels)
Soya bread (commercial)
Spaghetti
Stews
Tomato sauce
Turkey stuffing
Vegetables in sauces
Waffles
Weelbix
Wheaties
Wheat Flakes
Whole wheat
Vermicelli
Vegetables, creamed
Zweiback

NOTES

Chapter 1

1. Physicians for Automotive Safety, "Crash-Tested Devices Available—and How to Use Them" (copyrighted pamphlet, 10th Edition, 1976, 50 Union Avenue, Irvington, N.J. 07111) [Send $0.25 with a self-addressed, stamped, business-sized envelope.]
2. JAY M. ARENA, B.S., M.D., *Dangers to Children and Youth* (Durham, N.C. 27705: Moore Publishing Company, 1971) [$12.50].
3. Ibid.
4. BURTON L. WHITE, *The First Three Years of Life* (Englewood Cliffs, N.J.: Prentice-Hall, 1975) .

Chapter 3

1. MARY JANE KIBLER, "How to Map Out a Meal," Council on Foods and Nutrition, American Medical Association, *Today's Health* (March 1960) , p. 48.
2. Council on Foods and Nutrition, "Zen Macrobiotic Diets," *Journal of the American Medical Association,* Vol. 218, no. 3 (October 18, 1971) .
3. WILLIAM G. CROOK, M.D., *Are You Bothered By Hypoglycemia?* (Box 3494 Jackson, Tenn. 38301: Professional Books, 1977) [$5.50 ppd].

Chapter 4

1. Editorial, "Antibiotic Sugar Pills," reprinted by permission. From *The New England Journal of Medicine,* Vol. 273, no. 15, pp. 825–26 (October 7, 1965) .

Chapter 5

1. Copyright © 1972 by Jack G. Shiller, M.D. From the book CHILDHOOD ILLNESS: A Common Sense Approach. Reprinted with permission of Stein

and Day/Publishers and George Allen & Unwin Ltd., Book Publishers, Park Lane, Hemel Hempstead HP2 4TE England.
2. Ibid.
3. Ibid.

Chapter 9

1. The American Lung Association, "The Facts About Pneumonia" (1740 Broadway, New York, N.Y. 10019), January 1977.

Chapter 10

1. WILLIAM G. CROOK, M.D., *Your Allergic Child* (Box 3494 Jackson, Tenn. 38301: Professional Books, 1975) [$5.50 ppd].

Chapter 11

1. WILLIAM G. CROOK, M.D., *Your Allergic Child* (Box 3494 Jackson, Tennessee 38301: Professional Books, 1975).

Chapter 15

1. WILLIAM G. CROOK, M.D., *Your Allergic Child* (Box 3494 Jackson, Tennessee 38301: Professional Books, 1975).
2. The Allergy Foundation of America, "Why Are Allergies A National Health Problem?" (Fact Sheet, 801 Second Avenue, New York, NY 10017, July 1971).
3. CROOK, *Allergic Child.*
4. CROOK, *Allergic Child.*

Chapter 17

1. The American Lung Association, "The Facts About The Common Cold," (1740 Broadway, New York, N.Y. 10019) May 1976.

Chapter 20

1. CLAUDE A. FRAZIER, M.D., *Insect Allergy* 508 pp. 207 ill., 20 tab., 332 ref. (St. Louis, Missouri: Warren H. Green, Inc., 1969).

Chapter 21

1. DR. KRAL, *Veterinary Dermatology* (Philadelphia, Pennsylvania: J. B. Lippincott Co., 1953), p. 108.

Chapter 23

1. JAMES W. HARDIN and JAY M. ARENA, M.D., *Human Poisoning from Native and Cultivated Plants* (Durham, N.C.: Duke University Press, 1974), Second Edition.

PART IV

1. Kenneth F. Lampe, Ph.D. and Rune Fagerstrom, Pharm.Dr., *Plant Toxicity and Dermatitis, A Manual for Physicians* (Baltimore: The Williams & Wilkins Company, 1968). James W. Hardin and Jay M. Arena, M.D., *Human Poisoning from Native and Cultivated Plants* (Durham, N.C.: Duke University Press, 1974), Second Edition. John M. Kingsbury, *Poisonous Plants of the United States and Canada* (Englewood Cliffs, New Jersey: Prentice-Hall, Inc., 1964).
2. Adapted from: Catherine F. Adams, Agriculture Research Service, United States Department of Agriculture, *Nutritive Value of American Foods* (Washington, D.C.: U.S. Government Printing Office, 1975), Agriculture Handbook No. 456.
3. Bernice K. Watt and Annabel L. Merrill, *Composition of Foods* (Washington, D.C.: U.S. Department of Agriculture, U.S. Government Printing Office, 1963), Agriculture Handbook No. 8.
4. Ruth M. Feeley, Patricia E. Criner, and Bernice K. Watt, Ph.D., R.D., Agriculture Research Service, U.S. Department of Agriculture, "Cholesterol content of foods," *Journal of the American Dietetic Association*, 61 (August 1972), 134–136.
5. Adapted from Rinkel, H. J.; T. G. Randolph; and Michael Zeller, *Food Allergy*. Courtesy of Charles C Thomas, Publisher, Springfield, Ill. and Hollister-Stier Laboratories.
6. Ibid.
7. Ibid.
8. Ibid.

INDEX

For easy use, the words in this index referring to SYMPTOMS, SIGNS, TREATMENT, *and* FIRST AID are in **bold print**. Page numbers referring to FIRST AID or EMERGENCY MEDICAL CARE are also shown in **bold print**.